Enabling Recovery:
The Principles and
Practice of Rehabilitation
Psychiatry

Enabling Recovery: The Principles and Practice of Rehabilitation Psychiatry

Edited by Glenn Roberts, Sarah Davenport, Frank Holloway and Theresa Tattan

Gaskell

© The Royal College of Psychiatrists 2006

Gaskell is an imprint of the Royal College of Psychiatrists, 17 Belgrave Square, London SW1X 8PG
http://www.rcpsych.ac.uk

British Library Cataloguing-in-Publication Data.
A catalogue record for this book is available from the British Library.
ISBN 1-904671-30-6

Distributed in North America by Balogh International Inc.

The views presented in this book do not necessarily reflect those of the Royal College
of Psychiatrists, and the publishers are not responsible for any error of omission or fact.

The Royal College of Psychiatrists is a registered charity (no. 228636).

Printed in the UK by Cromwell Press Limited, Trowbridge.

Contents

Part 2: Therapeutic practices

Part 3: Services and organisational perspectives

Tables, boxes and figures

Figures

Contributors

Pat Abbott, Consultant Psychiatrist in Rehabilitation, Ashworth Hospital, Liverpool L31 1HW

Matthew Allin, Peggy Pollak Research Fellow in Developmental Psychiatry and Honorary Specialist Registrar in Psychiatry, Division of Psychological Medicine, Box 063, Institute of Psychiatry, De Crespigny Park, London SE5 8AF

Renuka Arjundas, Consultant Psychiatrist in Cognitive–Behavioural Therapy, South Tyneside Hospital, Harton Lane, South Shields NE34 0PL

Dominic Beer, Consultant Psychiatrist, Oxleas NHS Trust, Bracton Centre, Bracton Lane, Dartford DA2 7AF

Jed Boardman, Senior Lecturer in Social Psychiatry, PO Box 33, Health Services Research Department, Institute of Psychiatry, De Crespigny Park, London SE5 8AF

Irene Cormac, Consultant Forensic Psychiatrist, with a special interest in physical healthcare, Nottinghamshire Healthcare NHS Trust, Rampton Hospital, Retford DN22 0PD

Tom Craig, Professor of Social and Community Psychiatry, PO Box 33, Health Services Research Department, Institute of Psychiatry, De Crespigny Park, London SE5 8AF

Sarah Davenport, Consultant Psychiatrist, Lancashire Care Trust, Guild Lodge, Preston PR2 3AZ

Steffan Davies, Senior Lecturer in Forensic Rehabilitation Psychiatry, University of Nottingham, and Honorary Consultant Forensic Psychiatrist, Nottinghamshire Healthcare Trust, Rampton Hospital, Retford DN22 0PD

Gráinne Fadden, Consultant Clinical Psychologist, Birmingham and Solihull Mental Health Trust, Honorary Senior Research Fellow, Birmingham University Consultant Clinical Psychologist, Manager – The Meriden Family Programme, Birmingham & Solihull Mental Health NHS Trust, Tall Trees, Uffculme Centre, Queensbridge Road, Moseley, Birmingham B13 8QY

Alan Farmer, Consultant Psychiatrist, Assertive Outreach Service, Worcestershire North Team, 3 Millennium Court, Buntsford Park Road, Bromsgrove B60 3DX

Michael Ferriter, Senior Research Fellow, Nottinghamshire Healthcare NHS Trust, Rampton Hospital, Retford DN22 0PD

Simon Fleminger, Consultant Neuropsychiatrist, The Lishman Unit, Maudsley Hospital, Denmark Hill, London SE5 8AZ

Tom Harrison, Consultant Psychiatrist, Birmingham and Solihull Mental Health NHS Trust, Scarborough House Assertive Outreach Team, 35 Auckland Road, Birmingham B11 1RH

Frank Holloway, Croydon Integrated Adult Mental Health Services, Bethlem Royal Hospital, Monks Orchard Road, Beckenham, Kent BR3 3BX

Lindsey Kemp, Consultant for Rehabilitation and Continuing Care, Kent and Medway NHS and Social Care Partnership Trust, Priority House, Hermitage Lane, Barming, Maidstone ME16 9PH

Julian Leff, Emeritus Professor, Institute of Psychiatry, King's College, London, and Royal Free and University College Medical School, London; correspondence: 1 South Hill Park Gardens, London NW3 2TD

David Martin, Information, Audit and Development Manager, Coventry Teaching Primary Care Trust, Gulson Hospital, Gulson Road, Coventry, West Midlands CV1 2HR

Alan Meaden, Consultant Specialist Clinical Psychologist in Rehabilitation, Psychology Services, Birmingham and Solihull Mental Health NHS Trust, 208 Monyhull Hall Road, Kings Norton, Birmingham B30 3QJ

Rachel Perkins, Director of Quality Assurance and User/Carer Experience, South West London & St George's Mental Health NHS Trust, Springfield Hospital, Glenburnie Road, London SW17 7DJ

Paddy Power, Lead Consultant and Honorary Senior Lecturer, Lambeth Early Onset (LEO) service, South London & Maudsley NHS Trust, 108 Landor Road, London SW9 9NT

Glenn Roberts, Consultant in Rehabilitation Psychiatry, Wonford House Hospital, Exeter, Devon EX2 5AF

Brian Robinson, Consultant Psychiatrist, Susan Britton Wills Centre, Guinea Street, Bristol BS1 6SY

Geoff Shepherd, Director of Partnerships and Service Development, Cambridgeshire and Peterborough Mental Health Partnership NHS Trust, Kingfisher House, Kingfisher Way, Hinchingbrooke Business Park, Huntingdon PE29 6FH (visiting Professor of Mental Health Rehabilitation, Department of Health Services Research, Institute of Psychiatry, University of London)

David Shiers, General Practitioner, GP Advisor to Care Services Improvement Partnership and Joint Lead to NIMHE/Rethink National Early Intervention Programme, c/o Stackstones, School Lane, Longsdon, Stoke on Trent ST9 9QS

Jo Smith, Consultant Clinical Psychologist and Joint Lead to NIMHE/Rethink National Early Intervention Programme, c/o Worcestershire Mental Health Partnership NHS Trust, Psychology Department, Newtown Hospital, Worcester WR 5 1JG

Neill Simpson, Consultant in Learning Disabilities Psychiatry, NHS Greater Glasgow and Clyde, and Medical Advisor to Glasgow Learning Disability Partnership, 1055 Great Western Road, Glasgow G12 0XH

Melinda Sweeting, Consultant Rehabilitation Psychiatrist, Maudsley Hospital, Denmark Hill, London SE5 8AZ

Theresa Tattan, Consultant Psychiatrist, Women's Medium Secure Service, Fromeside, Blackberry Hill, Stapleton, Bristol BS16 1EG

Douglas Turkington, Professor of Psychosocial Psychology, Newcastle University, Newcastle NE1 4LP

Peter Tyrer, Professor of Community Psychiatry, Imperial College, Department of Psychological Medicine, St Dunstan's Road, London W6 8RP

Paul Wolfson, Consultant Psychiatrist in Rehabilitation and Assertive Outreach, Oxleas NHS Foundation Trust, The Lodge, Erith Community Mental Health Centre, Park Crescent, Erith DA8 3EE

Til Wykes, Professor of Clinical Psychology and Rehabilitation, Institute of Psychiatry, King's College, De Crespigny Park, London SE5 8AF

Rehabilitation and recovery now

Glenn Roberts, Frank Holloway,
Sarah Davenport and Theresa Tattan

The changing face of rehabilitation

Psychiatric rehabilitation offers a positive response to the problems, needs and aspirations of people with long-term, complex and life-limiting mental health problems. The central ambitions of contemporary rehabilitation services are to rekindle hope and to open routes to personal recovery, while accepting and accounting for continuing difficulty and disability. Best practice pivots on a mature and creative balance of optimism and realism, and requires the ability to tolerate protracted uncertainty and remain curious and hopeful. A core skill within rehabilitation is to keep doors and opportunities open, attending carefully both to the pace of change, so that it is neither too fast nor too slow, and to shaping expectations so as nurture hope and aspiration alongside an understanding of what is realistically possible.

The term rehabilitation is familiar, contested and occasionally confusing, given its broad application across fields such as severe mental illness, substance misuse, neurological disorders and beyond, to issues as diverse as renewing water mains and reintegrating political extremists. The recent history of resettlement of former in-patients during the era of 'deinstitutionalisation' has led some to feel that the term carries unhelpful and stigmatising associations with chronicity and the back wards of asylums. However, the word rehabilitation has been with us a long time, and there are interesting echoes between its historical usage to relate, for example, to the restoration of privileges and possessions, reinstatement in a previous position and vindication of reputation and our contemporary emphasis on social inclusion and recovery. In healthcare, there is not yet a satisfactory alternative and the current move is to extend the term rather than replace it, by speaking of 'rehabilitation and recovery services', a move anticipated some years ago by Pat Deegan (1988) in a paper in which rehabilitation is seen as a professional and service process and recovery as the aim and the desired outcome.

This book has grown out of the concerns and commitments of members of the Faculty of Rehabilitation and Social Psychiatry at the Royal College of Psychiatrists. It therefore centres on rehabilitation as a clinical philosophy and practical approach to people who have long-term and severe mental illnesses, in particular the psychoses. The relationship between rehabilitation services and recovery outcomes is a theme woven throughout the chapters. We have gathered in this volume a wide range of practice and experience that spans the current hierarchy of accepted evidence, from rigorous research to expert opinion and personal experience. This mirrors the reality of contemporary practice: each enlivens and enriches the other. Throughout the book, contributors emphasise both the value of evidence-based practice and the importance of the personal commitment and creativity of practitioners in reaching individualised solutions to complex and seemingly intractable problems.

In the quarter of a century since Wing & Morris (1981) published their multi-author Handbook of Psychiatric Rehabilitation Practice much has changed. The mental hospitals have, largely, closed. Traditional rehabilitation practices, which focused on the resettlement of long-stay institutionalised patients, have become less relevant (although the emerging specialty of forensic rehabilitation is engaged in precisely this process). Some dimensions have persisted and have been extended, for example rehabilitation has always required effective multidisciplinary and multi-agency working. There is an increasing emphasis on the importance of collaboration with service users and their carers, as 'partners in care' (see the Royal College of Psychiatrists Partners in Care campaign at http://www.rcpsych.ac.uk/campaigns/pinc). To some extent, previous 'disability language' has been replaced by new concepts such as empowerment and recovery, but there is an attendant need to ensure that a more optimistic orientation does not simply turn away from those with the greatest difficulties or deny the reality of enduring needs. All mental health professionals now pay lip service to collaborative working: the challenge is to put this into practice, taking account of the real dilemmas that professionals face in balancing the imperatives of empowerment and the management of risk. There have also, of course, been significant advances in evidence-based treatment technologies, which are documented in some detail in this book.

Why is psychiatric rehabilitation important?

It has been said that a society can be judged by how it treats those of its members who are most in need of its care and compassion. It would be invidious to suggest such a hierarchy of need, but those who are the central concern of rehabilitation services have fair claim to be near the top, and this book offers many useful suggestions for making community care a reality.

The National Service Framework (NSF) for Long-term Conditions (Department of Health, 2005) gives a very clear lead on the importance of rehabilitation principles and practice for people with chronic health problems, referring to rehabilitation more than 300 times. This NSF is clearly intended to have wide application and goes a long way to rectifying the scant mention of rehabilitation in the National Service Framework for Mental Health (Department of Health, 1999) which caused much puzzlement and concern.

Until recently rehabilitation appears to have been the forgotten need in mental health services (Holloway, 2005). There appears to have been a blind spot in fully accounting for the needs of people with enduring mental health problems which has been considered a 'denial of disability' (Holloway, 2005). In truth, many if not all people with psychotic and other severe mental illnesses do have 'long-term conditions' for which long-term thinking and strategies are appropriate. In his 5-year (half-way) review of the NSF for Mental Health, Appleby (2004) acknowledges the need for renewed emphasis on rehabilitation practice and a reinvestment in research and evaluation of rehabilitation services. We could beneficially combine the service framework for long-term conditions with that for mental health. Indeed, the former states in its executive summary:

'Although this NSF focuses on people with neurological conditions, much of the guidance it offers can apply to anyone living with a long-term condition. Commissioners are therefore encouraged to use this NSF in planning service developments for people with other long-term conditions' (Department of Health, 2005: p. 3).

We can only hope that they will, for its central emphasis on general, specialist and vocational rehabilitation is directly relevant to the principles and practices described here. Effective rehabilitation services can therefore deliver better outcomes for service users and their carers.

A further major concern for commissioners and rehabilitation psychiatrists alike are the burgeoning and uncontrolled costs associated with the rapid growth of out-of-area treatment and the need to develop constructive and collaborative relationships with independent and private providers of residential treatment and continuing care. This too has been the subject of a publication by the Royal College of Psychiatrists' Faculty of Rehabilitation and Social Psychiatry (Davies et al, 2005), which includes welcome good-practice guidelines that may have far-reaching consequences. Good-quality local rehabilitation services will undoubtedly be a cost-effective option for service commissioners.

What this book is, what it isn't and what's missing

This book is a milestone, marking how far we have come and where we have got to, but those hoping for a how-to-do it manual on setting up and running a rehabilitation service may be disappointed. At present there is no national or international consensus on what such a service, and therefore the accompanying book, would look like. There are core principles and practices but much diversity, and the journey continues.

Mental health professionals increasingly operate in a world of protocols, care pathways and standardised data-sets. In stark contrast, rehabilitation psychiatry values the stories people tell and have lived, and the work involves constant interaction with those stories, to which people are host or hostage. Accordingly we have organised this book with a narrative structure in mind. There are three major sections. In Part 1 we set out our beginnings, the core principles and values of rehabilitation that serve as the foundations of rehabilitation psychiatry. Part 2 consists of a rich description of therapeutic interventions, and Part 3 contains the ends that these achieve, the diverse approaches to service provision that have evolved. Part 4 addresses the special considerations of applying rehabilitation practice in the context of acquired brain injury, learning disability and forensic settings. The book concludes, in Part 5, with a chapter by the editors looking ahead, and is followed by Appendices containing a compendium of useful resource material.

This book aims to reach a wide audience, embracing psychiatrists, colleagues in companion disciplines, service users and carers. We have also sought to tackle the more difficult task of gathering the many different voices and values that collectively constitute contemporary rehabilitation psychiatry and will be active in guiding its continuing development.

Scientific writing has made a virtue of presenting dispassionate and apparently objective accounts, fashioned in a way that almost entirely conceals the presence of the author. This collection of chapters and positions is different. The authors have been chosen precisely because of their passion, commitment and authority in their fields. It is a book written by practitioners for practitioners. There is clearly a great deal on offer from these multiple perspectives: effective rehabilitation practice requires discussion, tolerance of disagreement and creative synthesis. In retaining a lively sense of who has written what, the reader should not passively accept what is written, but should take up the challenge of interacting with these insights and approaches and of choosing what to incorporate within their practice. We are all involved in a continuing process of adult learning.

Reviewers often struggle with multi-author books and are troubled by any sign of inconsistency, as though a key editorial task is to homogenise contributions and contrive to make them sound as though they were of the same voice. Our approach has been different. We asked contributors to produce something of similar size and shape, so that each gets a fair 'turn' and their chapters sit well together. However, we positively value the different voice of each and appreciate these differences, an approach that is fully consistent with the diverse sources and resources that contribute to rehabilitation practice. What we have produced is not so much a textbook, as a family gathering around the core concerns of rehabilitation and recovery. Each author has been encouraged to draw on their experience and tell it as they see it. This resulting account is inevitably incomplete, although full of the well-considered contributions of innovators, mature clinicians and expert commentators.

Some will doubtless disagree on our choice of chapters and contributors, in particular on what they feel should have been given more emphasis. We debated whether there should be separate chapters on ethics, spirituality and ethnicity, but decided to ask all our authors to keep these concerns in mind and regard them as interweaving threads to any and all considerations. We felt that there could be something lost by separating them out – we expect some to disagree with this integrationist approach, feeling instead that they are sufficiently important and neglected to warrant particular emphasis – and it was a close call.

We are also aware of particular shortfalls. We have not systematically addressed the issue of comorbid substance misuse, although references are scattered throughout the book. Practitioners and carers will be well aware of the impact of substance misuse, notably of alcohol, cannabis and cocaine. Individuals with serious mental illnesses accompanied by substance misuse often find themselves in locked or forensic settings and there is very robust evidence that comorbidity increases the risk of violence (indeed much of the small but significant excess of societal violence attributable to people with schizophrenia is due to those who misuse drugs or alcohol). Substance misuse is also a consistent predictor of relapse in psychosis and there is evidence that continuing cannabis consumption results in longer hospital stays.

Despite these stark facts, substance misuse, very common among inner-city users of psychiatric services, is often an exclusion criterion for accessing rehabilitation services, and mental illness is almost invariably an exclusion criterion for long-term drug rehabilitation. Unfortunately, at the time of writing, there is no UK-based published data on effective service interventions for substance misuse comorbid with mental illness, despite the current fashion for 'dual-diagnosis workers' and encouragement to train all members of local mental health teams to deal with substance misuse. The present state of knowledge requires us to be 'cautious about assuming that substance misuse interventions are unambiguous, evidence-based strategies with a high success rate' (Burns & Firn, 2002: p. 203). Any future edition of this book should be able to provide more solid evidence-based advice on the management of comorbidity.

We were not able to recruit as broad a contribution as we would have wished from service users to give a view about user-led services. At present we can look in vain for a mental health equivalent of the League of Friends that characterises patient involvement in general hospitals. Much of the energy and incentive for establishing service user groups has arisen from the traumas and griefs that sit at the heart of mental health problems and the sense of failure and disappointment in the response of services to such needs. Service user and carer movements are therefore characterised by an energetic diversity and iconoclasm. These are hard-won strengths that almost by definition locate such influences outside of the institution they need to challenge. At present this book may represent that institution, and we have a way to go before we realise our aspiration of developing true partnership working. We hope that any future revision will find a way to offer user-authors an acceptable invitation to take more of a place among new chapters, thereby making their voices more clearly heard and valued.

Finally, we are aware that some issues have escaped particular mention because they are so obvious, but we fully acknowledge that they are also prerequisites to any more complex or sophisticated therapeutic endeavour. It is common for people referred to rehabilitation services to have considerable difficulties with self-care and in sorting out the practical necessities of day-to-day living. This then raises such familiar, mundane but essential issues such as how to get someone out of bed, how to get day and night in their proper places, how to ensure that the person is dressed appropriately, has adequate personal hygiene and is taking necessary medication. This often extends to ensuring that personal finances are secure, 'friendships' are non-exploitive and sexual relationships are accompanied by both capacity and choice. It is simple and day-to-day issues such as these that carry the full weight of ethical concerns over human rights, personal choice, autonomy and diversity. These taken-for-granted matters of everyday practice are often conducted by highly experienced but unqualified workers. This needs to be understood and celebrated, for they constitute the core of what staff and patients do in the slow and difficult task of recovering the dignity of an ordinary lifestyle and personal care. The introduction of training for 'support time and recovery' (STR) workers to 'help service users to have an ordinary life [by] assisting them with their everyday, practical needs in whatever setting they find themselves to facilitate recovery' (Department of Health, 2003: p. 7) may significantly support both patients and staff in these practical, time-intensive, recovery-oriented skills.

Service principles

In its report on rehabilitation and recovery the Royal College of Psychiatrists puts it thus:

'Most rehabilitation services have a developmental history that bridges de-institutionalisation, reprovision in its many forms, community care and now social inclusion, working to reduce the impact of stigma and to promote recovery. Embracing the concept of recovery, and promoting the recovery ethos throughout rehabilitation service provision, probably represents a clear new direction ...

New ways of working with service users and their carers lie at the heart of the specialty. The journey towards individual recovery while respecting individual disabilities must inform rehabilitation service development. The perspective of service users and their families, together with their many partners in care, can provide a powerful force for development and should be the starting-point for new work' (Royal College of Psychiatrists, 2004: p. 5).

However hard they may be to fully achieve, the emerging watchwords are about collaboration, partnership, choice and recovery.'

Service models

Mental health rehabilitation services are present throughout England, but what they have to offer and how they are configured varies greatly (Killaspy *et al*, 2005). To embrace the full range of rehabilitation it is now necessary to reach wide, and invite between these covers many contributors who would not call themselves rehabilitation practitioners but who none the less represent skills, knowledge, and experience which is at the heart of contemporary rehabilitation practice. Internationally there are few coherent, comprehensive and integrated models of rehabilitation. Those that do exist are usually associated with specific individuals or departments and are often the fruit of a professional lifetime. Such isolated models of good practice are useful to learn from but difficult if not impossible to reproduce.

In practice every rehabilitation service is different. Each has strengths and weaknesses, and much is determined by their local history. Most if not all services are also in a process of active change and continuing development. It is a particular concern that some have been dismantled or relabelled to fulfil local requirements to meet targets and restrictions governing new functional services such as assertive outreach or even early intervention required by the NSF for Mental Health and the National Health Service Plan (Department of Health, 2000) (for a positive account of progress to date see Appleby, 2004). In other areas the emergent emphasis on recovery is providing the spark to rekindle, and sometimes recommission, rehabilitation services as recovery-based practice. The new functional services are associated with specific models (Department of Health, 2001) and are expected to be commissioned with high 'fidelity' to these 'evidence-based' blueprints. Although there may be merit in pursuing such conformity, rehabilitation psychiatry has a close affinity with the other common usage of fidelity relating to loyalty, faithfulness and allegiance, for without a certain stubborn persistence, dogged determination and holding of hope in sometimes prolonged situations of hopelessness, there would be no rehabilitation. With such fidelity, and eyes to see and value small but significant changes, remarkable things can happen.

Part of this future hope hinges on how we recognise and cultivate professionalism, which has been under attack for some years. Professionals of all kinds have become distrusted and have come to live in a structured and accountable world of governmental goals and targets, stars and traffic lights. There are signs that this is changing, and rehabilitation psychiatry needs a certain sort of professionalism – which may be provided by both lay and qualified people. Minzberg (1983) helpfully defined professionalism as 'the exercise of discretion, on behalf of another, in a situation of uncertainty', and over the past two decades the literature has reaffirmed that professionals deal with 'indeterminate' problems – ones that often lack a clear solution and are inherently complex and unpredictable. These require professionals to 'read the situation', to improvise and be flexible.

Schon (1984) evocatively described professional practice as more a matter of negotiating the 'swampy lowlands', than peering down from 'the heights of academe', and the significant movement towards supporting the development of the 'expert patient' (Cooper & Clarke, 2005) is, in effect, support for the growth of lay professionals.

Looking to the future

It may seem contradictory to anticipate the limited lifespan of a book at its birth. However, we hope and expect that the present volume will need to be rewritten within 10 years as the field continues to develop and there is more that can be said with confidence.

With the exception of research into some specific interventions such as cognitive–behavioural therapy and clozapine, the current evidence base for much of rehabilitation practice is poorly developed. We anticipate that a future edition will provide better data on outcomes for service configurations, clear models of user and carer integration and well-developed applications of recovery-based approaches, including a means of evaluating the recovery orientation of these services. It may also offer an evaluation of different housing and social care options, and a map of therapeutic interventions that are phase- and stage-specific. We will soon have a clearer picture of the value of early-intervention services and assertive outreach teams, and may be able to make confident statements about the best configuration of psychosis services across the lifespan. We hope that a succeeding edition will report unanticipated findings that show how outcomes and recovery for people with severe and enduring mental illnesses can be improved.

We must also expect governmental policy agendas to move on, hopefully from an obsession with service structures and targets towards making real and measurable difference to the daily lives of people with severe and enduring mental illness and their carers. There is much work to be done in tackling the multiple forms of social exclusion suffered by people with mental illnesses (Office of the Deputy Prime Minister, 2004): this work, to be effective, requires collaboration across agencies and into local communities.

Using this book

Those wishing to take time and care to reconsider a contemporary service for people with complex and persistent mental health problems that compromise and limit their lives will find abundant materials, models and inspiration from a remarkable set of chapters from innovators and champions in many disciplines. Above all, this book aims to be useful to practitioners, and from the outset the aim has been to bear witness to a much broader range of important contributions than just those of psychiatrists. Through them we have also aspired to speak to the interests and needs of the whole multidisciplinary team.

We asked our authors to write in plain English and at a length such that each chapter can reasonably be digested in a single sitting. Each chapter could form a summary or handout for teaching sessions on each topic. We also asked that the references should encompass the key contributions in the field, so that each chapter is a doorway for those wishing to pursue further study. We have concluded the book with Appendices of sources and resources in which you will hopefully find many more useful leads.

Within this text there are many examples of cross-disciplinary and collaborative work, but there is no one unifying model, except perhaps the care programme approach (Chapter 16), which provides an overarching structure for all secondary mental health services in England. The task of the reader is similar to that of the clinician: to take all the intersecting threads and customise what is offered to their particular circumstances, constraints and opportunities. This is not so much a handbook, still less a cookbook, but an offer of example and experience as a companion for your own personal, professional and service developments.

References

Appleby, L. (2004) *The National Service Framework for Mental Health – Five Years On* London: Department of Health.

Burns, T. & Finn, M. (2002) *Assertive Outreach in Mental Health: a Manual for Practitioners.* Oxford: Oxford University Press.

Cooper, J. M. & Clarke, A. (2005) *Expert Patients: Who are They? Lay-led Self-Management Programmes: An Additional Resource in the Management of Chronic Illness.* London: Long-Term Medical Conditions Alliance. http://www.lmca.org.uk/docs/article.htm

Davies, S., Mitchell, S., Mountain, D., *et al* Faculty of Rehabilitation and Social Psychiatry Working Group (2005) *Out of Area Treatments for Working Age Adults with Complex and Severe Psychiatric Disorders: Review of Current Situation and Recommendations for Good Practice.* London: Royal College of Psychiatrists. http://www.rcpsych.ac.uk/PDF/Reccomendations05.pdf

Deegan, P. E. (1988) Recovery: the lived experience of rehabilitation. *Psychosocial Rehabilitation Journal*, **11** (4), 11–19.

Department of Health (1999) *National Service Framework for Mental Health. Modern Standards and Service Models.* London: Department of Health. http://www.dh.gov.uk/assetRoot/04/07/72/09/04077209.pdf

Department of Health (2000) *The NHS Plan. A Plan for Investment, A Plan for Reform.* London: Department of Health.

Department of Health (2001) *The Mental Health Policy Implementation Guide.* London: Department of Health.

Department of Health (2003) *Mental Health Policy Implementation Guide: Support, Time and Recovery (STR) Workers.* London: Department of Health. http://www.dh.gov.uk/assetRoot/04/01/94/56/04019456.pdf

Department of Health (2005) *National Service Framework for Long-term Conditions.* London: Department of Health. http://www.dh.gov.uk/assetRoot/04/10/53/69/04105369.pdf

Holloway, F. (2005) *The Forgotten Need for Rehabilitation in Contemporary Mental Health Services: A Position Statement from the Executive Committee of the Faculty of Rehabilitation and*

Social Psychiatry, Royal College of Psychiatrists. London: Royal College of Psychiatrists. http://www.rcpsych.ac.uk/pdf/frankholloway_oct05.pdf

Killaspy, H., Harden, C., Holloway, F., *et al* (2005) What do mental health rehabilitation services do and what are they for? A national survey in England. *Journal of Mental Health*, **14**, 157–165.

Office of the Deputy Prime Minister (2004) *Mental Health and Social Exclusion. Social Exclusion Unit Report*. London: Office of the Deputy Prime Minister.

Minzberg, H. (1983) *Structures in Fives*. New York: Prentice Hall.

Royal College of Psychiatrists (2004) *Rehabilitation and Recovery Now* (Council Report CR121). London: Royal College of Psychiatrists.

Schon, D. (1984) *The Reflective Practitioner*. New York: Basic Books.

Wing, J. K. & Morris, B. (eds) (1981) *Handbook of Psychiatric Rehabilitation Practice*. Oxford: Oxford University Press.

Part 1

Foundations

CHAPTER 1

What is psychiatric rehabilitation?

Tom Craig

Rehabilitation has been defined by the World Health Organization as the application of measures aimed at reducing the impact of disabling and handicapping conditions and enabling disabled people to achieve social integration (World Health Organization, 1980). Implicit in this definition are two components. First, an active process through which a person adapts or acquires the skills needed to mitigate the constraints of disease, and second, an acknowledgement that there may also need to be changes in the environment, including the attitudes of non-disabled people, if optimal social integration is to be achieved.

For Anthony, product champion of psychiatric rehabilitation in the USA, rehabilitation involves 'improving the psychiatrically disturbed person's capabilities and competence' by bringing about 'behavioural improvement in their environment of need' (Anthony et al, 1984: p. 140). In subtle contrast Bennett (1978), whose views have strongly influenced UK practice, emphasised helping the individual adapt to their deficits in personal skills by 'making best use of his residual abilities in order to function in as normal environment as possible'.

Psychiatric rehabilitation is frequently defined as the activity of a set of specialist services. An alternative formulation would be in terms of the needs or characteristics of people who would benefit from rehabilitation interventions. Wykes & Holloway (2000) defined the potential client group as 'people with severe and long-term mental illnesses who have both active symptomatology and impaired social functioning as a consequence of their mental illness'. From this definition they argued that rehabilitation services should have the joint aims of minimising the symptoms of illness and promoting social inclusion.

In contrast to the concept of social inclusion, rehabilitation is deeply unfashionable and the term does not appear in any of the many mental health policy documents produced in the UK over recent years. Although the majority of mental health services in England have one or more dedicated rehabilitation in-patient unit and community team (Killaspy et al, 2005), the development of specialist rehabilitation services is very patchy.

Box 1.1 Simon's journey into a rehabilitation service

Simon is in his early 40s. He has had a diagnosis of schizophrenia for 15 years. He has been hospitalised five times, being compulsorily detained three times. A prominent feature of his illness is his unshakeable conviction that he is under constant surveillance by a government organisation. He believes he is followed wherever he goes and frequently sees people whom he believes to be these agents on the street and in local shops. Partly through fearfulness and partly through apathy, he spends most of his time alone in his flat. He takes no interest in his appearance or hygiene and has serious problems managing the upkeep of his flat, on which he owes a considerable amount of unpaid rent. He has not worked for many years. The view of some clinicians is that his is a pretty hopeless case. In the course of the long illness, he has received all the usual (and some not so usual) pharmacological and available psychosocial interventions, to apparently little effect.

Simon's view is just as bleak, if not more so. In the past 10 years he has had two consultant psychiatrists, whom he has seen mostly during his spells in hospital, and a string of trainee psychiatrists, seen fleetingly in an out-patient clinic. His main contact has been with a community psychiatric nurse but she moved away just as he was beginning to believe someone might have had his interests at heart. Conversations with mental health staff have mainly concerned medication or been disapproving of his lifestyle. He has picked up the air of hopelessness that surrounds his case, noticing that the enthusiastic promises of new treatments and new referrals (in which he had little faith anyway) have long since dropped away. Having been out of unemployment for many years, he does not believe that he is employable or, indeed, able to work and cannot see the point of attending a day centre to mingle with strangers or to work without reward. He feels quite powerless to do anything himself and has come to the view that there is little anyone else can do for him.

Following the psychiatric hospital closure programme, there is also now a much larger de facto system of continuing care within generic mental health and social care services: a 'virtual asylum'. Typically the contemporary pathway to a rehabilitation service involves many years of illness and disability (see Simon's story, related in Box 1). By this time the individual, their family and the supporting services at best will have low expectations and at worst may have lost hope altogether.

It is against this background of mutual hopelessness and mistrust that many specialist rehabilitation services come into play. And yet, it is the common experience of every professional with an interest in rehabilitation that such apparently intractable situations can be turned around to a surprising degree. The ingredients for this success are:

- the development of a culture of empowerment, healing and hope
- the provision of interventions to limit the impact of disability
- making adjustments to the environment that ease the burden of handicap.

This chapter will provide a brief and critical outline of how these three key ingredients can be provided; specific elements of the rehabilitation process are described in more detail throughout this book. The 'what is rehabilitation?' of the chapter title is clarified by answering 'how can we best carry out rehabilitation?'. Throughout the chapter the focus is on rehabilitation services. It is important to emphasise that the task of rehabilitation can, of course, be undertaken in a wide range of alternative services and settings, or indeed in no particular setting at all. To an important extent rehabilitation is as much an approach or attitude of mind as it is a treatment technology.

Promoting a culture of healing and instilling hope

Rediscovering recovery

Long before the discovery of effective medical and psychological treatments for psychosis it was known that better outcomes could be obtained if people were treated with respect and dignity and in settings that emphasised collaboration between staff and patients. This understanding was seen in the moral treatment provided in the best early 19th-century asylums and in the social psychiatry revolution of the 1950s. It has re-emerged in the current 'recovery' paradigm, which has its origins in the consumer/ ex-patient empowerment movement (see Roberts & Wolfson, Chapter 2, this volume). In this latest formulation, a distinction is drawn between the technologies of rehabilitation and the process of recovery: 'the lived or real life experience of persons as they accept and overcome the challenge of the disability' (Deegan, 1988: p. 11). This recovery process is understood to be unique to the individual. In large part it is the discovery of a purpose and meaning to life. It calls for active involvement in daily life, the assumption of personal responsibility, the exercise of choice and a degree of risk-taking. The individual may find purpose and meaning through work, in personal relationships or even through political action or advocacy on behalf of others. Importantly, there is no assumption of 'cure' in the sense of entirely escaping symptoms or impairments; instead, the emphasis is on achieving a fulfilling existence despite enduring disability.

From a service delivery perspective, these ideas emphasise the critical importance of collaboration in therapy, of choice rather than coercion, positive reinforcement of success rather than punishment for failure and a shared involvement with professionals in how the service is provided. From a staff perspective, this is the difference between viewing a patient as a person who happens to have schizophrenia and labelling him or her 'a schizophrenic'. This is a subtle but important distinction as it opens the door for conversations about what might be attempted or achieved despite the diagnosis or such and such symptom or experience. This focus and emphasis on the possibility of success rather than of failure, looking forward rather than back and making much of small steps are the ingredients of hope that in turn fuel self-esteem and self-respect.

Empowerment

In addition to instilling hope, a core task of psychiatric rehabilitation is empowerment. Empowerment is both something provided externally by the way services are structured and an internal psychological state of self-worth, self-confidence and courage to take calculated risks and to take responsibility for them. In terms of how services are structured, empowerment is facilitated both by ensuring that therapeutic interventions are collaborative, negotiated and their purpose transparent and by encouraging people with mental illnesses to take more personal responsibility for setting goals, working to achieve these and making decisions.

Much of what is involved in recovery is the business of picking up lost social roles – as tenant, employee, friend and so forth. In this respect, dependency is not an entirely bad word. It is typically the starting point of recovery, although it is not without risks, both in terms of being let down by those on whom the individual depends and in sapping initiative and self-directed action. In the recovery model, the aim is to move from dependency towards progressively more personal responsibility for choices and goals and their associated risks.

Principles into practice

In the case of someone entering a typical rehabilitation service, changes in the person's experience might begin the moment he (or she) is admitted to the unit. Instead of a frantic acute ward here is a relaxed, even-paced setting with a clear purpose to the day. Staff are interested in him as a person, his views are taken seriously and therapeutic arrangements occur when they are scheduled. He is expected to contribute to the life of the unit and it is clear that his contribution is valued and matters. Although he may not be entirely convinced that treatment is likely to be helpful, he might be pleased none the less that its purpose is explained and it is delivered at a pace that he can manage. During the course of his stay his experiences are listened to seriously and as much, if not more, attention is paid to the successes in his life than to the consequences of his illness. It is within this context that technical interventions that may have been tried and failed in the past may now succeed.

Limiting disability: processes and services

Impairment, disability and handicap

The recovery paradigm within mental health services is fashionable. Much less fashionable is an analysis of the complex effects of mental illness on the individual. It is helpful in understanding these effects to make a distinction between impairment, disability and handicap. In the context of severe mental illness, impairments comprise the positive and negative affective and cognitive symptoms of the illness (e.g. distressing auditory hallucinations, social withdrawal, depression and impaired concentration, all commonly experienced by someone with schizophrenia). Disabilities are the difficulties an individual experiences in performing everyday tasks (e.g. shopping, cooking and functioning at work) as a result of impairment. Handicap is the disadvantage and exclusion from social roles as a consequent of impairments and disabilities but also of external factors such as stigma, alienation from friends and family, unemployment, homelessness and poverty. (People with severe mental illnesses have also commonly experienced significant social disadvantage before becoming ill.) An additional and important issue is the individual's personal reaction to the impairments, disabilities and social disadvantage they experience as a result of an episode of illness. This often comprises depression and despair or, conversely, denial that there are problems that need to be addressed. Adverse personal reactions can compound and amplify the effects of illness on an individual.

Simon (Box 1.1), for example, suffers severe disabilities in terms of self-care, occupational functioning and social skills as a consequence of the symptomatic and cognitive impairments of his illness. Even if the severity of the symptomatic impairments could be reduced, there would remain much work to do in order to rebuild Simon's self-esteem, confidence and day-to-day coping skills. Handicaps from the illness will already have arisen – perhaps debt, unemployment and alienation of friends and family. Thus, it should come as little surprise that managing symptomatic impairment alone is not enough. The stigma, shabby accommodation and poverty Simon has experienced will erode self-esteem, destroy confidence and promote disability: instilling hope becomes a central requirement for Simon's chances of recovery from his illness.

Vulnerability, stress, coping and competence

Another useful way of conceptualising the focus of psychiatric rehabilitation is to consider the vulnerability–stress–coping–competence model (Anthony & Liberman, 1986). In this model, biological vulnerabilities predispose to illness when the person is exposed to environmental stress (e.g. interpersonal tensions or life events). Even if the biological vulnerability is impervious to intervention, the triggering and maintaining stressors can be mitigated by medication or by interventions that teach skills to cope with arousal or that provide buffering support. Rehabilitation can aim to reduce exposure to stress, to optimise protective factors and to develop living and coping skills.

Organising rehabilitation services

The ideal rehabilitation service provides a comprehensive, continuous, coordinated, collaborative and patient-oriented approach. Interventions

7

are linked to individualised needs assessments and to the personal goals of patients, each step negotiated and aiming at end-points that are personally meaningful and desired.

A key aspect of effective rehabilitation is the recognition that peoples' behaviour varies substantially from one situation to another. In general, task performance is more stable than social behaviour, and simple skills are more transferable than complex ones. Many of the improvements seen in a narrow rehabilitation setting are transient responses to the particular characteristic of that environment and do not readily transfer or generalise to more complex settings and situations. Therefore, rehabilitation assessment should focus more on an individual's capacities rather than fixed behaviours and should ideally be carried out across a wide spectrum of settings and conditions, in an attempt to work out what may be achieved under optimal conditions and what problems are likely in suboptimal conditions. People should be prepared for the environments in which they will be expected to function, and in general it is better to rehabilitate in the real situation than in the contrived setting of the hospital clinic.

It is also worth distinguishing long-term targets from short-term goals. The former are often couched in fairly broad terms, whereas the latter are the stepping stones to take the person where they want to go. Short-term goals need to be 'SMART' (specific, measurable, achievable, realistic and time-limited) and set in collaboration with the patient, relatives and other relevant people. With these short-term goals in mind specific interventions can then be devised that aim to produce a series of consistent, if modest, achievements backed up by frequent praise, encouragement and support. Watts & Bennett draw attention to the need to avoid setting goals that are unrealistically high or demoralisingly low. It is important to emphasise the individual's positive capacities and achievements, not only for the good this does self-esteem but also as 'the most effective antidote to the paternalistic attitudes that develop when psychiatric services try merely to care for long term patients' (Watts & Bennett, 1991: p. 12).

The judicious combination of pharmacological and psychological treatments is, of course, an essential ingredient of rehabilitation practice. These topics are covered in detail elsewhere in this volume. Here we will just outline important approaches to treatments that will reduce impairment and disability and services that address key areas of handicap, housing and employment.

Minimising impairment and disability

Pharmacological management

The past decade has seen many advances in the pharmacological treatment of severe mental illness (see Sweeting, Chapter 10, this volume). Currently, the vogue is to use the newer atypical antipsychotics. These drugs are as effective, at least in the short term, as traditional treatments, but have fewer troublesome extrapyramidal side-effects (Davis *et al*, 2003). (The exception is clozapine, which is undoubtedly more effective than other anti-psychotics.) The initial enthusiasm with which the atypicals were greeted by many rehabilitation psychiatrists has waned somewhat now that the majority of patients have already received these 'new' drugs before their first contact with rehabilitation services.

We have also seen the emergence of longer-term side-effects of atypical antipsychotics with protracted use. Of these, weight gain is probably the feature of most concern to patients. It is difficult to predict for the individual but sadly it is associated with a younger age and a good clinical response to treatment (Jones *et al*, 2001). The prevalence of diabetes in people with schizophrenia is almost twice that in the general population and may be further increased by some antipsychotic drugs (Baptista *et al*, 2002). These caveats aside, there is clearly an important role for the expert management of psychotropic medication in severe and enduring mental illness, not only for the control of symptoms but also for the management of co-occurring depression and cognitive impairment.

Cognitive–behavioural interventions

Cognitive–behavioural interventions have wide applicability for enduring mental illness (see Turkington & Arjundas, Chapter 12, this volume). For schizophrenia, for example, their main aim is to reduce distress and disability, and to help patients develop an understanding of their illness (Fowler *et al*, 1995). Individuals are encouraged to re-evaluate their beliefs through a gradual process of reviewing the evidence and constructing alternative explanations and to identify and manipulate factors that contribute to symptom maintenance. The therapist works collaboratively, taking an active enquiring stance towards the patient's account of their experiences. Direct confrontation of delusions is avoided, as this has been shown to be counterproductive. Moderately severe thought disorder can be tackled by disentangling the most emotionally relevant themes and helping the individual focus on these using thought-linkage techniques. The therapist encourages the patient to develop and use a variety of coping strategies, including anxiety management, activity scheduling and attention control, to reduce the occurrence and duration of hallucinations and of distressing experiences of anxiety or suspiciousness (Tarrier, 1992). An impressive number of randomised controlled trials have now been carried out, from which it appears that the approach reduces both positive symptoms and the risk of relapse (Pilling *et al*, 2002*a*).

Family interventions

In the UK, there has been a long-standing interest in the effect of the family environment on major mental illness. This has led to the development of family interventions of established efficacy in terms of preventing relapse and readmission and increasing adherence to pharmacological treatment.

It appears that interventions carried out with a single family at a time have superior outcomes at 1–2 years than those delivered to several families together (Pilling *et al*, 2002a), regardless of whether the single-family interventions are based explicitly on a behavioural model or on more systemically oriented approaches. By and large, later studies have produced less positive results than the earliest investigations, possibly because the early studies were led by charismatic enthusiasts (Mari & Streiner, 1994) or there has been increasing use of the less-potent delivery of the interventions to groups of families (Pilling *et al*, 2002a). It remains a challenge for family interventions to put this research into routine clinical practice (see Fadden, Chapter 11, this volume).

Skills training

Interventions aimed at correcting deficits in daily living skills such as poor personal hygiene, problems managing the home or dealing with finances are ubiquitous in rehabilitation practice, forming the basis for the daily work of nurses and occupational therapists in most if not all services. Many of these interventions involve simple advice, coaching and modelling. The more elaborate schemes draw on operant conditioning theory. In the most elaborate but now largely defunct approach, programmes were developed in which patients collected tangible rewards ('tokens') for performing desired behaviours. These were hugely complex programmes that were very difficult to implement and have proven untenable outside of very specialised settings. Furthermore, the skills acquired in the hospital or clinic often failed to generalise to daily living situations, and the latter had far more complexity than could be managed by a simple contingency-based reward system.

One skills training approach with a well-developed research base is the modular programme developed by Liberman and his colleagues at the UCLA Clinical Research Center for Schizophrenia and Psychiatric Rehabilitation in Los Angeles, California. This behavioural programme teaches a variety of skills, including medication self-management, basic conversation skills, grooming and self-care, job-finding and interpersonal problem-solving. A broad range of interventions are employed, including videotaped demonstrations, role-play, exercises in real situations and homework practice (Wallace *et al*, 1985). Numerous clinical trials have shown benefits over standard care in terms of improved conversational skills, assertiveness and medication management (Heinssen *et al*, 2000). These methods have been successfully employed with patients on acute wards, individuals with residual symptoms and individuals with severe and persistent illness. Not surprisingly, given the focus on specific social behaviours, social skills training has only modest impact on symptoms, relapse and hospitalisation. Some studies have found no significant advantage over more traditional occupational therapy or group-based supportive psychotherapy. Evidence on the extent to which new skills learnt in specific programmes generalise across settings or fade with time is sparse, although what there is points to a severe problem in generalisation from the classroom to real life. Some research indicates a benefit of including 'top-up' sessions and of carrying out some training away from the initial treatment setting (Eckman *et al*, 1992).

These formal programmes have proven much less popular in Europe than in the USA. A meta-analysis of randomised controlled trials of skills training found no consistent evidence for any benefit on relapse rate, global adjustment, social functioning or quality of life (Pilling *et al*, 2002*b*). There is, however, little reason to expect that an intervention aimed at improving self-care should have any effect on the incidence of relapse or rehospitalisation. Perhaps the prevailing view in the UK reflects a more widespread shift in recent years towards the cognitive end of the cognitive–behavioural spectrum of psychological interventions. Whatever the reason, it is striking that the interventions that comprise so much of nursing, occupational therapy and psychological practice in rehabilitation settings is so underresearched in the UK.

Cognitive remediation

Cognitive impairment in schizophrenia predicts poor rehabilitation outcomes. It is therefore an appealing thought that the remediation of the impairments of memory and executive function commonly seen in people with severe mental illnesses might facilitate skills training and contribute to improved social functioning (see Wykes, Chapter 14, this volume). Cognitive remediation seeks to retrain and improve processes of memory, attention and speed of information processing using a variety of 'exercise' programmes that were originally developed for neurological rehabilitation (after head injury or stroke, for example). In a study Wykes *et al* (1999) randomised individuals with chronic schizophrenia who had documented cognitive impairment to intensive cognitive remediation or to an 'intensive occupational therapy' control condition. Those receiving the intensive cognitive remediation attended for individual, daily, 1 h sessions that focused on executive functioning deficits (cognitive flexibility, working memory and planning). Some improvement in cognitive function was seen with both therapies, but a differential effect in favour of cognitive remediation was found for tests of cognitive flexibility and memory. Social functioning also tended to improve in those whose cognitive flexibility scores improved with treatment.

Benefits achieved in research settings do not necessarily transfer easily to routine care. An attempt was subsequently made to introduce cognitive remediation as a routine intervention within a rehabilitation team. A total of 23 staff received training but of these 13 subsequently moved to new jobs where it is unlikely that their cognitive remediation skills were used. Of the 16 clients who had been identified as suitable for cognitive remediation only 5 were willing and able to participate and only 2 completed the course, one of whom was thought to have benefited substantially (Cupitt *et al*, 2004). In routine practice it would appear that many staff and clients find the course too demanding and would rather be doing something else.

Addressing handicap

A home of one's own?

Throughout the 1970s and early 1980s, rehabilitation came to be regarded as synonymous with resettlement of the long-stay hospital population. This narrow view was rightly criticised at the time, not least because of the danger that once resettled, the job of rehabilitation might be seen to be over. A range of accommodation options, from highly staffed residential homes to independent flats with visiting support, forms an essential ingredient of any modern psychiatric service (see Wolfson, Chapter 17, this volume). However, there is surprisingly little research into the relative benefits of different configurations of housing and support.

Perhaps the best-known British research was carried out into the closure of Friern Hospital (the former Colney Hatch Asylum) in North London and re-provision for its patients (for a summary of the main findings see Leff, 1997). Most of the former in-patients were placed in group homes with shared facilities. These settings were less regimented and restrictive than the hospital and were preferred by patients to the hospital ward. Living in the community had some advantages: low rehospitalisation rates and, for some, the opportunity to develop friendships with ordinary members of the public. Although individuals showed large fluctuations in symptoms over the follow-up, there was no overall change in psychiatric state for the whole sample and behavioural problems also remained stable. There was little difference in cost between hospital and community care once account was taken of the few patients with particularly challenging behaviours who could not be immediately discharged to the community.

Comparable outcomes of hospital closure programmes have been reported both elsewhere in Britain and internationally (for a comprehensive review see Fakhoury & Priebe, 2002)). The number of residents living in such shared accommodation has risen substantially in the past decade, in line with Europe-wide trends in psychiatric care (Priebe *et al*, 2005). Thus, the hospital asylum has come to be replaced by a 'virtual asylum' comprising a patchwork of residential and nursing home care, long-stay hospital accommodation and private-sector medium and low secure services (Holloway, 2004). These at best replace the asylum ward with more 'homely' environments but at worst substitute one order of neglect with another (Geller, 2000).

An alternative model might rely more on a partnership between the providers of ordinary public housing and mental health services, the latter coordinating and providing a range of training and treatment. Such 'mobile support' models are preferred by service users and carers (Carling,

1993). But this is not to say that such an approach guarantees a better outcome.

The default approach is not to provide continuing monitoring and care through a specialist rehabilitation service; rather, it is to leave the case management to already overstretched generic community teams or to inexperienced housing support workers who may have little appreciation of the complexity of severe mental illness. Without close attention there are real risks of neglect, abuse and institutionalisation in these settings (Carling, 1995).

No substantial evaluations of the mobile support model have been carried out in the UK. Limited evidence is available from the USA. In one thought-provoking study Susser et al (1997) randomised 96 homeless mentally ill men who were being rehoused to receive either 9 months of a 'critical time' service (comprising intensive case management, including tenancy support) or care as usual. At 18-month follow-up, the average number of homeless nights was 30 for the 'critical time' group and 91 for the group receiving usual services. Overall costs of care were similar in both groups (Jones et al, 2003). Attempts have also been made to implement and evaluate city-wide programmes. One such effort was sponsored by the Robert Wood Johnson Foundation and the US Department of Housing and Urban Development. This brought together housing and health authorities in nine US cities to provide and evaluate a comprehensive system of housing subsidy and mobile support for people with severe mental illnesses. The success of this programme varied widely from city to city, with some benefits in terms of quality of life but no substantial effect on clinical outcomes or rehospitalisation (Goldman et al, 1994). Social isolation and the lack of recreational opportunities were frequently cited problems in these programmes, any expansion in social contacts often being confined to health professionals and fellow residents (Friedrich et al, 1999).

A job to do

The importance of meaningful occupation and employment to recovery has been recognised since the dawn of 'moral treatment' (see Boardman & Robinson, Chapter 19, this volume). Shockingly, employment rates for people with severe mental illnesses in the UK are far lower now than in the 1950s (Marwaha & Johnson, 2004). There are many reasons for this, not least the profound changes in the nature of available work and the performance demands made on employees and employers in the modern economy. Mental health professionals may tend to overestimate the negative impact of employment on mental health and to underestimate their clients' capacity (Secker et al, 2001). Negative symptoms of schizophrenia, poor social skills and neuropsychological impairments have all been shown to impair performance at work. Medication side-effects can also be problematical: sedation can be a particular difficulty, although this is less of an issue in contemporary practice, where high-dose regimens are avoided.

The earliest models in the post-asylum era in the UK involved the transfer of the industrial therapy units and work crews into smaller, community-based offices on the high street that provided part-time poorly paid or unpaid occupation. Movement from these 'sheltered workshops' to competitive employment in the open labour market was rare and the model has fallen out of favour, although the risks of dependency and institutionalisation can be minimised by an emphasis on market orientation, employee involvement and regularly reviewed action plans. The better sheltered workshop still has a limited part to play in modern rehabilitation services for people with the most severe disabilities, who would not be accepted in any more open setting (O'Flynn & Craig, 2001).

One development of the sheltered workshop theme worth mentioning is the 'clubhouse' model. This emerged in America in the 1950s as a setting for support and preparation for employment. Clubhouse members are expected to participate in all aspects of the organisation, sharing responsibility with staff for maintaining the building, preparing meals, working in the office and greeting visitors. Following a period of pre-vocational training, employment placements are arranged in a variety of temporary jobs with mainstream employers, the employment contract being held by the clubhouse organisation and shared between members (Beard et al, 1982). The model has been criticised on the grounds that pre-vocational training is of limited value and that the shared job placements are largely limited to unskilled, low-grade positions (Bond et al, 1997).

Clubhouse and more traditional sheltered employment schemes have been overtaken in popularity by approaches that support people in finding and retaining ordinary 'open' employment. In Europe, many of the sheltered workshops have evolved or transformed into 'social firms' – small market-oriented business ventures that are run by and/or employ significant numbers of disabled people. There is some evidence for their commercial viability, high user satisfaction and reduced use of mental health services (Grove & Drurie, 1999).

In North America there has been considerable interest in programmes in which people with severe mental illnesses are placed and supported in open employment, an approach hailed as the most important development in vocational rehabilitation. Placements may involve a subsidy to the employer or modification of the job to take account of particular needs. The approach achieves high rates of competitive employment without increasing hospitalisation (Bond et al, 1997). On the downside, however, job turnover is high, the majority of placements are in low-paid unskilled occupations and a continuing high level of support is essential to job retention. A follow-up of an earlier research programme found that only a quarter of those whose support had terminated at the end of the programme remained in employment, compared with three-quarters of those whose support was maintained over the year (McHugo et al, 1998).

There have been several successful programmes in which people with mental illnesses have been employed in front-line caring roles, typically as case managers or case manager aids, both in the USA (Solomon & Draine, 1995; Mowbray et al, 1998) and in the UK (Craig et al, 2004). Despite these model programmes most services have a poor record in explicitly recruiting people who have mental health problems.

The evaluation of the various models of employment is methodologically difficult as they often involve small schemes with different local circumstances, patient populations and programme details. Nevertheless, there is now a fair amount of evidence available on what works and practice guidelines are beginning to emerge. These essentially boil down to managing the tension between the individual's rehabilitation needs on the one hand and the market-oriented demands of the job on the other. For example, coping strategies such as taking frequent short breaks to maintain concentration or minimise intrusive hallucinations can be problematical in the workplace and viewed poorly by employers (Cook & Razzano, 2000). Also, although a comprehensive assessment of an individual's suitability for a particular post may take several weeks, many employers demand maximum productivity from the outset. Finally, no one model is likely to be sufficient for all rehabilitation needs. Each approach is likely to be helpful to different people at different times in their recovery (O'Flynn & Craig, 2001).

Conclusions

It should be obvious that, although the thrust of this chapter has concerned people with chronic and persistent mental illness, the principles and ingredients of psychiatric rehabilitation are just as applicable to earlier stages of illness, when they may play an important role in preventing disability. The 2 or 3 years following first onset of severe mental illness have been identified as a critical period for intervention (Birchwood et al, 1998). It is during these early years that much damage is done to self-esteem and social networks, and education and employment opportunities may be lost for ever (see Power et al, Chapter 9, this volume).

Depression and anxiety are major causes of disability worldwide. The specific interventions for the management of severe neuroses and personality disorder are likely to be rather different from those described in this book, which is devoted to services for people with psychotic illnesses. However, the guiding principles of psychiatric rehabilitation – delivery of goal-directed therapy managed in partnership and provided in real situations in a culture of empowerment and optimism – remain the cornerstone of all branches of mental health care. These principles are therefore appropriate not just to services with a designated 'rehabilitation' label: they are applicable to all mental health services at any stage in an individual's contact with the mental health system.

References

Anthony, W. A. & Liberman, R. P. (1986) The practice of psychiatric rehabilitation: historical, conceptual and research base. *Schizophrenia Bulletin*, **12**, 542–559.

Anthony, W. A., Cohen, M. R. & Cohen, B. F. (1984) Psychiatric Rehabilitation. In *The Chronic Mental Patient. Five Years Later* (ed. J. A. Talbott), pp. 137–157. New York: Grune & Stratton.

Baptista, T., Kin, N., Beaulieu, S., *et al* (2002) Obesity and related metabolic abnormalities during antipsychotic drug administration. Mechanisms, management and research perspectives. *Pharmacopsychiatry*, **35**, 205–219.

Beard, J. H., Propst, R. N. & Malamud, T. J. (1982) The Fountain House model of rehabilitation. *Psychosocial Rehabilitation Journal*, **5**, 47–53.

Bennett, D. H. (1978) Community psychiatry. *British Journal of Psychiatry*, **132**, 209–220.

Birchwood, M., Jackson, C. & Todd, P. (1998) The critical period hypothesis. *International Clinical Psychopharmacology*, **12**, 27–38.

Bond, G. R., Drake, R. E., Mueser, K. T., *et al* (1997) An update on supported employment for people with severe mental illness. *Psychiatric Services*, **48**, 335–346.

Carling, P. J. (1993) Housing and supports for persons with mental illness: emerging approaches to research and practice. *Hospital and Community Psychiatry*, **44**, 439–449.

Carling, P. (1995) *Returning to Community, Building Support Systems for People with Psychiatric Disabilities*. New York: Guilford Press.

Cook, J. A. & Razzano, L. (2000) Vocational rehabilitation for persons with schizophrenia: recent research and implications for practice. *Schizophrenia Bulletin*, **26**, 87–103.

Craig, T., Doherty, I., Jamieson-Craig, R., *et al* (2004) The consumer-employee as a member of a mental health assertive outreach team. 1. Clinical and social outcomes. *Journal of Mental Health*, **13**, 59–69.

Cupitt, C., Byrne, L. & Tompson, N. (2004) Delivering cognitive remediation therapy in a clinical setting. *Clinical Psychology*, **37**, 10–14.

Davis, J. M., Chen, N. & Glick, I. D. (2003) A meta-analysis of the efficacy of second-generation antipsychotics. *Archives of General Psychiatry*, **60**, 553–564.

Deegan, P. E. (1988) Recovery: the lived experience of rehabilitation. *Psychosocial Rehabilitation Journal*, **11**, 11–19.

Eckman, T. A., Wirshing, W. C., Marder, S. R., *et al* (1992) Technique for training schizophrenic patients in illness self-management: a controlled trial. *American Journal of Psychiatry*, **149**, 1549–1555.

Fakhoury, W. & Priebe, S. (2002) The process of deinstitutionalisation: an international review. *Current Opinion in Psychiatry*, **15**, 187–192.

Fowler, D., Garety, P. & Kuipers, E. (1995) *Cognitive Behaviour Therapy for People with Psychosis*. Chichester: John Wiley and Sons.

Friedrich, R. M., Hollingsworth, B., Hradek, E., *et al* (1999) Family and client perspectives on alternative residential settings for persons with severe mental illness. *Psychiatic Services*, **50**, 509–514.

Geller, J. L. (2000) The last half century of psychiatric services as reflected in 'Psychiatric Services'. *Psychiatric Services*, **51**, 41–67.

Goldman, H. H., Morrissey, J. P. & Ridgely, M. S. (1994) Evaluating the Robert Wood Johnson Foundation program on chronic mental illness. *Milbank Quarterly*, **72**, 37–47.

Grove, B. & Drurie, S. (1999) *Social Firms: An Instrument for Economic Empowerment and Inclusion*. Redhill: Social Firms UK.

Heinssen, R. K., Liberman, R. P. & Kopelowicz, A. (2000) Psychosocial skills training for schizophrenia: lessons from the laboratory. *Schizophrenia Bulletin*, **26**, 21–46.

Holloway, F. (2004) Reprovision for the long-stay patient. *Psychiatry*, **3**, 5–9.

Jones, B., Basson, B. R., Walker, D. J., *et al* (2001) Weight change and atypical antipsychotic treatment in patients with schizophrenia. *Journal of Clinical Psychiatry*, **62** (suppl. 2), 41–44.

Jones, K., Colson, P. W., Holter, M. C., et al (2003) Cost-effectiveness of Critical Time Intervention to reduce homelessness among persons with mental illness. *Psychiatric Services*, **54**, 884–890.

Killaspy, H., Harden, C., Holloway, F., et al (2005) What do mental health rehabilitation services do and what are they for? A national survey in England. *Journal of Mental Health*, **14**, 157–165.

Leff J. (ed.) (1997) *Care in the Community – Illusion or Reality?* Chichester: John Wiley & Sons.

Mari, D. J. & Streiner, D. (1994) An overview of family interventions and relapse on schizophrenia: meta-analysis of research findings. *Psychological Medicine*, **24**, 565–578.

Marwaha, S. & Johnson, S. (2004) Schizophrenia and employment: a review. *Social Psychiatry and Psychiatric Epidemiology*, **39**, 337–349.

McHugo, G. J., Drake, R. E. & Becker, D. R. (1998) The durability of supported employment effects. *Psychiatric Rehabilitation Journal*, **22**, 55–61.

Mowbray, C. T., Moxley, D. P. & Collins, M. E. (1998) Consumers as mental health providers: first-person accounts of benefits and limitations. *Journal of Behavioural Health Services and Research*, **25**, 397–411.

O'Flynn, D. & Craig, T. (2001) Which way to work? Occupations, vocations and opportunities for mental health service users. *Journal of Mental Health*, **10**, 1–4.

Pilling, S., Bebbington, P., Kuipers, E., et al (2002a) Psychological treatments in schizophrenia I: Meta-analyses of family intervention and cognitive behaviour therapy. *Psychological Medicine*, **32**, 763–782.

Pilling, S., Bebbington, P., Kuipers, E., et al (2002b) Psychological treatments in schizophrenia. II. Meta analyses of randomized controlled trials of social skills training and cognitive remediation. *Psychological Medicine*, **32**, 783–791.

Priebe, S., Badesconyi, A., Fioritti, A., et al (2005) Reinstitutionalisation in mental health care: comparison of data on service provision from six European countries. *BMJ*, **330**, 123–126.

Secker, J., Grove, B. & Seebohm, P. (2001) Challenging barriers to employment, training and education for mental health service users: the service users perspective. *Journal of Mental Health*, **10**, 395–404.

Solomon, P. & Draine, J. (1995) The efficacy of a consumer case management team: 2–year outcomes of a randomised trial. *Journal of Mental Health Administration*, **22**, 135–146.

Susser, E., Valencia, E., Conover, S., et al (1997) Preventing recurrent homelessness among mentally ill men: a 'critical time' intervention after discharge from a shelter. *American Journal of Public Health*, **87**, 256–262.

Tarrier, N. (1992) Management and modifciation of residual positive psychotic symptoms. In *Innovations in the Psychological Management of Schizophrenia* (eds M. Birchwood & N. Tarrier), pp. 147–169. Chichester: John Wiley & Sons.

Wallace, C. J., Boone, S. E., Donahoe, C. P., et al (1985) The chronic mentally disabled: independent living skills training. In *Clinical Handbook of Psychological Disorders: A Step-by-Step Treatment Manual* (ed. D. Barlow), pp. 147–168. New York: Guilford Press.

Watts, F. & Bennett, D. (1991) The concept of rehabilitation. In *Theory and Practice of Psychiatric Rehabilitation* (eds F. N. Watts & D. H. Bennett), pp. 3–14. Chichester: John Wiley & Sons.

World Health Organization (1980) *International Classification of Impairment, Disabilities and Handicaps: A Manual of Classification Relating to the Consequences of Disease*. Geneva: WHO.

Wykes, T. & Holloway, F. (2000) Community rehabilitation: past failures and future prospects. *International Review of Psychiatry*, **12**, 197–205.

Wykes, T., Reeder, C., Corner, J., et al (1999) The effects of neurocognitive remediation on executive processing in patients with schizophrenia. *Schizophrenia Bulletin*, **25**, 291–307.

CHAPTER 2

New directions in rehabilitation: learning from the recovery movement[†]

Glenn Roberts and Paul Wolfson

'The goal of recovery is not to become normal. The goal is to embrace the human vocation of becoming more deeply, more fully human.'

Deegan (1996)

To ask whether someone will recover is often our first response when we are confronted with any severe health problem, and helping people to recover is a fundamental goal for any service or practitioner. It has long been assumed that people with severe mental illnesses do not recover, and this belief leads to low expectations that tend to erode hope and collude with chronicity (Harrison & Mason, 1993). Advances in psychiatric practice usually involve an improvement of existing treatments or a new method of service delivery. The present interest in developing recovery-oriented services does involve changes in practice but in response to a new clinical philosophy that enables old problems to be thought of in a different way.

In ordinary usage, 'recovery' is thought of as broadly equivalent to 'cure', a return to how things were before the injury occurred or the illness began. By these standards, as Whitwell (1999) has observed, few people with severe mental illnesses recover. At the heart of the growing interest in recovery is a controversial redefinition of what recovery means to people with severe mental health problems. The experience of recovery has been reconceptualised as a personal process of learning how to live, and how to live well, with enduring symptoms and vulnerabilities. Through this the possibility of recovery becomes available to all. The implications of people with long-term conditions redefining themselves from 'chronically ill' to 'in recovery' can be pivotal and profound.

As psychiatrists continue to debate their roles and responsibilities, service users are developing a model in which people can recover without the help of doctors, and sometimes even despite them. The recovery movement may superficially look like the latest reincarnation of the anti-psychiatry movement, but it is potentially the opposite, a focus for

[†]This chapter is a modified version of Roberts, G. & Wolfson, P. (2004) The rediscovery of recovery: open to all. *Advances in Psychiatric Treatment*, **10**, 37–49.

collaboration between all those with strong motivation and commitment to improved services and outcomes for individuals and families.

The origins of recovery

Over 200 years ago, a critical appraisal of contemporary psychiatric practice inspired the Tukes at York to establish a clinical philosophy and therapeutic practice that became known as moral treatment. This was based on kindness, compassion, respect and hope of recovery (Tuke, 1813). Today, visitors to the Royal College of Psychiatrists in London are greeted by an image of William Tuke as they pass through the entrance lobby. In the latter half of the 20th century some of the principles of moral treatment were rediscovered, through deinstitutionalisation, the physical disability movement, anti-discriminatory and disability legislation and the growth of consumerism (Anthony, 1993; Allott et al, 2002), which all played a part in the development of recovery as a clinical philosophy.

In the UK, as in the USA, mental health professionals have made significant contributions to the growing number of moving and instructive personal accounts of recovery from severe mental illness (North, 1988; Jamison, 1995; Fisher, 2001; May, 2004), and there is a process analogous to 'coming out' in combating stigma. When a recent President of the Royal College of Psychiatrists sought election with the usual brief CV detailing his qualifications for the job, unusually this included his personal experience of depression. There seems to have been an acknowledgement within the profession that people can become 'experts by experience' as well as by training (Crane, 2003).

Recovery emerged as a guiding vision for mental health services in the USA during the 1990s (Ralph *et al*, 2002), and since 1998 New Zealand mental health services have been based on the recovery-centred 'Blueprint' (O'Hagan, 2001). In the UK, increasing convergence between a recovery perspective and mental health policy is reflected in *The Journey to Recovery* (Department of Health 2001*b*), a summary of the NHS Plan and National Service Framework for Mental Health, and support for initiatives such as the Expert Patient programme (Department of Health, 2001*a*; Cooper & Clarke, 2005). There are also striking parallels between practices that US service users have identified as pivotal to recovery (Ohio Department of Mental Health, 2003) and clinical guidelines for schizophrenia published by the National Institute for Clinical Excellence (now the National Institute for Health and Clinical Excellence, NICE, 2002) (Box 2.1).

What is meant by 'recovery'?

Definition and redefinition

The word 'recovery' appears to have a simple and self-evident meaning, but within the recovery literature it has been variously used to mean an

---

Box 2.1 Comparison of the highest-ranking recovery-oriented practices from the Ohio outcomes initiative (Ohio Department of Mental Health, 2003) and the NICE clinical guidelines for schizophrenia (National Institute for Clinical Excellence, 2002)

Ohio	Encourage my independent thinking
NICE	Discuss preferences, record advance directives (p. 39)
Ohio	Treat me in a way that helps my recovery process
NICE	Offer help in an atmosphere of hope and optimism (1.1.1)
Ohio	Treat me as an equal in planning my services
NICE	Foster a collaborative working relationship (1.1.5)
Ohio	Give me the freedom to make my own mistakes
NICE	Service-user preferences are central (1.4.5)
Ohio	Treat me like they believe I can shape my own future
NICE	Patients have the right to be fully informed and share in decision-making (p. 50)
Ohio	Listen to me and believe what I say
NICE	Encourage patients to write their own account of their illness in their notes (1.3.3); record your treatment preferences (p. 39)
Ohio	Look at and recognise my abilities
NICE	Include assessment of occupational status and potential (1.4.6)
Ohio	Work with me to find the resources or services I need
NICE	Comprehensive care coordination (p. 46)
Ohio	Be available to talk to me when I need to talk to someone
NICE	Professionals who work with you should be engaging and kind, in constructive partnership (p. 38)
Ohio	Teach me about the medications I am taking
NICE	Give patients clear intelligible information, full discussion, choice (1.4.5)

approach, a model, a philosophy, a paradigm, a movement and a vision. To the sceptical, a definition of recovery that significantly departs from the commonsense equation with 'cure' can even seem to be perpetuating a damaging myth (Whitwell, 2005). Two main perspectives on outcome have generated very different kinds of data. The first focuses on traditional dimensions of clinical and social recovery, measured objectively through reduced symptoms, disability and use of services, and expressed as approximations to cure. The second focuses on the personal and existential dimensions of recovery, taking the form of subjective and self-evaluated accounts of what an individual has regained in their life and how they have learned to accommodate their illness experience. These have become the founding stories of the recovery movement (Chamberlin, 1978; Lovejoy, 1984; Deegan, 1988, 1996; Leete, 1989; Unzicker, 1989; Clay, 1994; Coleman, 1999; Ridgeway, 2000). Anthologies of these personal stories have been used by professions and governments as a means of combating stigma and reasserting the importance of a personal perspective (Leibrich, 1999; Lapsley et al, 2002; Ramsay et al, 2002).

For example, Daniel Fisher, as a psychiatrist and co-director of the National Empowerment Center in the USA, illustrates the power of the personal account through his challenge in the *Washington Post*, which begins

'I have recovered from schizophrenia. If that statement surprises you – if you think schizophrenia is a lifelong brain disease that cannot be escaped – you have been misled by a cultural misapprehension that needlessly imprisons millions under the label of mental illnesses'. The evidence-based clinician will also be aware that a general theory and expectation cannot be based on a single case history' (Fisher, 2001).

Anthony (1993) is credited with the most widely accepted definition of recovery. He argues that the *person* with a mental illness can recover even when the *illness* is not cured, and that the process of recovery can proceed in the presence of continuing symptoms and disabilities. From this viewpoint 'wellness' and 'illness' may be considered as independent variables. A person's health is not wholly determined by their illness and, conversely, having symptoms that are well controlled by medication is no guarantee of greater autonomy or better quality of life. In recovery I can become progressively more robust, and my life richer and more rewarding, even when my illness and symptoms continue to fluctuate or, as the Stanford University self-management course puts it, 'living a healthy life with chronic conditions' (Cooper & Clarke, 2005). Thus, recovery involves:

'a deeply personal, unique process of changing one's attitudes, values, feelings, goals, skills and roles. It is a way of living a satisfying, hopeful, and contributing life even with limitations caused by the illness. Recovery involves the development of new meaning and purpose in one's life as one grows beyond the catastrophic effects of mental illness' (Anthony, 1993).

Anthony's definition celebrates our experience of people who have overcome suffering by personal and spiritual growth, but at the same time can produce a feeling of unease for some. For example, Oyebode (2004) suggests that 'the involvement of governments in this endorsement of a peculiar departure in ordinary language use demonstrates that we are here dealing with the politics of healthcare and not the clinical aspects'.

Recovery and cure: the significance of long-term outcome studies

Many authors cite Harding *et al*'s (1987) pioneering long-term studies of schizophrenia, which found that half to two-thirds of patients significantly improved or recovered, including 'some very chronic cases'. The criteria for recovery are impressive: no current medication, working, relating well to family and friends, integrated into the community and behaving in such a way that no one could detect that the individual had ever been hospitalised for a psychiatric problem.

However, the applicability of these findings to other clinical settings has been questioned on the grounds of selection bias and the unusual comprehensiveness of the patients' treatment. An inherent difficulty in interpreting long-term outcome studies is that the 'outcomes' can say as much about the sampling of patients admitted to these studies as about the illnesses studied (Harrison and Mason, 1993). Furthermore, a critique based on selection bias seems reasonable but one based on evidence of particularly comprehensive treatment seems perverse. Warner's (1994) review of 85 studies over the past 100 years led him to observe that 'few topics in psychiatry have been researched as frequently, and over as long a period of time, as has recovery from schizophrenia', but despite this volume of work, 'a clear picture of long-term outcome has not emerged'. He attributes this to the limited validity of schizophrenia as a diagnostic entity.

The International Study of Schizophrenia (Harrison *et al*, 2001), which is probably the most substantial long-term follow-up study to date, included 1633 participants from 14 culturally diverse areas, studied at 15 years and 25 years after diagnosis. The results were in line with previous studies. Global outcomes at 15 years and 25 years were favourable for over half of all people followed up. There was evidence of a 'late recovery' effect, which supported the case for therapeutic optimism and suggested that these findings should 'join others in relieving patients, carers and clinicians of the chronicity paradigm which dominated thinking throughout much of the 20th century'. But the authors concede that 'the criteria *most pertinent to patients'* personal recovery have still not been evaluated, nor have the instruments yet been developed that could measure these' (emphasis added). Until the core concepts of recovery have been carefully operationalised, its estimation may not be greatly helped by current models of outcome research.

Recovery and the medical model

It is a largely non-medical assertion that medical practice is governed by something called 'the medical model', and the largely non-medical recovery literature yields a strong and clear view that psychiatric thought and practice are almost entirely hostage to it. It is often depicted as narrowly focused on disease, treatment and biological reductionism, underwritten by evidence-based medicine. This is contrasted with the broader, person-centred focus of recovery models (Ralph et al, 2002), which assert the validity of evidence largely comprising personal narrative, and the views of 'experts by experience'. At present, these two perspectives, their values and language stand in significant tension with one another (Table 2.1).

The recovery literature often characterises psychiatrists as risk averse and wedded to a relapse-prevention and maintenance model of care ('warehousing') that compounds disability and fosters dependency. Critics further emphasise that time, much time, can pass without benefit. Deegan (1988) has poignantly recollected that she stood 'drugged and stiff in the hallways of a mental hospital while my classmates went off to college. We experienced time as a betrayer. Time did not heal us.'

Table 2.1 Differences in concepts, language and values between the recovery and the medical models

Recovery model	Medical model
Distressing experience	Psychopathology
Biography	Pathography
Interest centred on the person	Interest centred on the disorder
Pro-health	Anti-disease
Strengths-based	Treatment-based
Experts by experience	Doctors and patients
Personal meaning	Diagnosis
Understanding	Recognition
Value-centred	(Apparently) value-free
Humanistic	Scientific
Growth and discovery	Treatment
Choice	Compliance
Modelled on heroes	Underpinned by meta-analysis
Guiding narratives	Randomised controlled trials
Transformation	Return to normal
Self-management	Expert care coordinators
Self-control	Bringing under control
Personal responsibility	Professional accountability
Within a social context	Decontextualised

After Ralph *et al* (2002), May (2004), Allott *et al* (2002).

The process of recovery

In contrast with the emphasis on the struggle for cure, Deegan (1988) defines recovery as 'a process, a way of life, an attitude, and a way of approaching the day's challenges.' The recovery literature (Ralph *et al*, 2002; Allott *et al*, 2002) similarly describes being 'in recovery' as an ongoing process, which involves gaining or regaining many aspects of life that are usually taken for granted and may have been lost or severely compromised by mental illness. Recovery may involve many stages, and inevitably setbacks and uncertainty, so that it becomes 'an uncharted, unpredictable, and personal journey' (Sheehan, 2002).

The experience of recovery is often described as having a defining moment or turning point (Allott *et al*, 2002), sometimes at a particularly low time (Rakfeldt & Strauss, 1989). Before this moment the user feels stuck, perhaps denying the illness because of anxiety or unresolved grief for loss of health and future. It has been claimed that recovery is often further delayed by a state of learned helplessness induced by the low expectations of mental health professionals, especially when they remove a person's choice and responsibility. But these need not be so. Even in circumstances that begin with compulsory admission, a recovery perspective could involve progressive handing back of control, so that choice and self-direction are supported at the earliest opportunity.

The experience of entering the process of recovery may come out of the blue, but is more often described as arising from talking to others, and commonly service users rather than professionals. It is experienced as regaining a sense of self, of taking control and responsibility, often combining optimism for the future with acceptance of the past. Service users describe a wide range of transitions at work in the recovery process. Finding meaning in and for psychotic experiences can be empowering (Roberts, Chapter 7, this volume), as can the emphasis on spirituality that is common in patients' accounts (Faulkner, 2000; Leibrich, 2002) and of increasing interest to psychiatrists (http://www.rcpsych.ac.uk/info/spirituality.asp).

From within the user movement, Coleman (1999) has emphasised that recovery depends far more on self-help and collaboration than on being treated:

'Recovery is not a gift from doctors but the responsibility of us all . . . We must become confident in our own abilities to change our lives; we must give up being reliant on others doing everything for us. We need to start doing these things for ourselves. We must have the confidence to give up being ill so that we can start becoming recovered'.

And although this risks formulating recovery as 'simply' an act of faith, it is apparent that it will be difficult to recover without faith and hope in the possibility, which my be gained as much from fellow travellers as from professionals.

How can we know what influences recovery?

The need for measurement

Liberman & Kopelowicz (2002), after a decade of witnessing the promotion of recovery in the USA, insist on the need to

'go beyond the hype, vague "vision" and glittering generalities . . . and move into the realm of empirically supported validation of an operationally defined concept of recovery'.

They suggest a list of the dimensions that could be used to derive such an operational definition (Box 2.2).

The measurement of recovery is at an early stage, and the need to strengthen the evidence base is potentially a major area for collaboration between service users and providers. Narratives of recovery offer service users relief from alienation, validation of unusual experience and a social context in which coping strategies can be exchanged. Meta-analyses of randomised controlled trials, although important, provide psychiatrists with little guidance on matters such as these, on what might make a difference to an individual patient entering the service or how to develop their own service to be more effective in supporting recovery. Research methods that integrate the essence of subjective accounts with the rigour

Box 2.2   Dimensions for operationalising recovery from schizophrenia

1 Remission of both positive and negative psychotic symptoms and signs
2 Working or studying in normative employment or educational settings
3 Independent living without supervision of money, self-care and medication
4 Social activities with peers
5 Cordial family relations and contacts
6 Recreational activity in normative settings (i.e. not in psychosocial clubhouses or day treatment programmes)
7 Resilience and capacity for problem-solving when faced with stressors or challenges in everyday life
8 Subjective satisfaction with life
9 Self-esteem and stable self-identity
10 Participation as a citizen in voting, self-advocacy, neighbourliness and other civic arenas

(Liberman & Kopelowicz, 2002.
Reproduced with permission from Taylor & Francis Ltd)

of objective measures are much needed. As the former US Secretary of State Robert McNamara is reputed to have said, 'the challenge is to make the important measurable, not the measurable important'. There is a continuing process of working to design tools that aim to be simple but valid measures of both individual progress in recovery and recovery as a service outcome. A recent service user-led evaluation of current measures (Campbell-Orde *et al*, 2005) includes the Ohio Consumer Assessment, recommended by the National Institute for Mental Health in England's (NIMHE's) Experts by Experience Group as a valid way of measuring progress in personal recovery, and the Developing Recovery Enhancing Environments Measure (DREEM, Ridgeway & Press, 2004), which is being piloted by NIMHE as a user-led service outcome measure (Dinniss, *et al*, 2006).

Steps towards a recovery-oriented psychiatric practice

The appliance of science: ensuring that we use the evidence base

The development of evidence-based guidelines has not been accompanied by allocation of resources to permit their implementation. There is a duty on all doctors to practise in conformity with NICE guidelines, but it does not appear to be anyone's responsibility to ensure that services are equipped to do so. One rather obvious way to promote recovery, in the traditional sense, would be to ensure universal access to services and treatments of proven effectiveness. Falloon *et al* (2004) have reported the 2-year outcomes of a 5-year international collaborative programme seeking to do just that. Their

---

> **Box 2.3** Optimal treatment with evidence-based strategies
>
> A combination of :
> - optimal dose antipsychotics
> - strategies to educate himself and his carers to cope more effectively with environmental stresses
> - cognitive behavioural therapy to enhance work and social goals and reduce residual symptoms
> - assertive home-based management to help prevent and resolve major social needs and crises, including recurrent symptoms
>
> (From Falloon *et al*, 2004)

---

concept of 'optimal treatment' (Box 2.3) is a close correspondence to what is specified in the NICE schizophrenia guidelines (National Institute for Clinical Excellence, 2002). This interim report on over 600 patients from 10 countries finds that 'on all measures the evidence-based Optimal Treatment Project approach achieved more than double the benefits associated with current best practice and one half of recent cases had achieved full recovery from clinical and social morbidity'. However, it also notes that 'One in four cases of recent onset and first episode cases and 40% of chronic cases showed no improvement after 2 years of optimal treatment'. More than three-quarters of the 'centres of excellence' that initially joined the study dropped out of the long-term follow-up because they were unable to sustain 'optimal treatment' for more than a year. There are considerable gains to be had from the application of evidence-based practice, but significant limitations in the real-world effectiveness of both treatments and services. The recovery movement is a positive response to these shortcomings.

A shift of professional role: from authority to coach

A change in the role of the psychiatrist is required, from someone who is perceived as a remote expert or authority to someone who behaves more like a coach or personal trainer, offering their skills and knowledge, while learning from and valuing their patients, who are experts by experience. There are striking stories of how effective it can be when 'seeing a psychiatrist' is experienced as having alongside you an experienced and committed person, who believes in you and your future (Ramsay *et al*, 2002).

Focusing on the core significance of hope and optimism

Being met with hope and optimism, especially at the initial contact, is important in many peoples' accounts of recovery, and 'offering help, treatment and care in an atmosphere of hope and optimism' is the first and overarching principle of the NICE schizophrenia guidelines (National

---

Box 2.4 Dimensions of hope-inspiring relationships

1 Valuing people as human beings
2 Acceptance and understanding
3 Believing in the person's abilities and potential
4 Attending to people's priorities and interests
5 Accepting failures and setbacks as part of the recovery process
6 Accepting that the future is uncertain
7 Finding ways of sustaining our own hope and guarding against despair
8 Accepting that we must learn and benefit from experience

(From Repper & Perkins, 2003)

Institute for Clinical Excellence, 2002: 1.1.1.1). This has implications for the selection and training of staff who will be able to engage in hope-inspiring relationships (Box 2.4) and acquire 'recovery competencies' (see p. 30). The NHS Institute for Innovation and Improvement has published new training strategies for the whole of the mental health workforce, building on 'ten essential shared capabilities'. Among the ten is 'promoting recovery' (Hope, 2004).

Timing responses: what helps when?

McGorry (1992) describes the need to carefully match explanations of illness to the individual's readiness to accept them. He advises us 'to avoid adding insight to injury', for denial of illness, especially early on, may have a self-protective function (Deegan, 1988). Although a 'sealing over' recovery style predicts poor engagement, a shift from 'integration' to 'sealing over' in the first 6 months is associated with symptomatic improvement (Tait *et al*, 2003). Symptoms have meanings, and the process of recovery may be accompanied by complex losses and powerful realisations (Roberts, 2000; Roberts, Chapter 7, this volume; Box 2.5). It follows that working *with* psychotic symptoms may be more helpful than attempting to demonstrate their falseness (Romme & Escher, 2002).

Medication and medicating: more than compliance

Many service users have considerable problems with the need to take medication. It is often not just the drugs themselves, and their unwanted effects, but the implications of taking something for a 'broken brain' and the atmosphere of persuasion or compulsion that often surrounds them. Many patients associate being well with getting off medication, even when there are recurring adverse consequences.

If decisions about prescription take place by negotiation, so that risks can be taken within safe parameters and lessons learned from experience,

> **Box 2.5** 'The end of empire'
>
> And so I walked, beside the canal,
> plans and policies talked out so far
> only silence remained, enemies everywhere,
> none greater than those closest,
> news from the frontier forgotten as soon as it is told,
> spies lost in their own ciphers.
> In this way an empire crumbles,
> aimlessly, along the canal, a walk,
> the swans that can at least fly this place,
> a chill wind blowing from the Alps.
> Soon, all this will be desolation,
> The banks broken, the ducks caught
> for starving troops. Alone, I walked,
> aimless, with the strange lethargy
> of total defeat, and memories of other days
> stirring the silence with fanfares.
>
> Graeme Hobbs (undated),
> 'written after 3 years of schizophrenia and *a few days before I recovered my sanity*'
> (reproduced with permission from Hobbs, 1998; emphasis added)

a service user may be more likely to value medication as a tool in pursuit of their recovery. The NICE schizophrenia guidelines (National Institute for Clinical Excellence, 2002: 1.4.5 and p. 48) emphasise choice based on a thorough search for the most effective medication at the lowest dose, and include recognition that, for some, the experience of taking medication can be worse than the disorder. It is clearly possible for some to recover and stay well without medication, but there is as yet no reliable way of knowing who these will be, and at present stopping medication is probably the most common reason for relapse, leading to breakdown.

Working with risk: a shift from risk avoidance to risk-sharing

Deegan's rallying call that 'professionals must embrace the concept of the dignity of risk, and the right to failure if they are to be supportive of us' (Deegan, 1996) seems completely at odds with the risk-averse climate in which we live and work, where, for instance, patients may have to be medically vetted before an occupational therapist can take them for a cycle ride. And yet risk is inevitable, and healthy. We begin to take risks with our first few steps in life, and without risk there is no progress or development. However, balancing risk avoidance with creative risk-taking is not an easy task and it cannot be handled responsibly without good team work. Every candidate taking the Royal College of Psychiatrist's Membership examinations is now trained to formulate a systematic risk assessment. But there is a considerable art in turning what can be a decontextualised checklist focused on how to ensure that problematic behaviours will not recur into a negotiated recovery-oriented risk management strategy that aims to support safe risk exposure in the service of promoting recovery.

For psychiatrists, the risk associated with stopping a patient's medication can epitomise the tensions involved in implementing a recovery model. Ceasing medication may well be the most common reason for relapse leading to readmission, but May (2004) speaks for many service users in finding medication intolerable, especially as, in his experience, the medication induced 'psychic indifference' towards psychotic symptoms that carried over into every aspect of his life. When he stopped taking his medication he went into hiding from family and services for weeks and experienced what he describes as a withdrawal syndrome that was quite different in quality from previous episodes of psychosis and resolved spontaneously. He subsequently took a psychology degree and trained as a clinical psychologist. He has remained medication free ever since and has become a highly respected witness and advocate for recovery.

A single and heroic story cannot support 'non-compliance' as a route to recovery, but if an individual were determined to stop medication, a recovery-oriented approach would aim to negotiate a phased reduction, during which contact and relationship is maintained. This would reduce the risk of relapse through awareness of early signs, and enable both patient and prescriber to learn from the experience. We know that there are many people previously diagnosed with psychotic illness who are well and medication free, but we know little about how to identify them prospectively. Not much more is known about how to work successfully towards living well without medication, although some guidance on how to more safely experiment with 'coming off' is emerging (Mind, 2005; Holmes, 2006).

What would a recovery-based service look like?

Anthony (1993, 2000) has emphasised that effective service development must be based on what people in recovery have found to be helpful, even when this differs from standard textbook practice (Faulkner, 2000; Baker & Strong, 2001; Mental Health Foundation, 2002). Some services are beginning to train staff in 'recovery competencies' (O'Hagen, 2001; Hope, 2004; Box 2.6).

Promoting self-management

There is increasing awareness of the value of self-management strategies that empower individuals to take control of their lives (Repper & Perkins, 2003). The Wellness Recovery Action Plan (WRAP; Copeland, 2002) is one of the most popular and established recovery tools. The individual user identifies actions, thoughts and behaviours that, in their own experience, are associated with staying well and reducing symptoms. These 'personal wellness tools' are then incorporated into a written plan that includes daily

---

Box 2.6 New Zealand guidelines on recovery competencies for mental health workers

A competent mental health worker:

1　understands recovery principles and experiences in the national and international contexts
2　recognises and supports the personal resourcefulness of people with mental illness
3　understands and accommodates the diverse views on mental illness, treatments, services and recovery
4　has the self-awareness and skills to communicate respectfully and develop good relationships with service users
5　understands and actively protects service users' rights
6　understands discrimination and social exclusion, its impact on service users and how to reduce it
7　acknowledges different cultures and knows how to provide a service in partnership with them
8　has comprehensive knowledge of community services and resources and actively supports service users in accessing them
9　has knowledge of the service-user movement and is able to support its participation in services
10　has knowledge of family perspectives and is able to support the family's participation in services

(Adapted from O'Hagan, 2001, with permission.)

---

maintenance, triggers and how to avoid them, warning signs and how to respond to them, and a crisis plan (for sample WRAPs go to http://www.recoverydevon.co.uk/ and follow the links from the 'A to Z and Search Facility'). It is not hard to envisage how this perspective could eventually replace the care programme approach.

The hospital redesigned as a 'springy safety net'

Although May (2004) acknowledged that hospital was a useful safety net for him and his family, his main complaint was 'the lack of springiness in the net to allow me to get back on the tightrope'. Service users want rapid access to help in a crisis, but once it has resolved they do not necessarily wish to be caught up in long-term involvement and monitoring, however well intentioned. What they do want is to be able to renew contact with services as soon as problems arise, without having to wait for complex referral processes to be instigated.

The expert patient

There is a progressive move across the NHS to value patients as 'experts in their own experience' (Department of Health, 2001a), but an associated need to reconcile the preservation of autonomy with a duty of care for some of the most vulnerable people in society. A recovery-based service would centre staff training on the lived experience of service users, but would still need to find safe and respectful ways of addressing the issues raised by reduced capacity. Such training would also typically cover the history of recovery and its social context, the language used by clinicians, the importance of complementary therapies and the use of the WRAP. Mental health workers may also reveal their own experience of mental illness (C. Willey, Clinical Nurse Manager, Black Country NHS Trust, personal communication, 2003). Learning benefits include focusing on life rather than illness, changes in the use of language and greater emphasis on what patients value most: safe and satisfactory accommodation, sufficient money, supportive relationships, work and meaningful activity. It is also possible to bridge the gap between service users and providers by recognising that many are both.

Valuing ethnicity and diversity

The North American recovery literature has been criticised (Deegan, 1988) for an approach that sidelines ethnicity and its social consequences for users, and 'projects traditional American values onto disabled people, such as rugged individualism, competition, personal achievement and self-sufficiency', coupled with a lack of appreciation that, for some users, 'independent living amounts to the loneliness of four walls in some rooming house'. Celebrating the small achievements of ordinary living (Leibrich, 1999) is more productive than dwelling on failure to match up to heroic ideals. The New Zealand approach, particularly in the context of Maori people (Fenton & Te Koutua, 2000; O'Hagan, 2001; Lapsley et al, 2002), has illustrated the importance of valuing a person's cultural origins and personal meanings as reference points around which to combat stigma and support their citizenship. Recovery is based on 'knowing who you are, and where you come from, and re-integrating yourself with your own people in your own way' (Lapsley et al, 2002).

Making recovery worthwhile: what is there to recover for?

Traditional medical approaches attempt to relieve symptoms but give insufficient consideration to what will happen next. Butterworth & Dean (2000) describe how a survey of mental health service users in the Bristol area found that less than half the participants were engaged in any form of occupational activity. In 1997, a Work Development Team was created within mental health services, which then became a Beacon site. By 2003, this team had helped over 200 people to return to full-time employment, and its job retention service was helping over 50 people to remain in their jobs and 19 to explore other career paths before successfully returning to the labour market (R. Butterworth, personal communication, 2003).

Work and employment have such a pivotal role in recovery that there is a clear case for drawing occupational therapists back from generic roles in community teams. Mental health trusts could also put their own house in order by developing supported employment schemes and supporting the development of support, time and recovery (STR) worker posts for people whose qualification is their personal experience (Repper & Perkins, 2003).

Difficulties over diagnosis and steps towards a common language

The development of a professional language and identity can be seen as part of a 'tribal' induction, so that membership of a group follows a formal exhibition of proficiency to its elders (Sims, 1999). Somewhat in contrast, mental health workers have been advised to share their specialist knowledge in such a way that it can easily be understood by those it concerns (National Institute for Clinical Excellence, 2002, 1.1.7) as a step towards evidence-based patient choice (Hope, 2002). In common with all doctors, they must now copy all letters to patients and should therefore write in a way patients can readily understand (Department of Health, 2003) and also consider whether what they have written supports recovery or chronicity.

Diagnosis is a recurrent concern. It can be perceived as a 'life sentence', reducing a person's expectations of the future to one saturated with problems, with all the associated pessimism and stigma. There can be an overwhelming eclipse of personal identity such that people who have psychotic illnesses become 'schizophrenics'. Davidson & Strauss (1992) found that a key correlate of favourable long-term outcome in schizophrenia was the individual's ability to differentiate the self from the diagnosis and the illness experience, to have a secure sense of a 'me' separate from an 'it'. It is noteworthy that Leibrich's (1999) anthology of personal recovery stories was commissioned by the New Zealand Government as part of their national anti-stigma campaign. Reading or hearing stories about people with severe illnesses can carry hope and significantly influence one's own experience. Describing oneself as being 'in recovery' has very different implications from being defined by others as 'chronically ill' (see also Kleinman, 1988).

Although diagnostic caution is commendable when considering a severe mental illness such as schizophrenia, avoidance or denial may risk an unhealthy collusion with a patient or their relatives, provoking divisions within a family and becoming a barrier to desperately needed treatment and support. Practitioners need to understand what a diagnosis is and is not, and ensure they are at least as aware as their patients of the continuing debate over the diagnosis of schizophrenia (van Os & McKenna, 2003).

Medical notes are often taken by the courts as an objective and accurate record of what has happened and why, although they are clearly a medical interpretation of events. In an interesting development, professionals are now required to support individuals in writing their own account of their illness for their notes (National Institute for Clinical Excellence, 2002: 1.3.3). The explicit aim is to help patients understand what has happened to them and to give an account of it in their own words, but the implications are much broader. There will no longer be a single 'medical' version. Current guidance promotes the preservation of a diversity of viewpoints within the official record.

Looking ahead

Hope and caution

As in many movements for change, some proponents readily take up extreme or hostile positions. Collaboration between service users and NHS planners has been likened to 'supping with the devil' (Jackson, 2003). The growing involvement and influence of professionals, academics, managers and government within what began as a user movement has provoked understandable anxieties about a takeover.

Some service users have little affinity with the recovery movement and do not believe they will ever recover. The reasons for such 'resistance' vary from realism to pessimism, or even fear of the challenge they would face if they were seriously to consider resuming control of and responsibility for their lives. Here as much as anywhere there is a need for sensitivity and support for informed choice.

Growing professional enthusiasm for recovery principles has raised concerns about the implications of recovery on service provision. At a recent consultation between service providers and users about the introduction of a recovery-oriented service, one of us (P.W.) discovered that there are widespread fears that day services, i.e. provision for those in continuing need of support, would be stopped entirely. Among mental health workers it is suspected that services will respond to the challenge to become recovery-oriented simply by changing their names and headed notepaper, without fully embracing the implications. The need to spend more time in direct contact with individual service users and their supporters has serious resource implications that may not be acknowledged. Redefinition also carries a responsibility to adopt a clinical philosophy that may be significantly at odds with other strands of NHS thinking, especially in the area of risk. Clinicians may wonder whether, when things go wrong, the principle of risk-sharing will extend to the trust board, and it may be a wise early step to seek endorsement from senior management in developing recovery-based services where choice and risk are significant issues.

Many psychiatrists remain sceptical about the redefinition of recovery, concerned that it equates to colluding in a false hope that could engender unrealistic expectations in patients and families. In the context of a progressive dementia, for example, the victory over disease implied by 'recovery' can seem a hollow example of society's need to sanitise the distress caused by events beyond our control. The National Institute for

---

Box 2.7 Contacts and resources for the recovery movement

Department of Health's Expert Patient Programme	http://www.ohn.gov.uk/ohn/people/expert.htm http://www.lmca.org.uk/docs/expert.htm
Long-term Medical Conditions Alliance (LMCA)	http://www.lmca.org.uk
Manic Depression Fellowship's self-help resources	http://www.mdf.org.uk
Mary Ellen Copeland's mental health recovery self-help strategies (including WRAP)	http://www.mentalhealthrecovery.com
National Empowerment Center (USA)	http://www.power2u.org
New Zealand Mental Health Commission	http://www.mhc.govt.nz
Ohio Department of Mental Health's guiding principles of the recovery model and outcomes	http://www.mh.state.oh.us/initiatives/outcomes/ outcomes.html
Rethink's self-management project	http://www.rethink.org/recovery/self-management/index.htm
Scottish Recovery Network	www.scottishrecovery.net

Mental Health in England (2004) has attempted to reach out to doctors by promoting a new classification of recovery based on familiar diagnostic categories, but it is doubtful whether this will resolve the feeling of unease. In the UK, the Royal College of Psychiatrists' Faculty of Rehabilitation and Social Psychiatry is probably the branch of medicine that has become most closely associated with the recovery movement, redefining rehabilitation for the 21st century as 'rehabilitation and recovery now' (Royal College of Psychiatrists, 2004). There are many sources of further information and support on developing recovery perspectives (Box 2.7) and not only is the Royal College of Psychiatrists joining with the Care Services Improvement Partnership (CSIP) and the Social Care Institute for Excellence (SCIE) to develop a joint statement on recovery, but the College's annual meeting in 2007 will largely focus on recovery.

At present, both professionals and patients have some misunder-standings and misgivings about what is meant by recovery. Much of this concern can be resolved by being clear that recovery is not about an unrealistic hope of magical transformation. It is an open-ended and cautiously optimistic process of developing a hopeful and personal path forward alongside whatever remains of the individual's illness. A great deal is yet to be learned about what prevents and what promotes and sustains recovery. There is even more uncertainty about why some people enter into a recovery process and others do not. However, an overarching emphasis on recovery offers a broad, inclusive, humanistic philosophy, which could give direction and ambition to professionals, service users, managers and others in working together for better lives for those who experience severe mental health problems.

References

Allott, P., Loganathan, L. & Fulford, K. W. M. (2002) Discovering hope for recovery: a review of a selection of recovery literature, implications for practice and systems change. *Canadian Journal of Community Mental Health*, **21**(2), 13–34.

Anthony, W. A. (1993) Recovery from mental illness: the guiding vision of the mental health service system in the 1990s. *Psychosocial Rehabilitation Journal*, **16**, 11–23.

Anthony, W. A. (2000) A recovery-oriented service system: setting some system level standards. *Psychiatric Rehabilitation Journal*, **24**, 159–168.

Baker, S. & Strong, S. (2001) *Roads to Recovery: How People with Mental Health Problems Recover and Find Ways of Coping*. London: Mind.

Butterworth, R. & Dean, J. (2000) Putting the missing rungs into the vocational ladder. *Life in the Day*, **4**, 5–9.

Campbell-Orde, T., Chamberlin, J., Carpenter, J., *et al* (2005) *Measuring the Promise: A Compendium of Recovery Measures. Volume 2*. Cambridge, MA: Evaluation Center@HSRI. http://www.tecathsri.org/pub_pickup/pn/pn-55.pdf

Chamberlin, J. (1978) *On Our Own: Patient Controlled Alternatives to the Mental Health System*. New York: McGraw-Hill.

Clay, S. (1994) The wounded prophet. In *Recovery: The New Force in Mental Health*. Columbus, OH: Ohio Department of Mental Health.

Coleman, R. (1999) *Recovery: An Alien Concept*. Gloucester: Hansell Publishing.

Cooper, J. M., Clarke, A. (2005) 'Expert Patients: who are they? Lay-led self-management programmes: an additional resource in the management of chronic illness'. London: Long-term Medical Conditions Alliance. http://www.lmca.org.uk/docs/article.htm

Copeland, M. E. (2002) Overview of WRAP: Wellness Recovery Action Plan. *Mental Health Recovery Newsletter*, **3**, 1–9.

Crane, H. (2003) Depression. Doctors as patients. *BMJ*, **326**, 1324–1325.

Davidson, L. & Strauss, J. (1992) Sense of self in recovery from severe mental illness. *British Journal of Medical Psychology*, **65**, 131–145.

Deegan, P. E. (1988) Recovery: the lived experience of rehabilitation. *Psychosocial Rehabilitation Journal*, **11**, 11–19.

Deegan, P. (1996) Recovery as a journey of the heart. *Psychiatric Rehabilitation Journal*, **19**, 91–97.

Department of Health (2001a) *The Expert Patient: A New Approach to Chronic Disease Management for the 21st Century*. London: Department of Health.

Department of Health (2001b) *The Journey to Recovery – The Government's Vision for Mental Health Care*. London: Department of Health.

Department of Health (2003) *Copying Letters to Patients. Good Practice Guidelines*. London: Department of Health.

Dinniss, S., Roberts, G., Hubbard, C., *et al* (2006) A user-led assessment of the recovery orientation of a rehabilitation service using DREEM: the Developing Recovery Enhancing Environments Measure. *Psychiatric Bulletin*, in press.

Falloon, I. R. H., Montero, I., Sungar, M., *et al* (2004) Implementation of evidence-based treatment for schizophrenic disorders: two year outcome of an international field trial of optimal treatment. *World Psychiatry*, **3**, 104–109.

Faulkner, A. (2000) *Strategies for Living: A Summary Report of User-Led Research into People's Strategies for Living with Mental Distress*. London: Mental Health Foundation. http://www.mentalhealth.org.uk/html/content/s4lreportsum.pdf

Fenton, L. & Te Koutua, T. W. (2000) *Four Maori Korero about Their Experience of Mental Illness*. Wellington: The Mental Health Commission. http://www.mhc.govt.nz/publications/2000/Recovery_Maori.pdf

Fisher, D. B. (2001) We've been misled by the drug industry. *Washington Post*, 19 August, p. B03. Also at http://www.power2u.org/articles/recovery/misled.html

Harding, C. M., Brooks, G. W., Asolaga, T., *et al* (1987) The Vermont longitudinal study of persons with severe mental illness. 1: Methodological study sample and overall status 32 years later. *American Journal of Psychiatry*, **144**, 718–726.

Harrison, G. & Mason, P. (1993) Schizophrenia – falling incidence and better outcome? *British Journal of Psychiatry*, **163**, 535–541.

Harrison, G., Hopper, K., Craig, T., *et al* (2001) Recovery from psychotic illness: a 15- and 25-year international follow-up study. *British Journal of Psychiatry*, **178**, 506–517.

Hobbs, G. (1998) *From My Madness*. Nottingham: Poetry Monthly Press.

Holmes, G. (2006) Helping people to come off neuroleptics and other psychiatric drugs. *Clinical Psychology Forum*, **163**, 21–25.

Hope, R. (2004) *The Ten Essential Shared Capabilities: A Framework for the Whole of the Mental Health Workforce*. London: Department of Health. http://www.scmh.org.uk/80256FBD004F3555/vWeb/flPCHN6FRLEK/$file/essential+shared+capabilities.pdf

Hope, T. (2002) Evidence-based patient choice and psychiatry. *Evidence-Based Mental Health*, **5**, 100–101.

Jackson, C. (2003) Service users say they are sick of being used by the NHS. *Mental Health Today*, February, 8–9.

Jamison, K. R. (1995) *An Unquiet Mind: A Memoir of Moods and Madness*. New York: Alfred A. Knopf.

Kleinman, A. (1988) *The Illness Narratives: Suffering, Healing and the Human Condition*. New York: Basic Books.

Lapsley, H., Waimarie, L. N. & Black, R. (2002) *Kia Mauri Tau! Narratives of Recovery from Disabling Mental Health Problems*. Wellington: Mental Health Commission.

Leete, E. (1989) How I perceive and manage my illness. *Schizophrenia Bulletin*, **8**, 605–609.

Leibrich, J. (1999) *A Gift of Stories: Discovering How to Deal with Mental Illness*. Dunedin: University of Otago Press.

Leibrich, J. (2002) Making space: spirituality and mental health. *Mental Health, Religion and Culture*, **5**, 143–162.

Liberman, R. P. & Kopelowicz, A. (2002) Recovery from schizophrenia: a challenge for the 21st century. *International Review of Psychiatry*, **14**, 245–255. http://www.tandf.co.uk/journals/titles/09540261.html

Lovejoy, M. (1984) Recovery from schizophrenia: a personal odyssey. *Hospital and Community Psychiatry*, **35**, 809–812.

May, R. (2004) Making sense of psychotic experience and working towards recovery. In *Psychological Interventions in Early Psychosis: A Treatment Handbook* (eds J. F. M. Gleeson & P. D. McGorry), pp. 245–260. Chichester: John Wiley & Sons.

McGorry, P. D. (1992) The concept of recovery and secondary prevention in psychotic disorders. *Australian and New Zealand Journal of Psychiatry*, **26**, 3–17.

Mental Health Foundation (2002) *Something Inside So Strong: Strategies for Surviving Mental Distress*. London: Mental Health Foundation.

Mind (2005) *Making Sense of Coming off Psychiatric Drugs*. London: Mind. http://www.mind.org.uk/NR/rdonlyres/62EBF683-E845-459C-914E-BFF57556737C/0/comingoffpsychdrugs2005.pdf

National Institute for Clinical Excellence (2002) *Schizophrenia: Core Interventions in the Treatment and Management of Schizophrenia in Primary and Secondary Care. Clinical Guideline 1*. London: NICE. http://www.nice.org.uk/pdf/CG1NICEguideline.pdf

National Institute for Mental Health in England (2004) *Emerging Best Practices in Mental Health Recovery*. London: NIMHE.

North, C. (1988) *Welcome, Silence: My Triumph over Schizophrenia*. London: Simon & Schuster.

O'Hagan, M. (2001) *Recovery Competencies for New Zealand Mental Health Workers*. Wellington: Mental Health Commission. http://www.mhc.govt.nz/publications/2001/Recovery_ Competencies.pdf

Ohio Department of Mental Health (2003) Ohio Mental Health Recovery and Consumer Outcomes Initiative. http://www.mh.state.oh.us/oper/outcomes/outcomes.index.html

Oyebode, F. (2004) Invited commentary on: The rediscovery of recovery. *Advances in Psychiatric Treatment*, **10**, 48–49.

Rakfeldt, J. & Strauss, J. (1989) The low turning point. A control mechanism in the course of mental disorder. *Journal of Nervous and Mental Disease*, **177**, 32–37.

Ralph, R. O., Lambert, D. & Kidder, K. A. (2002) *The Recovery Perspective and Evidence-Based Practice for People with Serious Mental Illness: A Guideline Developed for The Behavioural Health Recovery Management Project*. http://bhrm.org/guidelines/Ralph%20Recovery.pdf

Ramsay, R., Page, A., Goodman, T., *et al* (2002) *Changing Minds: Our Lives and Mental Illness*. London: Gaskell.

Repper, J. & Perkins, R. (2003) *Social Inclusion and Recovery*. London: Baillière Tindall.

Ridgeway, P. A. (2000) Re-storying psychiatric disability: learning from first person narrative accounts of recovery. *Psychiatric Rehabilitation Journal*, **24**, 335–343.

Ridgeway, P. A. & Press, A. (2004) *Assessing the Recovery-commitment of your Mental Health Service: A User's Guide for the Developing Recovery Enhancing Environments Measure (DREEM) UK Pilot Version 1*. Further information from Piers.Allott@eastmidlands.csip.nhs.uk and Hugh.Middleton@eastmidlands.csip.nhs.uk

Roberts, G. A. (2000) Narrative and severe mental illness: what place do stories have in an evidence-based world? *Advances in Psychiatric Treatment*, **6**, 432–441.

Romme, M. & Escher, S. (2002) *Making Sense of Voices. A Guide for Mental Health Professionals Working with Voice Hearers*. London: Mind Publications.

Royal College of Psychiatrists (2004) *Rehabilitation and Recovery Now* (Council Report CR121). London: Royal College of Psychiatrists.

Sheehan, A. (2002) Preface. In *A Calendar of Recovery* (Ed. National Institute of Mental Health in England). London: National Institute of Mental Health in England.

Sims, A. (1999) Sacred tales. In *Healing Stories: Narrative in Psychiatry and Psychotherapy* (Eds G. Roberts & J. Holmes), chapter 6. Oxford: Oxford University Press.

Tait, L., Birchwood, M. & Trower, P. (2003) Predicting engagement with services for psychosis: insight, symptoms and recovery style. *British Journal of Psychiatry*, **182**, 123–128.

Tuke, S. (1813) *Description of The Retreat*. Reprinted (1996) with an introduction by K. Jones. London: Process Press.

Unzicker, R. (1989) On my own: a personal journey through madness and re-emergence. *Psychosocial Rehabilitation Journal*, **13**, 70–77.

van Os, J. & McKenna, P. (2003) *Does Schizophrenia Exist?* (Maudsley Discussion Paper no. 12). London: Institute of Psychiatry Media Support Unit.

Warner, R. (1994) *Recovery from Schizophrenia: Psychiatry and Political Economy* (2nd edn). New York: Routledge.

Whitwell, D. (1999) The myth of recovery from mental illness. *Psychiatric Bulletin*, **23**, 621–622.

Whitwell, D. (2005) *Recovery beyond Psychiatry*. London: Free Association Books.

CHAPTER 3

The social context of mental illness

Julian Leff

For many decades schizophrenia and manic–depressive illness (now more commonly known as bipolar affective disorder or simply bipolar disorder) were known as endogenous psychoses, with the implication that their origin and course were entirely driven from within the individual. However, in the latter half of the 20th century evidence accumulated for the influence of the social environment on the course of these illnesses, and theories were proposed that social factors also contributed to their origin. The evidence for this has been hard to establish, but recent research findings have buttressed this idea and will be discussed in this chapter.

'Natural history' of severe mental illness

The sense that schizophrenia pursued a downward course from its onset to a final stage of mindlessness was inherent in the first diagnostic label of dementia praecox. However, even Kraepelin, who coined this term, was aware of patients whose illness was much more benign. Long-term follow-up studies of cohorts of people with schizophrenia have revealed a variety of courses, ranging from a single episode with full recovery to persistent symptoms from the first manifestation of the illness that show little amelioration throughout the rest of the person's life. It was Bleuler's belief that schizophrenia is not a homogeneous illness but that the diagnosis covers several distinct conditions, which is why his book on the subject is entitled *Dementia Praecox or The Group of Schizophrenias* (Bleuler, 1911). To date there is no convincing evidence for this view, although DSM–IV (American Psychiatric Association, 1994) has a separate diagnostic category of schizophreniform psychosis for people with symptoms of schizophrenia whose illness is less than 6 months in duration. This is a dubious distinction for the following reason: there are medical illnesses that show considerable variation in outcome. For example, many people are infected with tuberculosis without ever developing symptoms or being aware that they are ill; others present with respiratory symptoms that recover with or without treatment, whereas yet others develop a generalised infection that may end in death. These different outcomes are not made the basis for arguing that these are distinct illnesses, because the same pathological agent can be identified in all patients. The variation in course is ascribed to the virulence of the organism interacting with host factors such as the state of the person's nutrition and the response of their immune system. Although we remain ignorant about the pathological basis of schizophrenia, it is premature to subdivide this category according to duration of symptoms before contact with services. Furthermore, studies have shown that it is possible to considerably reduce the duration of untreated psychosis by the administrative measure of early intervention (Larsen *et al*, 2001).

On the other hand, the distinction between schizophrenia and bipolar disorder that is seen in the different symptom patterns is substantiated by their varied courses. Although people with bipolar disorder generally have better clinical and social outcomes than those with schizophrenia, a small proportion develop a chronic condition, particularly those who experience rapid cycling of manic and depressive states. A survey of long-stay patients in two London psychiatric hospitals in the 1980s revealed that 7% carried a diagnosis of manic–depressive psychosis (bipolar disorder with psychotic symptoms) compared with over 80% whose diagnosis was schizophrenia.

Although the role of inheritance in the aetiology of schizophrenia is no longer in question, the magnitude of the genetic contribution is still a matter of dispute. Adoption studies that have been conducted over many years in Finland have now produced evidence that the appearance of schizophrenia-spectrum disorder in adopted people at high risk through being born to a mother with schizophrenia depends on the nature of the adoptive family environment (Tienari *et al*, 2004). This important conclusion emphasises the need to focus on the social environment of patients, which is potentially remediable, whereas at present we can do nothing about a person's genetic constitution.

Chronicity in severe mental illness

The multinational study by the World Health Organization (WHO) on the course of psychoses in patients making first contact with services yielded valuable insights into the development of chronicity (Jablensky *et al*, 1992). In each of the nine centres the proportion of patients whose illness took a chronic course from the start showed a narrow range between 10 and 15% of the total sample. A wide range of societies and cultures were represented in this study, including Nagasaki in Japan, Chandigarh in northern India and Nottingham in the UK. The relative uniformity in the proportion of individuals who failed to recover from the first episode of their illness suggests that social and cultural factors have very little influence over the phenomenon. Rather, it is likely to stem from the nature of the psychosis, representing the most biologically determined of its manifestations. Of course this does not indicate the futility of rehabilitation for people with first-onset psychosis. On the contrary, they need the most specialised and focused of programmes (Leff & Szmidla, 2002). But it does suggest that there is little room for the prevention of clinical chronicity in this group.

The current interest in early-intervention programmes for people with schizophrenia is based on the premise that they will be successful in preventing the development of chronicity. However, the evidence for this optimism is not yet forthcoming, since none of the controlled trials of these programmes has been completed. There is a general consensus among clinicians that the first 10 years of a schizophrenic illness are the most turbulent and that after this period individuals become more stable and hence easier to engage in programmes of rehabilitation. Nevertheless, attempts have been made recently to use cognitive–behavioural approaches with people in an acute episode of psychosis. Not only have these proved feasible, but there appears to be a long-standing benefit (Turkington & Arjundas, Chapter 12, this volume).

In considering the evolution of chronicity it is useful to distinguish between positive and negative symptoms. As noted above, patients who develop persistent delusions and/or hallucinations at the first onset of psychosis are on the way to chronicity. The optimism that infused asylum staff on the return of military psychiatrists from the Second World War was manifested in the conviction that negative symptoms were a consequence of custodial practices. Once released from the deadening environment of the psychiatric hospital, patients were expected to regain their energy, motivation and zest for life. This view was promulgated in the influential book by Russell Barton inaptly entitled *Institutional Neurosis* (Barton, 1959). In a UK study by the Team for the Assessment of Psychiatric Services (TAPS) of nearly 700 long-stay patients discharged from two psychiatric hospitals in north London, the first few groups to be discharged into the community did show a significant reduction in negative symptoms over time (Leff *et al*, 1994). However, the total sample did not show any improvement in negative symptoms (Leff & Trieman, 2000). This disappointing finding may be explained by the patients' length of exposure to an institutional environment: on average, 20 years. It is possible that, after a certain length of time, the damage done by poor institutional care is irreversible, underlining the need for stimulation early on in the illnesses. These findings also suggest that negative symptoms are an intrinsic feature of schizophrenia and will need to be the focus of rehabilitation after the disappearance of asylums.

Social consequences of severe psychiatric illness

These can be baldly stated as: loss of employment, loss of status, loss of family support, loss of friends, loss of self-respect and loss of liberty. It may be contested that loss of personal freedom is only temporary, until the person responds to treatment. But it must be acknowledged that, taking a global view, there are many people with severe psychiatric illnesses whose rights are unprotected since they live in countries without any mental health law; Chile, for example, is such a country. In some low- and middle-income countries without adequate psychiatric personnel and facilities, patients can be kept in chains for much of their life. The other adverse consequences also vary in intensity according to availability of appropriate resources and to societal attitudes. Thus, the ability to fulfil an occupational role depends on the local unemployment situation, the availability of sheltered work and the existence of family enterprises in which disabled relatives can cope with undemanding tasks. As an example of the influence of local conditions, a comparison of individuals with schizophrenia in Bologna, Italy, and Boulder, Colorado (USA), revealed that twice as many in the Italian city were employed.

The lack of paid employment results in a series of losses. Many people feel that their job contributes to the definition of who they are. In most social encounters, the next question after asking your name is 'What do you do?' This conversation opener is not available to the unemployed, who may have little of interest to talk about to a new acquaintance if they have few leisure activities or none at all. The absence of a wage or salary is never adequately compensated for by state benefits and patients in this position are severely hampered by lack of money from pursuing hobbies or leisure interests. A job also enables a person to feel that they are making a contribution to society, and jobless patients complain of lack of self-esteem. Work embeds a person in a social matrix separate from their home life and friends and confers the added advantage of increasing their network of friends (Boardman & Robinson, Chapter 19, this volume).

Friends can provide emotional support to a person with psychosis, but few will understand the experience the individual is going through and most will be alarmed that the person is confiding in them. A natural reaction is to distance oneself from such disturbing revelations and it becomes increasingly difficult to sustain the relationship when the person is repeatedly admitted to hospital. Visitors to a psychiatric admission ward often have to negotiate a locked entrance door and once inside are rarely greeted by a welcoming environment. The presence of acutely disturbed patients is upsetting to the lay person and it is not surprising that visits tail off over time. Even after discharge, encounters with the ill person may yield little pleasure, partly because of the restricted emotional responsiveness of many people with psychosis and partly because the usual topics of conversation between friends are overshadowed by events linked to the illness.

Support from the immediate family is likely to outlast friendships, but even family members can become worn down by the stress of caring for a person with persistent symptoms and problematic behaviour. In the absence of help from skilled professionals, the inadequate coping styles of relatives with high expressed emotion (see next section) fuel tension between them and the ill person and have a deleterious effect on their own mental health and on that of the patient (Raune *et al*, 2004). Conflict often arises when relatives are critical or hostile, and if the ill person is aggressive in response it is likely that she or he will be ejected by the family or will leave the home spontaneously. The loss of family support is particularly devastating, since no professional is able to substitute for the dedicated care and emotional responsiveness that relatives often provide.

Social determinants of outcome

It has been established by many studies that the outcome of schizophrenia is worse for men than for women, for those with an early onset of symptoms and for those with an insidious as opposed to an acute onset. It is also regularly found that the onset in men is about 5 years earlier than in women. An early onset may be a manifestation of biological determinants of the illness, but it has obvious social effects. If onset is in early adolescence, the individual has not had time to negotiate crucial steps to maturity: completing studies or training for a job, establishing an adult sexual relationship and at least initiating the process of independence from parents. The impact of schizophrenia is much less devastating in later life, when the person has a fully formed personality, an established role as a worker or homemaker and a long-standing social network. Hence, the social consequences compound the effects of whatever biological substrate is responsible for an early onset.

It is unknown why schizophrenia has an earlier onset in men than in women, although there has been speculation about the protective effects of oestrogen. It has also been suggested that men are exposed to the demands of society to perform adult roles earlier than women. Little convincing evidence has been advanced to support either of these hypotheses. However, as we have discussed above, the earlier onset in men could readily account for their poorer outcome. An insidious onset may also exert its malign influence through social effects. Prospective cohort studies often reveal a decline in social performance years before the onset of frank symptoms. It is common to find that academic performance in school falls off at around the age of 12 even though the illness may not declare itself until the late teens or early twenties. Once again this may be a manifestation of an underlying biological fault, but it has serious social consequences.

One of the most potent predictors of outcome of severe mental illness is the expressed emotion (EE) of the family carers. The key measures from the Camberwell Family Interview, which is given to relatives at the time of a patient's relapse or admission to hospital, are critical comments, hostility, over-involvement and warmth. The three negative emotions are used to determine the EE level of the carers. People with schizophrenia who live in high EE households have nearly three times the risk of relapse over 9 months than those in low EE households. These findings have been replicated in over 30 studies conducted in a wide range of cultures and in many different languages. A meta-analysis of some of these studies confirmed the strong relationship between EE and relapse (Butzlaff & Hooley, 1999). A few similar studies have been conducted on bipolar disorder and these also found a link between EE and relapse of this illness. In fact, Butzlaff & Hooley found that EE was an even more powerful predictor of relapse in major depression than in schizophrenia. The fact that EE is related to relapse in a variety of psychiatric and also non-psychiatric conditions indicates that it cannot be a specific aetiological factor for schizophrenia. Rather, it is one measurable source of environmental stress that can precipitate an episode of schizophrenia.

Whereas EE represents long-term environmental stress, sudden happenings in the patient's life cause acute stress and have also been implicated in relapses. The work of George Brown on developing measures of life events is well-known and began with a focus on schizophrenia, although much of the subsequent research was concerned with depression. In collaboration with Jim Birley, he showed that there was an excess of life events in the 3 weeks before an episode of schizophrenia (Brown & Birley, 1968). This result was replicated in a large-scale cross-national study mounted by the World Health Organization (WHO). Although the EE findings stimulated the development of family intervention programmes, which have been proved efficacious in randomised controlled trials, it is not so evident how one could moderate the impact of unexpected life events. However, the demonstration of the sensitivity of people with schizophrenia to stress originating in the social environment substantiated the formulation by John Wing that over-stimulation could be as dangerous for such people as under-stimulation.

The importance of social factors in the course and outcome of severe psychiatric disorders has been given a considerable boost by the international studies of psychosis conducted by the WHO. Prior to these, research in Mauritius and Sri Lanka suggested a better outcome for people with schizophrenia in these countries than in the West. However, similar studies in Hong Kong and India failed to confirm these findings. The first WHO study, the International Pilot Study of Schizophrenia (IPSS), compared the outcome over 1 year and 5 years of samples from nine centres in high-income and in low- and middle-income countries. At both time points patients in low- and middle-income countries had a considerably better clinical outcome than those in high-income countries (Leff, 1988: pp. 151–162). However, the fact that this was a prevalence sample clouded the interpretation of these findings. The next step was to mount an incidence study (Jablensky et al, 1992) that might give a more definitive result, even though it was difficult to complete successfully in low- and middle-income countries with a relatively deficient infrastructure. The opportunity was grasped to examine whether differences in the levels of EE might partially account for differences in outcome between the centres. This measure was incorporated in assessments in Chandigarh, northern India, which had a long tradition of rigorous research.

The study of Determinants of Outcome of Severe Mental Disorders (DOSMeD) produced usable data from 10 of the 11 participating centres, including Chandigarh. This incidence study confirmed previous research by showing that a much higher proportion of people with schizophrenia recovered completely and remained well for at least 2 years in India than in the centres in high-income countries (Jablensky *et al*, 1992). It is unfortunate that the centre in Nigeria did not produce viable data, since this left only a single centre in a low- or middle-income country for comparison. Nevertheless the EE data from Chandigarh were very informative. Urban relatives living in Chandigarh had much lower levels of EE than their counterparts in London, while rural Indian relatives had even lower levels (Wig *et al*, 1987). Overall, twice as many Chandigarh relatives as London relatives were rated as low EE, and twice as many Chandigarh patients as London patients fell into the category of the best outcome over the first year since contact. Hence, variation in EE levels largely accounted for the differential prognosis of patients in London and Chandigarh. There are obvious implications for working with families of people with first-episode schizophrenia, and some current early-intervention programmes include attention to the family's needs.

Issues of ethnicity

Following the Second World War there was a period of intensive immigration to the UK, predominantly from the Caribbean and the Indian subcontinent. It soon came to the attention of psychiatric services that there were a surprisingly high number of first admissions for schizophrenia among people of African–Caribbean origin. Successive studies of increasing sophistication confirmed this clinical impression and produced incidence rates between two to fourteen times the rate for the White population. Epidemiological studies in Barbados, Trinidad and Jamaica failed to find high rates in these sending islands, rendering a genetic explanation unlikely, while elevated incidence rates in UK-born African–Caribbeans ruled out the migratory process as an aetiological factor. At the same time, comparative studies of Indian migrants revealed a slightly higher incidence than for Whites, but nowhere near the excessive rates affecting the UK African–Caribbean population (Mallett *et al*, 2002; Cantor-Graae & Selten, 2005). Studies have also shown a very high incidence of bipolar disorder in this group and in immigrants to the UK from Africa (Lloyd *et al*, 2005).

A focus on the social environment of the patients has identified several factors that may contribute to the ethnic variations in incidence. One of these is social isolation, which emerged from early ecological studies of schizophrenia, such as Hare's (1956) research in Bristol. This feature may also account for the recent finding that African–Caribbeans living in areas where few of their people reside have a higher risk for schizophrenia than those living in areas of high ethnic density (Boydell *et al*, 2001). Two other factors that emerged from a multi-ethnic study by Mallett *et al* (2002) are unemployment and separation from parents. The unemployment rate among first-contact African–Caribbean patients was found to be dramatically higher than for comparable Indian and White patients. However, a causal link between unemployment and schizophrenia remains to be established. Separation in childhood from one or both parents for more than 4 years had occurred much more commonly in the histories of African–Caribbean patients than in their matched controls or the other two ethnic groups. This was not due to delayed migration of the children, since most were born in the UK. It may be explained by the fact that a high proportion had been taken into care, and this possibility is currently being explored within the Aetiology and Ethnicity in Schizophrenia and Other Psychoses (AESOP) study.

Stigma and self-image

Psychiatric conditions are regarded with fear and rejecting attitudes by the general public. In this respect psychiatric illness differs from most other diseases (AIDS is a clear exception). Within the ambit of psychiatry, depression is less heavily stigmatised than the psychoses, while substance misuse, including alcoholism, and personality disorders rank between depression and schizophrenia. The distinctive presence of the old psychiatric hospitals and their custodial function, often exercised over many decades of patients' lives, undoubtedly contributed to the stigma surrounding psychiatry. However, the demise of these institutions has hardly lessened the stigma, which attaches not only to patients but also to their family and to the professionals involved in their care.

Stigma affects people with severe psychiatric illnesses in all aspects of their lives. Friends and neighbours keep their distance from identified users of psychiatric services. Relatives outside the household may cease to visit. Healthy siblings within the household may opt to spend as little time as possible in the home. Mental health service users can suffer harassment and exploitation by youths in their neighbourhood. Private landlords may attempt to evict them. Applying for a job in the open market raises the dilemma of how to explain gaps in the employment record. Being open about having schizophrenia or bipolar disorder usually forfeits the job. Misrepresenting the condition as depression raises the chances of employment slightly but still invokes stigma. Concealing psychiatric illness entirely places the individual in a false position and risks dismissal when the truth emerges at the next relapse.

Even the psychiatric services are not immune from this problem. Psychiatrists hold stigmatising attitudes towards their patients (Crisp *et al*, 2000). Service users themselves can be prejudiced against other users. It is

45

not uncommon for service users to reject admission to a psychiatric ward on the grounds that they 'don't want to be among mad people'. This raises the issue of the acceptance by patients of the diagnosis given by psychiatric staff. The professional stance is that it is beneficial for patients to have full insight, since they will then be more likely to cooperate with treatment. This entails as a first step accepting that they have a psychiatric illness and, further, taking on board the diagnosis given by their psychiatrist. This level of acceptance does not invariably have a positive effect on outcome. Some people become depressed with the knowledge of their diagnosis, while others embrace the sick role and become very passive, expecting others to wait on them hand and foot. Some more recent research has contradicted the conventional professional view of insight by showing that people with a first onset of psychosis retain higher self-esteem if they have little insight into the nature of their illness (Morgan, 2003). It is possible that a determination to continue living as though the illness did not exist leads to a more positive outcome. Nevertheless, the persistence of unrealistic expectations often results in repeated experiences of failure, particularly in the face of stigmatising attitudes from potential employers and social contacts.

The effect on self-image of exclusion from social life and from employment is conveyed vividly in the words of a service user who found a job through a supported employment project:

'My own sense of worth has improved beyond measure ... I feel a worthwhile member of society now. I am no longer ostracised by the feeling of chronic failure, unable to find work because of my mental problems' (Perkins *et al*, 1997).

Conclusions

Although a genetic basis to the psychoses has been firmly established, the individual's social environment plays a major part in determining the course of these illnesses. There is also increasing evidence of social influences in the genesis of the functional psychoses (Cantor-Graae & Selten, 2005). In the present state of knowledge there is no possibility of therapeutic changes to the human genome, but social interventions to improve the course, outcome and consequences of severe psychiatric disorders have a long history. Increased understanding of the role of the social environment in these conditions enables more focused and effective interventions to be mounted. The deinstitutionalisation movement is an example of major social engineering applied to people with psychotic illnesses. Although many benefits to mental health service users have accrued, their position in society is still largely one of disadvantage. There are enormous barriers impeding the gaining of full-time paid work, a supportive social network and the respect of their fellow citizens. Removing these impediments is properly the remit of rehabilitation, the scope of which has necessarily broadened with the closure of the asylums in which it first developed.

References

American Psychiatric Association (1994) *Diagnostic and Statistical Manual of Mental Disorders* (4th edn) (DSM–IV). Washington, DC: APA.

Barton, R. (1959) *Institutional Neurosis*. Bristol: John Wright & Sons.

Bleuler, E. (1911) *Dementia Praecox or the Group of Schizophrenias*. Reprinted 1950 (trans. and ed. J. Zinkin). New York: International University Press.

Boydell, J., van Os, J., McKenzie, K., *et al* (2001) Incidence of schizophrenia in ethnic minorities in London: ecological study into interactions with environment. *BMJ*, **323**, 1336–1337.

Brown, G. W. & Birley, J. L. T. (1968) Crises and life changes and the onset of schizophrenia. *Journal of Health and Social Behaviour*, **9**, 203–214.

Butzlaff, R. & Hooley, J. (1999) Expressed emotion and psychiatric relapse: a meta-analysis. *Archives of General Psychiatry*, **55**, 547–552.

Cantor-Graae, E. & Selten, J.-P. (2005) Schizophrenia and migration. A meta-analysis and review. *American Journal of Psychiatry*, **162**, 12–24.

Crisp, A. H., Gelder, M. G., Rix, S., *et al* (2000) Stigmatisation of people with mental illnesses. *British Journal of Psychiatry*, **177**, 4–7.

Hare, E. H. (1956) Mental illness and social conditions in Bristol. *Journal of Mental Science*, **102**, 349–357.

Jablensky, A., Sartorius, N., Ernberg, G., *et al* (1992) Schizophrenia: manifestations, incidence and course in different cultures: a World Health Organization 10-country study. *Psychological Medicine, Monograph Supplement*, **20**, 1–97.

Larsen, T. K., McGlashan, T. H., Johannessen, J. O., *et al* (2001) Shortened duration of untreated first episode of psychosis: changes in patient characteristics at treatment. *American Journal of Psychiatry*, **158**, 1917–1919.

Leff, J. (1988) *Psychiatry around the Globe: A Transcultural View*. London. Gaskell.

Leff, J. & Szmidla, A. (2002) Evaluation of a special rehabilitation programme for patients who are difficult to place. *Social Psychiatry and Psychiatric Epidemiology*, **37**, 1–5.

Leff, J. & Trieman, N. (2000) Long-stay patients discharged from psychiatric hospitals. Social and clinical outcomes after five years in the community. The TAPS Project 46. *British Journal of Psychiatry*, **176**, 217–223.

Leff, J., Thornicroft, G., Coxhead, N., *et al* (1994) The TAPS Project 22: A five-year follow-up of long-stay psychiatric patients discharged to the community. *British Journal of Psychiatry*, **165** (suppl. 25), 13–17.

Lloyd, T., Kennedy, N., Fearon, P., *et al* (2005) Incidence of bipolar affective disorder in three UK cities. Results from the AESOP study. *British Journal of Psychiatry*, **186**, 126–131.

Mallett, R., Leff, J., Bhugra, D., *et al* (2002) Social environment, ethnicity and schizophrenia. A case control study. *Social Psychiatry and Psychiatric Epidemiology*, **37**, 329–335.

Morgan, K. (2003) *Insight and Psychosis: An Investigation of Social, Psychological and Biological Factors*. PhD thesis. London: King's College London.

Perkins, R., Buckfield, R. & Choy, D. (1997) Access to employment. A supported employment project to enable mental health service users to obtain jobs within mental health teams. *Journal of Mental Health*, **6**, 307–318.

Raune, D., Kuipers, E. & Bebbington, P. (2004) Expressed emotion at first-episode psychosis: investigating a carer appraisal model. *British Journal of Psychiatry*, **184**, 321–326.

Tienari, P., Wynne, L. C., Sorri, A., *et al* (2004) Genotype–environment interaction in schizophrenia-spectrum disorder. Long-term follow-up study of Finnish adoptees. *British Journal of Psychiatry*, **184**, 216–222.

Wig, N. N., Menon, D. K., Bedi, H., *et al* (1987) Expressed emotion and schizophrenia in North India. II: Distribution of expressed emotion components among relatives of schizophrenic patients in Aarhus and Chandigarh. *British Journal of Psychiatry*, **151**, 160–165.

CHAPTER 4

The physical healthcare of patients in rehabilitation services[†]

Irene Cormac, David Martin & Michael Ferriter

Many psychiatric patients continue to need long-term care, whether in institutions in the public or private sector, or in supported accommodation in the community. Rehabilitation services vary in size, level of security, facilities and type of care provided. Patients are usually regarded as long-stay if they are in an institution for more than a year. Some individuals in rehabilitation services become long-stay and experience limitations to their freedom, personal choice and activity, usually compounded by a low income and relative isolation from the community.

Psychiatrists caring for patients in long-term care settings have a duty to care for all aspects of these individuals' health and welfare, whether psychological, social or physical. However, few psychiatrists have up-to-date skills in primary care or health promotion. This chapter seeks to address this deficit, documenting major areas where improvements can be made, highlighting some of the most successful practice and providing references for further reading and research.

Improving the physical health of patients is now a priority for all mental health services. The principles outlined in this chapter are relevant to psychiatric patients in rehabilitation services in the community who receive physical healthcare from general practitioners and other specialists. Whatever the setting, mental health professionals should recognise their responsibility for ensuring that their more vulnerable patients receive adequate physical healthcare.

Physical health

Epidemiological studies have consistently shown increased standardised mortality ratios in people with mental disorders. In a review of 152 studies,

---

[†]This chapter is a modified version of Cormac, I., Martin, D. & Ferriter, M. (2004) Improving the physical health of long-stay psychiatric patients. *Advances in Psychiatric Treatment*, **10**, 107–115.

Harris & Barraclough (1998) found that over 27 forms of mental disorder were associated with an increased risk of premature death, with 60% of deaths due to natural causes. They attributed the causes of increased mortality to the effects of the mental disorder and to the patient's altered lifestyle.

The excess mortality in schizophrenia is well-known. Brown *et al* (2000) found that the standardised mortality ratios, compared with those of the general population, were increased three-fold for all causes, particularly for diseases of the circulatory, respiratory, digestive, endocrine and nervous systems. Modifiable health risk factors are common in people with schizophrenia (Connolly & Kelly, 2005). Mood disorders are associated with increased mortality due to cardiovascular disorders in men and respiratory disorders in women (Joukamaa *et al*, 2001). People with learning disabilities have been found to have twice the rate of health problems as the general population (van Schrojenstein Lantman-De Valk *et al*, 2000). Hollins *et al* (1998) found that people with learning disabilities are 58 times more likely to die before they are 50 years old.

In Australia, new long-stay patients, who had been in hospital for over 1 year and less than 3 years, were found to have significant medical problems from their psychiatric illnesses, together with concomitant physical illnesses and disabilities (Richards *et al*, 1997). In the USA, a study of 330 long-stay psychiatric patients found an array of medical problems and nursing needs in 84% of the sample (Fisher *et al*, 2001). They concluded that the presence of significant medical problems is one of the barriers to the discharge of such patients. In a high secure hospital in England, 54% of patients had one or more physical health problems (Cormac *et al*, 2005).

Improving health in England and Wales

The Government has produced a number of policies and targets for improving the health of the population of England and Wales. These include the National Service Frameworks (NSFs) for Mental Health (Department of Health, 1999), Coronary Heart Disease (Department of Health, 2000b), Cancer Services (Department of Health, 2000c), Diabetes (Department of Health, 2001a) and Older People (Department of Health, 2001b). In 1997, the Government introduced the concept of clinical governance, by which National Health Service (NHS) organisations are accountable for continuous improvement in the quality of services (Department of Health, 1997). The National Institute for Health and Clinical Excellence (NICE; formerly the National Institute for Clinical Excellence) has produced guidance on the most cost-effective forms of treatment for certain conditions, many of which are relevant to the care of patients in rehabilitation (for websites see Box 4.1). Local strategies for health services are implemented by primary care trusts, and staff are expected to deliver services according to predetermined performance indicators.

Box 4.1 Useful web addresses

ASH (Action on Smoking and Health)	http://www.ash.org.uk
Cancer screening	http://www.cancerscreening.nhs.uk
Department of Health	http://www.doh.gov.uk
Department of Health's 'essence of care'	http://www.doh.gov.uk/essenceofcare
Department of Health's Expert Patients Programme	http://www.expertpatients.nhs.uk
Food Standards Agency	http://www.foodstandards.gov.uk
Health Development Agency	http://www.hda-online.org.uk
Malnutrition Universal Screening Tool	http://www.bapen.org.uk/the-must.htm
Maudsley guidelines	http://www.iop.kcl.ac.uk/main/publications/prescribing_guidelines.html
National electronic Library for Health	http://www.nelh.nhs.uk
NHS Recipe Book	http://www.betterhospitalfood.com/downloads/recipe_book.pdf
NHS screening	http://www.nelh.nhs.uk/screening
NICE guidance	http://www.nice.org.uk
Improving the Patient Experience	http://patientexperience.nhsestates.gov.uk/content/home/home.asp
Tobacco control policies	http://www.hda-online.org.uk/wheredowego.pdf
US National Heart, Lung and Blood Institute	http://www.nhlbi.nih.gov
US Preventive Services Task Force Guidelines	http://www.ahrq.gov/clinic/uspstfix.htm

The Government has also produced a resource pack for improving the quality of a patient's experience of care. Developed primarily as a nursing initiative, *The Essence of Care* (Department of Health, 2001c) takes a structured approach to identifying standards of care and practice, using 'benchmarks'. After best standards of care have been identified, action plans are developed to remedy poor practice. The system is applied to eight areas affecting patient care (Box 4.2). Benchmarking can be used in conjunction with the NSFs, NICE guidance, audit and clinical governance to improve the quality of care and the physical health of patients in contact with mental health services.

Box 4.2 The essence of care: benchmark topics

- Principles of self-care
- Personal and oral hygiene
- Food and nutrition
- Continence, bladder and bowel care
- Pressure ulcers
- Safety of people with mental illness
- Record-keeping
- Privacy and dignity

Clinicians and management have realised that this is an important area to get right, both for the benefit of patients and to avoid repercussions later. Any project on health improvement will be more likely to succeed if it has leadership, sufficient resources and the support of decision-makers. A multiprofessional health promotion group can coordinate and organise interventions for health promotion, including smoking cessation, physical activity and weight management.

Health promotion

The major causes of death in England and Wales are cardiovascular disease, cancer and respiratory disease. Modifiable lifestyle behaviours associated with these conditions are tobacco smoking, physical inactivity, poor diet and nutrition (Department of Health, 2000b). Smoking causes 17% of deaths as a result of coronary heart disease, respiratory disease and many forms of cancer (Callum, 1998). The risks of smoking increase with the number of years of smoking and with the amount of tobacco consumed. Physical activity is important to maintain fitness and reduce the risk of coronary heart disease. It also reduces risks associated with obesity, hypertension and diabetes. Obesity contributes to excess morbidity and premature mortality, being associated with type 2 diabetes, coronary heart disease, hypertension and some forms of cancer. Research into nutrition has shown that a healthy diet promotes substantial health gains (James *et al*, 1997).

Although long-stay patients receive benefits from care in an institution, there is no room for complacency over the need to tackle modifiable health risk factors. Health promotion has an important role to play in reducing these risk factors and should be available to all psychiatric patients as part of their routine care.

Smoking

Tobacco smoking has been part of the culture of psychiatric institutions and 70% of psychiatric patients smoke. The highest prevalence (74%) is in those with psychotic disorders, 52% of whom are heavy smokers, consuming over 20 cigarettes per day (Meltzer *et al*, 1996). The Government has made smoking reduction a high priority for health improvement. A target has been set to reduce the rate of smoking in the general population of England and Wales from 28% to 26% by 2010 (West *et al*, 2003). Statistics from Action on Smoking and Health (ASH) in 2005 show that 28% of men and 24% of women in the UK smoke (Action on Smoking and Health, 2005).

In rehabilitation services, preparations for making changes to influence smoking behaviour might include surveying smoking facilities, smoking behaviour and the attitudes of staff and patients towards smoking (NHS Executive, 1999). Guidance about smoking facilities and policies has been published by the NHS Executive (1999) and the Health Development Agency (West *et al*, 2003). Priority has been given to providing smoke-free areas for non-smoking patients. Tobacco must not be used as a reward or incentive for patients. There are now pressures to make the entire NHS estate a smoke-free environment, with specific limited exceptions, for example in long-stay psychiatric facilities.

West *et al* (2000) have prepared smoking cessation guidelines for use by health professionals, based on a meta-analysis of research evidence. They concluded that such interventions are a cost-effective way of preserving life and reducing ill health. Brief advice from a general practitioner led 1–3% of patients to stop smoking for 6 months. Clinicians should therefore give advice about smoking cessation and document this in clinical records.

In trials, nicotine replacement therapy increased the chances of smoking cessation by 18%, compared with controls, whatever the setting and regardless of the type of replacement therapy used (Anonymous, 1999). All trials included some form of psychological support. Bupropion is an effective aid to smoking cessation, but it may interact with some forms of psychotropic medication. It is contraindicated for people with epilepsy and with bipolar affective disorder (Anonymous, 2000).

Specialist smoking cessation clinics increase the success rate of smoking cessation by combining behavioural and pharmacological therapies (West *et al*, 2000). Most success is achieved by clinics run by specially trained staff employed solely for this purpose. Clinics should offer individual and group treatments. Groups are most effective when there are 15–30 participants, meeting weekly for at least 6 weeks, and when patients take nicotine replacement therapy or bupropion (West *et al*, 2000). At the beginning of sessions, abstinence should be monitored by checking for expired carbon monoxide.

There is a paucity of research evidence on smoking cessation in psychiatric patients. In the USA, one non-controlled trial of 50 out-patients with schizophrenia found that 42 achieved smoking cessation and 12 were abstinent at 6-month follow-up (Addington *et al*, 1998). The ingested products of tobacco combustion may induce liver enzymes, which return to normal after smoking cessation. There is a risk that patients who stop smoking may develop side-effects to their psychotropic medication (e.g. clozapine), so that dose reduction may be necessary. Smoking is a serious risk to the health of psychiatric patients, so consideration should be given to supporting multiple attempts at smoking cessation.

Diet and nutrition

Diet plays a fundamental role in the development of many diseases, including coronary heart disease, obesity, diabetes and some forms of cancer. The Committee on the Medical Aspects of Food and Nutrition (Department of Health, 1994) has recommended a reduction in dietary fat and salt and an increase in complex carbohydrates. The Food Standards Agency recommends that at least five portions of fruit or vegetables should be consumed per day and at least two portions of oily fish should be eaten per week (Food Standards Agency, 2001). Patients should be given advice on healthy eating, be provided with healthy dishes on the menu and be encouraged to prepare healthy food to eat.

The NHS Plan has set standards for food in NHS hospitals (Department of Health, 2000*a*). All NHS institutions must provide the recommended nutritional intake in food and a range of popular dishes that are likely to be eaten (for website see Box 4.1). Menus should include clearly marked 'healthy options' of main course dishes with <15g of fat, desserts with <5g of fat and <10g of added sugar, and a daily salt intake of 4–6g.

Nutritional needs vary with gender, age and level of activity and are an important consideration in menu planning, timing of meals and portion size. Patients may have special dietary requirements (which should be noted in care plans) such as the need for texture-modified meals if they have chewing or swallowing problems. Health professionals and catering staff should work together to review the diet and make improvements. Those learning to prepare their own food should be taught about basic nutrition and be encouraged to prepare healthy, nutritious meals, within their budget.

Confectionery and carbonated drinks are the most common additions to the diet of psychiatric patients and may substantially increase energy intake. We recommend that patients are given the opportunity to make purchases at shops or recreational facilities that have a range of goods including healthy options. Thirst is a problem for many people taking psychotropic medication and they may consume large quantities of carbonated and caffeine-containing drinks. Patients should have access to drinking water throughout the day, unless there are contraindications such as polydipsia. Weight gain is a particular problem with some psychotropic medications, and people starting these treatments should be weighed prior to commencement and given specific dietetic advice.

Physical activity

Physical activity has many beneficial effects on health and improves cardio-respiratory fitness, body strength, flexibility, balance, body shape and posture (Department of Health, 2004). Regular exercise will alter body composition by increasing muscle and reducing body fat. Elderly people benefit from exercise with improved fitness, muscle strength and bone conservation, which contribute to the prevention of falls (Forwood & Larson, 2000). Other beneficial effects of exercise are improved self-esteem, socialisation and sleep (Honeybourne *et al*, 2000: pp. 199–233). Daley (2002) described the beneficial effects of exercise therapy on the mental state of people with depression and schizophrenia.

Exercise limits the proportion of lean tissue lost during dieting and assists with maintaining weight loss. It reduces the risk of cardiovascular disease and decreases the mortality rate in coronary heart disease. Regular exercise delays the onset of hypertension, reduces blood pressure, improves the control of diabetes and reduces the risk of colon cancer. The current recommended guideline for physical activity is 30 minutes of moderate-intensity activity such as brisk walking, heavy gardening and heavy housework on at least 5 days per week (Department of Health, 1996). Opportunities for exercise may be limited for some patients in rehabilitation and for others exercise may not be a realistic option. Ways of improving patients' physical activity are outlined in Box 4.3.

Staff enthusiasm plays a major role in encouraging patients to be more active. It is usual practice for fitness instructors to assess individuals before starting them on an exercise programme. The assessment may include measurements of resting pulse rate, blood pressure and body fat and calculation of body mass index (BMI), defined as weight divided by height squared, kg/m^2. Tests are also available for flexibility, strength and cardiorespiratory fitness. The fitness instructor may provide progress reports to the clinical team and for care programme approach meetings. Plans for physical activity should be incorporated into care plans.

Box 4.3 Ways to improve patients' physical activity

- Ask patients and staff for their views on exercise and fitness
- Use pedometers to measure exercise taken
- Arrange fitness assessments by appropriately trained fitness staff
- Offer a variety of exercise and activities, e.g. walking, swimming and gym-based exercise
- Arrange access to sports and leisure facilities
- Ensure that sportswear is available
- Develop exercise policies, procedures and risk assessments

Table 4.1 Weight classification

Classification	Body mass index (kg/m^2)
Underweight	<18.5
Normal	18.5–24.9
Overweight	25.0–29.9
Obese	30.0–39.9
Severely obese	>40

Many patients have been inactive for years, particularly those in long-stay settings. A pre-exercise group or individual sessions can give them the confidence, skills and knowledge to begin gentle exercise. Appropriate sportswear may be needed. A systematic review of strategies to promote physical activity found that interventions that encouraged walking were more likely to lead to increases in physical activity (Hillsdon et al, 1999). Physical activity may take place during occupational therapy and some forms of employment. An imaginative approach to exercise, with a range of available options, is most likely to be successful. Community teams often develop activities that encourage exercise, such as swimming, badminton and football groups, using generic recreational facilities.

Weight management

Obesity is defined as having a BMI ≥30 (Table 4.1) and it has reached epidemic proportions in the UK. Some people have a genetic predisposition to obesity, but the fundamental cause is excessive calorie intake. Obesity is a major risk to health, and mortality rises with increasing weight. Excess weight is associated with an increased incidence of cardiovascular, respiratory, gastrointestinal and metabolic disorders as well as certain forms of cancer. The health risks of obesity are increased with central deposition of adipose tissue, and waist size is a measure of the risk to health (Lean et al, 1995) (Table 4.2). An intentional weight loss of 10 kg in obese people can confer significant health benefits. According to Jung (1997) these include

Table 4.2 Waist sizes as a measure of health risk[1]

	Waist size (cm)	
	Male	Female
Increased health risk	>94	>80
Intervention needed to reduce risk to health	>102	>88

1. Figures obtained from Lean et al (1995).

55

Box 4.4 Physical health monitoring

History
- Current complaints
- Past medical history
- Nutritional screen
- Identify health risks, e.g. smoking
- Medication

Physical examination
- All systems
- Blood pressure
- Waist measurement
- Calculate BMI
- Extrapyramidal side effects
- Cardiovascular risk factors
- Senses: hearing and eyesight

Investigations as appropriate[1]
- Full blood count
- Renal function
- Liver function
- Thyroid function
- Fasting lipids
- Fasting glucose
- HbA_{1c} (glycosylated haemaglobin, type 1c)
- Prolactin level
- Urine analysis
- Electrocardiograph (ECG)

1. See the Maudsley Prescribing Guidelines (Taylor *et al*, 2005) for recommendations for monitoring requirements for patients taking psychotropic medication

---

a reduction in risk by 20% of total premature mortality, a 30% reduction in deaths due to diabetes, a 40–50% reduction in cancers due to obesity and up to 30% reduction in triglycerides.

Obesity is prevalent in many psychiatric patients and is exacerbated by physical inactivity and sometimes by medications with the side-effect of weight gain (Allison *et al*, 1999). Monthly monitoring of weight and waist size should alert staff to significant changes and the need for investigation of physical health (Box 4.4). More frequent monitoring is advisable when medication that carries a high risk of weight gain is given (e.g. clozapine, olanzapine, lithium carbonate and sodium valproate). The Maudsley Prescribing Guidelines (Taylor *et al*, 2005; for website see Box 4.1) contain useful information on psychotropic medication with the potential for causing weight gain.

Effective strategies for weight management include a combination of dietary restriction, increased physical activity, behavioural modification and psychological support. Guidelines for weight loss recommend a reduction of 0.5–1.0 kg per week to preserve muscle. The most reliable way of achieving weight loss is with a hypocalorific diet of 500–600 kcal/day (2090–2510 kJ/day) less than the person's estimated energy requirements, together with a modest increase in exercise (Anonymous, 1998). A reduction in energy intake may be achieved by reducing total dietary fat content and by increasing complex carbohydrates in the diet. The aim should be to change long-term eating habits. Support from others and weekly weighing are important factors in successful weight management.

Pharmacological treatments with sibutramine or orlistat should be considered for those who meet the criteria set by NICE (National Institute for Clinical Excellence, 2001a,b). Very low calorie dietary products can be used as substitutes for meals, but as a safeguard, they should be used only under the supervision of a physician, on selected patients with a BMI ≥30. High-protein diets restrict the consumption of healthy foods and generally do not meet nutritional requirements. Behavioural methods used by certain slimming clubs may not be suitable for vulnerable patients. Surgery is available to treat severe obesity but only as a last resort.

Nutritional screening is a useful way of identifying individuals who are undernourished or obese (Malnutrition Universal Screening Tool, for website see Box 4.1). Unexplained change in weight may be the first sign of an underlying serious illness that requires investigation. Patients who are under- or overweight should be given nutritional advice and support when needed.

Physical healthcare

It is important that psychiatrists retain their basic medical skills. Nursing staff working in rehabilitation must have competencies in physical healthcare. Clinical staff should be alert to the possibility that medical disorders can present as psychiatric disorders. Furthermore, psychiatric patients with physical disorders may not complain of symptoms or may have atypical symptoms.

Although many psychiatric patients have identified healthcare needs, they are not always referred to specialists and even when referred they may receive suboptimal treatment. Psychiatric patients should receive the same quality of physical healthcare as the general population. The quality of care can be improved by using systems with agreed aims, procedures and a preset timetable, including the timing of reviews at care programme approach meetings. Information on the patient's physical health should be stored in a designated section in the clinical records and should be readily available to the care team. Standard forms are useful for recording the physical examination, weight, height, BMI, waist size, and the smoking, substance misuse and past medical histories. Important information can be recorded on a medical alert card for use in an emergency. A rolling record of health events should be kept. Computer health records may improve data management.

Patients in rehabilitation settings should have an annual physical health check to monitor the progress of existing conditions and to identify previously undiagnosed disorders. The quality of data collection may be improved by the use of semi-structured or structured questionnaires such as the Cardiff Health Check for patients with learning disabilities (Department of Health, 2002). The physical examination should be preceded by a systemic enquiry (Garden, 2005). A history should be taken of current complaints, past medical history and family medical history, which will focus the doctor's attention on relevant areas of the physical examination. Routine haematological investigations and urine analysis should be undertaken. Infectious diseases such as hepatitis B and C and sexually transmitted diseases such as syphilis should be identified. Immunisations should be provided, for example against hepatitis B, tetanus and influenza. There should be properly equipped facilities for physical examinations, with adequate lighting, heating, furnishings and privacy. Equipment should include accurate weighing scales and a height measure.

Primary care

Many psychiatric patients receive physical healthcare from psychiatrists, who are not usually trained as general practitioners. Primary care services delivering acute and chronic disease management according to NSF standards should be arranged for psychiatric patients (Fisher & Roberts, 1998), including those in rehabilitation services. Initially, the focus should be on patients with a high-risk of coronary heart disease, for example men over 50 with a BMI ≥ 30, who are smokers. Patients who have a history of myocardial infarction, stroke, diabetes mellitus, hypertension and raised cholesterol should be identified and treated, when appropriate, according to nationally agreed protocols. Comorbid substance and alcohol misuse should be assessed and managed according to locally agreed procedures and policies.

Screening

Patients should be given relevant information about screening, be encouraged to take part and be given the opportunity to attend a screening facility. It is important to recognise the sensitivity of some patients to the gender of the medical practitioner or nurse carrying out the screening procedure. The NHS has screening programmes for cervical, breast, colon and prostate cancer, glaucoma and type 2 diabetic retinopathy. Details are available at http://www.nelh.nhs.uk/screening. Patients should be offered screening at appropriate intervals and, whenever possible, should be registered for automatic recall for screening. Patients may be taught self-examination techniques for the detection of breast or testicular masses. The Books

Beyond Words series is a source of information for patients with learning disabilities (http://www.rcpsych.ac.uk/publications/booksbeyondwords. aspx).

Other specialist services

Oral health affects comfort, eating, speech and appearance (Cormac & Jenkins, 1999). The dental status (decayed, missing and filled teeth) of psychiatric patients was found to be similar to that of the general population, but oral hygiene was not as good (Lewis et al, 2002). Oral hygiene should be part of routine care, along with regular visits to the oral hygienist and dentist. Eyes should be assessed regularly by an optician, for visual acuity and ocular problems such as glaucoma and cataracts. Specialist tests are available for those with learning disabilities (McCulloch et al, 1996). Hearing should be tested using audiometry, and hearing aids should be provided if needed.

The pharmacist has an important role in advising about medication, side-effects and monitoring, especially with complex regimens. A dietician should assess dietary needs and advise on the management of those who are under- or overweight. Speech and language therapists have expertise in the assessment and management of swallowing and speech problems. Chiropodists should see patients with foot conditions, and special care should be taken with the feet of individuals with diabetes. A physiotherapy service may be needed.

Occupational therapists may wish to use 'goal-setting' to help individuals make healthy choices about activities of daily living. They may encourage the development of interests such as gardening and physical exercise. Physical health is one of the key areas chosen for goal-setting by patients in rehabilitation (Lecomte et al, 2005; Box 4.5).

Vulnerable patients

People with cognitive or learning disabilities may need help to access care. Sensory impairments are common (Wilson & Haire, 1990), as are epilepsy, dental and skin problems. Women with learning disabilities tend to have an early menopause and menstrual problems (Martin et al, 2001). Physical disabilities may occur in association with underlying genetic disorders such as Down's syndrome. All patients with learning disabilities in residential care should have had an annual health check and a health action plan by June 2005 (Department of Health, 2002, 2006). Health action plans are designed to meet the individual's healthcare needs and are prepared by each individual, with help from staff when necessary.

Elderly psychiatric patients in rehabilitation have the same spectrum of health problems as other elderly people in the general population. The NSF for Older People (Department of Health, 2001b) addresses specific issues in relation to prevention of falls and strokes. Advice from the pharmacist

Box 4.5 Goal-setting for improving physical health

Self-care
- Clean teeth twice daily
- Bathe or shower daily
- Nail and foot care (as needed)
- Skincare – sunscreens, anti-fungal treatment (as needed)
- Monitor weight monthly
- Weight management

Health promotion
- Healthy eating
- Smoking cessation
- Exercise
- Avoid alcohol and substance misuse
- Sexual health
- Contraception

Access to healthcare services
- Register with a general practitioner
- Physical health check annually
- Register with a dental practitioner
- Dental check every 6 months
- Sight and hearing tests annually
- Preventive screening as required

(After Lecomte *et al*, 2005)

will be particularly useful, as pharmacokinetics change with age and drug interactions and side-effects are more likely.

For people with schizophrenia, the NICE guidance (National Institute for Clinical Excellence, 2002) sets standards for health promotion, regular health checks and screening for side-effects of medication. A review by Marder *et al* (2004) contains a useful schedule for monitoring the physical health of out-patients with schizophrenia.

Psychotropic medication

Psychotropic medication may increase health risks by direct or indirect pharmacological action. Medication side-effects may have serious consequences, for example prolongation of the QTc interval, which necessitates regular monitoring of the electrocardiogram. Women are at risk from antipsychotic-induced hyperprolactinaemia, which causes menstrual irregularities, galactorrhoea and sexual dysfunction. A significant proportion of premenopausal women taking antipsychotic medication may be at risk of premature bone loss and osteoporosis (Wieck & Haddad, 2003). Men with hyperprolactinaemia may experience sexual dysfunction and galactorrhoea.

Liaison

It is important for all services to develop good working relationships with staff from primary care and the local general hospital, especially for individuals who self-harm and frequently use the accident and emergency services. Sometimes there is a tendency to discharge psychiatric patients too quickly from hospital to psychiatric facilities that are not staffed or equipped to deal with physical illness.

Conclusions

Improving the physical healthcare of psychiatric patients in rehabilitation settings is an important task for the multiprofessional team. This chapter has documented the major areas where improvements can be made, highlighted some of the most successful practice, and provided references for further reading and research.

References

Action on Smoking and Health (2005) *Basic Facts: One. Smoking Statistics*. London: ASH. http://www.ash.org.uk/html/factsheets/html/basic01.html)

Addington, J., el-Guebaly, N., Campbell, W., *et al* (1998) Smoking cessation treatment for patients with schizophrenia. *American Journal of Psychiatry*, **155**, 974–975.

Allison, D. B., Mentore, J. L., Heo, M., *et al* (1999) Antipsychotic-induced weight gain: a comprehensive research synthesis. *American Journal of Psychiatry*, **156**, 1686–1696.

Anonymous (1998) When and how adults should lose weight. *Drug and Therapeutics Bulletin*, **36**, 89–92.

Anonymous (1999) Nicotine replacement to aid smoking cessation. *Drug and Therapeutics Bulletin*, **37**, 52–53.

Anonymous (2000) Bupropion to aid smoking cessation. *Drug and Therapeutics Bulletin*, **38**, 73–75.

Brown, S., Barraclough, B. & Inskip, H. (2000) Causes of the excess mortality of schizophrenia. *British Journal of Psychiatry*, **177**, 212–217.

Callum, C. (1998) *The Smoking Epidemic*. London: Health Education Authority.

Connolly, M., & Kelly, C. (2005) Lifestyle and physical health. *Advances in Psychiatric Treatment*, **11**, 125–132

Cormac, I. & Jenkins, P. (1999) Understanding the importance of oral health in psychiatric patients. *Advances in Psychiatric Treatment*, **5**, 53–60.

Cormac, I., Ferriter, M., Benning, R., & Saul, C. (2005) Physical health and health risk factors in a population of long-stay psychiatric in-patients. *Psychiatric Bulletin*, **29**, 18–20.

Daley, A. J. (2002) Exercise therapy and mental health in clinical populations: is exercise therapy a worthwhile intervention? *Advances in Psychiatric Treatment*, **8**, 262–270.

Department of Health (1994) *Nutritional Aspects of Cardiovascular Disease: Report of The Cardiovascular Review Group of the Committee on Medical Aspects of Food Policy*. London: HMSO.

Department of Health (1996) *Strategy Statement on Physical Activity*. London: Department of Health.

Department of Health (1997) *The New NHS, Modern and Dependable*. London: HMSO.

Department of Health (1999) *National Service Framework for Mental Health. Modern Standards and Service Models*. London: Department of Health.

Department of Health (2000a) *The NHS Plan. A Plan for Investment. A Plan for Reform*. London: TSO (The Stationery Office).

Department of Health (2000b) *National Service Framework for Coronary Heart Disease. Main Report*. London: TSO (The Stationery Office).

Department of Health (2000c) *National Service Framework for Cancer Services*. London: TSO (The Stationery Office).

Department of Health (2001a) *National Service Framework for Diabetes*. London: TSO (The Stationery Office).

Department of Health (2001b) *National Service Framework for Older People*. London: TSO (The Stationery Office).

Department of Health (2001c) *The Essence of Care. Patient-focussed Benchmarking for Health Practitioners*. London: TSO (The Stationery Office).

Department of Health (2002) *Choosing Health: Making Healthier Choices Easier*. London: TSO (The Stationery Office).

Department of Health (2004) *At Least Five a Week. Evidence on the Impact of Physical Activity and Its Relationship to Health. A Report of the Chief Medical Officer*. London: TSO (The Stationery Office).

Department of Health (2006) *Action for Health. Health Care Action Plans and Health Facilitation. Detailed Good Practice Guidance on Implementation for Learning Disability Partnership Boards*. London: Department of Health.

Fisher, N. & Roberts, R. (1998) Primary health care service for long-stay psychiatric in-patients. *Psychiatric Bulletin*, **22**, 610–612.

Fisher, W. H., Barreira, P. J., Geller, J. L., *et al* (2001) Long-stay psychiatric patients in state hospitals at the end of the 20th century. *Psychiatric Services*, **52**, 1051–1056.

Food Standards Agency (2001) *The Balance of Good Health. Information for Educators and Communicators*. London: FSA & Department of Health.

Forwood, M. R. & Larsen, J. A. (2000) Exercise recommendation for osteoporosis. A position statement of the Australian and New Zealand Bone and Mineral Society. *Australian Family Physician*, **8**, 761–764.

Garden, G. (2005) Physical examination in psychiatric practice. *Advances in Psychiatric Treatment*, **11**, 142–149.

Harris, E. C., & Barraclough, B. (1998) Excess mortality of mental disorder. *British Journal of Psychiatry*, **173**, 11–53.

Hillsdon, M., Thorogood, M. & Foster, C. (1999) A systematic review of strategies to promote physical activity. In *Benefits and Hazards of Exercise* (ed. D. MacAuley), pp. 25–26. London: BMJ Publications.

Hollins, S., Attard, M. T., von Fraunhofer, N., *et al* (1998) Mortality in people with learning disability: risks, causes, and death certification findings in London. *Developmental Medicine and Child Neurology*, **40**, 50– 56.

Honeybourne, J., Hill, M. & Moors, H. (2000) *Advanced Physical Education and Sport for A-Level* (2nd edn). Cheltenham: Nelson Thornes.

James, W. P. T., Nelson, N., Ralph, A., *et al* (1997) The contribution of nutrition to inequalities in health. *BMJ*, **314**, 1545–1549.

Joukamaa, M., Heliövaara, M., Kneckt, P., *et al* (2001) Mental disorders and cause-specific mortality. *British Journal of Psychiatry*, **179**, 498–502.

Jung, R. T. (1997) Obesity as a disease. *British Medical Bulletin*, **53**, 307–321.

Lean, M. E. J., Han, T. S. & Morrison, C. E. (1995) Waist circumference as a measure for indicating need for weight management. *BMJ*, **311**, 158–161.

Lecomte, T., Wallace, C. J., Perreault, M., *et al* (2005) Consumers' goals in psychiatric rehabilitation and their concordance with existing services. *Psychiatric Services*, **56**, 209–211.

Lewis, S., Jagger, R. G. & Treasure, E. (2002) The oral health of psychiatric in-patients in South Wales. *Special Care in Dentistry*, **21**, 182–186.

Marder, S., Essock, S. M., Buchanan, R. W., *et al* (2004) Physical health monitoring of patients with schizophrenia. *American Journal of Psychiatry*, **161**, 1334–1349.

Martin, D. M., Cassidy, G., Ahmad, F., *et al* (2001) Women with learning disabilities and the menopause. *Journal of Learning Disabilities*, **5**, 121–132.

McCulloch, D. L., Sludden, P. A., McKeown, K., *et al* (1996) Vision requirements among intellectually disabled adults: a residence-based pilot study. *Journal of Intellectual Disability Research*, **40**, 140–150.

Meltzer, H., Gill, B., Petticrew, M., *et al* (1996) *Economic Activity and Social Functioning of Residents with Psychiatric Disorders* (OPCS Surveys of Psychiatric Morbidity in Great Britain, Report 6). London: HMSO.

National Institute for Clinical Excellence (2001a) *Guidance on the Use of Sibutramine for the Treatment of Obesity in Adults* (Technology Appraisal Guidance no. 31). London: NICE.

National Institute for Clinical Excellence (2001b) *Guidance on the Use of Orlistat in the Treatment of Obesity in Adults* (Technology Appraisal Guidance no. 22). London: NICE.

National Institute for Clinical Excellence (2002) *Schizophrenia. Core Interventions in the Treatment and Management of Schizophrenia in Primary and Secondary Care* (Clinical Guideline 1). London: NICE.

NHS Executive (1999) *Been There, Done That. Revisiting Tobacco Control Policies in the NHS.* London: Health Education Authority.

Richards, J., Smith, D. J., Harvey, C.A., *et al* (1997) Characteristics of the new long-stay population in an inner Melbourne acute psychiatric hospital. *Australian and New Zealand Journal of Psychiatry*, **31**, 488–495.

Taylor, D., Paton, C., Kerwin, R., *et al* (2005) *The Maudsley 2005–2006 Prescribing Guidelines* (8th edn). London: Taylor & Francis.

van Schrojenstein Lantman-De Valk, H. M. J., Metsemakers, J. F. M., Haveman, M. J., *et al* (2000) Health problems in people with intellectual disability in general practice: a comparative study. *Family Practice*, **17**, 405–407.

West, R., McNeill, A. & Raw, M. (2000) Smoking cessation guidelines for health professionals: an update. *Thorax*, **55**, 987–999.

West, R., McNeill, A. & Raw, M. (2003) *Meeting Department of Health Smoking Cessation Targets. Recommendations for Primary Care Trusts.* London: Health Development Agency.

Wieck, A. & Haddad, P. M. (2003) Antipsychotic-induced hyperprolactinaemia in women: pathophysiology, severity and consequences. *British Journal of Psychiatry*, **182**, 199–204.

Wilson, D. & Haire, A. (1990) Health care screening for people with mental handicap living in the community. *BMJ*, **301**, 1379–1381.

CHAPTER 5

A comprehensive approach to assessment in rehabilitation settings

Alan Meaden and Alan Farmer

People who experience persistent and significant difficulties as a result of psychotic symptoms have complex and multiple needs. Mainstream primary and secondary care services often find it hard to provide a sufficiently intensive and sustained approach to addressing these. Referral to rehabilitation services generally represents a tacit admission of failure by acute mental health services and is often seen as such by those who are referred. Some individuals who enter rehabilitation services have received a comprehensive range of therapeutic interventions. Others, particularly those who have had a lengthy stay on an acute psychiatric ward, may have received a limited range of treatments and have experienced an impoverished social environment that has had low expectations of them. Unmet or unrecognised needs are common among people referred to rehabilitation services. This can result in increased risk, slow progress and greater probability of relapse.

Successful rehabilitation is partly about being thorough. Comprehensive assessment is an essential starting point to making the most effective use of the limited specialist resources available to people with enduring severe mental illness. As Wykes & Holloway (2000) note, despite powerful policies aimed at improving care planning and the assessment of outcome, there has been little agreement on what assessment procedures are most appropriate for identifying rehabilitation interventions and monitoring success. However, recent decades have witnessed a growth in multidisciplinary psychosocial approaches to treatment (Fowler *et al*, 1995) and the development of a range of assessment tools for identifying and evaluating the usefulness of specific interventions. More recently, policy and practice have recognised the importance of a collaborative approach that includes service users and carers as partners in the planning and provision of treatment and support and the adoption of a recovery perspective (Roberts & Wolfson, 2004). Assessments and the assessment process have been modified and developed to better inform and guide these approaches.

This chapter provides a broad overview of assessment in these contexts. The aim is to provide the clinician with a guide to areas for consideration when making a comprehensive assessment and lists a small number of potentially useful tools. (See Appendix 1 at the end of this book for a more detailed discussion of useful assessment schedules.) The process of conducting an assessment is considered and advice is presented on how findings can be used to devise a formulation that can guide treatment and care. Population needs assessment is also briefly discussed.

Why assess?

A comprehensive rehabilitation service should contain professionals with a wide range of skills, as well as having access to a variety of community resources. It is first and foremost vital to recall that, although people with long-term mental health problems have complex needs, they are also real people with real lives. To carry out an adequate assessment a great deal of information must be elicited, recorded and made useful. This requires a clear structure, which should be developed locally and continually revised.

Ongoing assessment forms the core of the rehabilitation process. Initially, we organise information about a person's complex needs and match that to a range of interventions. We may ask ourselves whether a person needs a specialist rehabilitation team (taking into consideration the particular inclusion and exclusion criteria that are in place) or whether advice and support from the existing care team may suffice. An evaluation of risk may indicate the need for urgency or a combination of approaches, inform the care plan and suggest the appropriate care setting. A process of formal review should monitor the effectiveness and acceptability of treatment, as well as providing an opportunity for further information-gathering and dialogue with the client (patient) and their carers. Assessment now embraces the concepts of recovery, strengths and empowerment. We strive to work with the whole person in their social setting rather than merely perceiving a client who presents with a combination of symptoms, demographic characteristics and diagnosis. Assessment must be collaborative. It should be undertaken sensitively and, if done properly, can be an engaging and therapeutic process in itself. People with long-term mental illnesses are often pleased, and sometimes rather surprised, to be offered the opportunity to talk about themselves, their past life and their future aspirations; indeed, it is often the staff who are reluctant to talk with people experiencing such difficulties.

The value of structured assessments

A full assessment of a person with complex needs requires more than completion of a checklist. However, some form of structure is important to ensure that major difficulties for the client and their carers, such as social anxiety and behavioural problems, are not overlooked. Rehabilitation teams develop special knowledge and skills in areas such as employment and accommodation: it is important that their assessments in these areas are not just about fitting people into available resources but are capable of identifying the need for changes in the organisation and provision of services.

We are in an era that demands the routine evaluation of the outcome of care using standardised measures. It is likely that routine outcome measures will also support research into the unfashionable area of rehabilitation and thus further the development of evidence-based practice. Routine outcome measurement within rehabilitation services can demonstrate to staff, clients and carers that the careful, undramatic efforts of these services can result in sustained clinical improvement.

The continuing relevance of diagnosis

Accurate diagnosis remains an important part of a fuller formulation. It guides evidence-based pharmacological and psychological treatments and provides information about the long-term nature of the illness and prognosis that we can share with the person concerned, their carers and other professionals. Rather than being just a label, diagnosis can guide the individual's own research and link them to other individuals and organisations such as the Manic Depression Fellowship (which acts under the name 'MDF The BiPolar Organisation') and Rethink (see Appendix 2 for more organisations and contact details) .

The importance of comorbid disorders

Many clients have more than one form of mental health problem. In the past, important comorbidity has been obscured by the label of psychosis. Problems and distress related to depression, anxiety, obsessional symptoms, substance misuse, personality disorder, learning disability, acquired brain injury and autistic-spectrum disorder will certainly colour the clinical picture and may require specific therapeutic intervention. Problems relating to some of these disorders may not be easily identified. Where such difficulties go unrecognised, rehabilitation efforts often fail. This can be frustrating for all concerned and may lead to reduced empathy among staff and earn the individual the label of a 'heart sink patient'.

Individuals diagnosed with schizophrenia present with an increased risk of substance misuse, which in turn is associated with greater risk of relapse, failure to follow medication regimens, aggression, depression, suicide, frequent changes of accommodation and family burden (Drake & Mueser, 2001). As substance misuse tends to go unreported, detection and screening are important in any assessment. Drake & Mueser (2001) offer a useful assessment approach consisting of several interconnected steps, beginning with detection and emphasis on active substance misuse and long-term observation by professionals using multiple sources of information, through to a more specialised assessment process involving behavioural analysis to identify appropriate treatment goals.

Impairments in social interaction and communication due to an autistic-spectrum disorder may be misinterpreted as evidence of both positive and negative symptoms of a schizophrenia-spectrum disorder (Fitzgerald & Corvin, 2001). If both disorders are present, individuals often fall between services. It is important therefore to obtain a good developmental history and assess as far as possible social interaction and communication difficulties.

Individuals presenting with personality difficulties often engender a degree of hostility in staff. To a certain extent, premorbid personality characteristics influence the way in which individuals cope with mental illness and how they respond to services and help-giving. However, for some this influence is more marked and significantly impairs the rehabilitation process. Certain personality disorders have been more closely associated with schizophrenia than others. People with paranoid, schizoid or schizo-typal personality disorder often present with psychosis-type symptoms (Derksen, 1995). Personality characteristics associated with schizoid and schizotypal personality disorder have also being implicated as potential vulnerability factors in the development of schizophrenia (Nuechterlein & Subotnik, 1998). Psychosis-type symptoms may also emerge in borderline personality disorder. It is important therefore to consider factors such as premorbid functioning and the persistence of psychotic symptoms when conducting an assessment. The use of a 'shared formulation' , as described later in this chapter, may be particularly relevant when working with people with psychosis and a comorbid personality disorder.

What should we assess?

Assessments should be meaningful, have a clear purpose, be targeted at the task at hand and be no more detailed or systematic than the circumstances require. Staff undertaking an assessment should have adequate experience and training (training being at least as important as experience when using specific assessment tools).

Assessment measures should reflect the aims of the service. If a team's rehabilitation approach is based on social recovery and quality of life, their assessments should reflect this. Assertive outreach teams, for example, might assess engagement on an ongoing basis. In residential care the focus might be on determining the level of support required of subsequent placements. Outcome assessments should also reflect the nature of the intervention: an occupational therapy intervention is not best assessed using a psychiatric rating scale.

Assessments should be sensitive to the individual's stage of illness (e.g. stable, in relapse or experiencing residual difficulties) and, wherever possible, should focus on recovery, incorporating personal goals, hopes, aspirations and motivation for self-management. One vital component of the assessment process within rehabilitation is assessment of the individual's functional skills. Often referred to as 'activities of daily living', these are basic life skills and include shopping, cooking, cleaning, budgeting and interacting with others. Assessment of functional skills is best undertaken in the environment where the individual is most likely to use them, and one that allows (and expects) the person to use their skills. Symptoms are less significant than function in planning for a person's future care needs, although some specific behavioural problems – forms of challenging behaviour – do have a marked impact on placement options. If not adequately assessed and planned for, these may result in placement failure, which can be demoralising for the person, their carers and staff alike.

The growth in psychological assessments has led to conceptualisation of approaches at different levels (Haddock & Tarrier, 1998). Assessment may be carried out at a symptom or syndrome level (e.g. eliciting whether a person is hearing voices) or at the level of dimensions of experience (e.g. frequency and severity of experiences) or it can be used to inform therapy (e.g. assessing antecedents and consequences of experiences or beliefs). Assessment of neurocognitive functioning, which is generally, if subtly, compromised in people referred to rehabilitation services, may have a role to play in planning rehabilitation interventions. Cognitive deficits have been linked to poor functional outcomes and may limit rehabilitation outcomes (Wykes & Holloway, 2000). Fowler *et al* (1995) offer a useful brief test battery which includes the National Adult Reading Test, the Wechsler Adult Intelligence Scale II, the Cognitive Estimation Test and the Probabilistic Reasoning Task. However, such assessments are likely to be time-consuming and, if only subtle impairments are present, they can be difficult to interpret owing to confounding factors such as test effort, test anxiety and medication side-effects. Briefer assessments that can reliably identify the cognitive deficits reported in the literature are sorely needed. The repeatable battery for the assessment of neurological status (Gold *et al*, 1999) may prove to be one such measure.

Assessment tools

A variety of assessment tools have been developed that aim to standardise direct observations and interviews. The advantage of a standardised method is that it allows comparisons between individuals and in an individual over time. Different professionals should record similar findings. Interviews can be structured – for example the Present State Examination (Wing *et al*, 1974) – or systematic, in the form of a rating scale such as the Brief Psychiatric Rating Scale (Lukoff *et al*, 1986) and the Health of the Nation Outcome Scales (HoNOS; Wing *et al*, 1996). Structured interviews are mainly used in research, whereas rating scales are more widely used in clinical practice.

Some clinicians and services find this standardisation helpful and embrace such methods. Others favour a less-structured approach, relying instead on an ongoing dialogue with service users and those involved in their care. In either case, a comprehensive view should be sought. The guidelines on the treatment of schizophrenia produced by the National Institute for Clinical Excellence (now the National Institute for Health and Clinical Excellence; NICE) in 2002 identify a number of assessment domains: degree of symptomatic recovery; quality of life; degree of personal autonomy; ability and access to work; stability and quality of living accommodation; degree and quality of social integration, degree of financial independence; and experience and impact of side-effects of treatment.

Box 5.1 shows a fuller list of areas for assessment. There is a plethora of assessment instruments that can provide measurements in each area. Within our own service (Birmingham and Solihull Mental Health NHS Trust) we make use of a number of instruments for both assessment and routine measurement of outcome. These include: the Beliefs about Voices Questionnaire – Revised; the Cognitive Assessment of Voices; the Beliefs and Convictions Scale; the Calgary Depression Scale; and the Beck Anxiety

---

Box 5.1 Assessment areas for rehabilitation clients

Snapshot assessments
- Current subjective problems
- Current mental state:
  - type of symptoms (include depressive symptoms)
  - severity of symptoms
  - impact on mood and behaviour
  - change in symptoms/mood/behaviour
- Current physical health:
  - weight
  - general physical symptoms
  - sensory impairment
  - sexual functioning
- Side-effects of medication
- Physical investigations:
  - metabolic syndrome
  - drug plasma levels
  - medication-dependent tests
- Risk:
  - of relapse
  - to self (including accidental harm and neglect)
  - to others
  - from others (exploitation)

History
- History and pattern of illness
- Duration of untreated psychosis (often an important predictor of longer-term outcomes)
- Previous treatments and treatment response
- Premorbid functioning

continued

Box 5.1 *continued*

Social functioning
- Non-psychotic symptoms/secondary difficulties, e.g. social anxiety
- Longitudinal picture of family and social networks (including family dynamics)
- Quality of life
- Finances

Lifestyle assessments
- Substance use
- Criminal convictions
- Cultural and spiritual issues
- Gender and sexual issues

Engagement
- Beliefs about and attitude to illness
- Attitudes towards services
- Attitudes towards treatment and treatment adherence

Accommodation needs
- Current needs
- Current risk
- Personal experience/preferences
- Plans for moving
- Finances

Employment and educational needs
- Education history
- Employment history
- Specific work rating scales
- Finances
- Educational attainment and needs

Personal coping
- Attempts to cope with difficulties
- Coping style
- Support systems
- Early-warning signs

Recovery factors
- Hopes and aspirations
- Valued roles and goals
- Personal strengths and preferences
- Understanding of difficulties/insight/attitude to illness
- Motivation for self-management

Carer assessment
- Burden of care/quality of life
- Psychiatric/psychological symptoms
- Unmet needs
- Personal strengths and preferences
- Valued roles and goals
- Motivation

Specialist assessments
- Neurocognitive assessment/psychometric assessment
- Electrocardiogram/computed axial tomography/magnetic resonance imaging

Inventory for assessment and monitoring of psychological interventions (full references for these assessments are supplied in Appendix 1 to this book). In addition, we have found Young's Schema Questionnaire and its companion assessments the Young Parenting Inventory, the Young–Rygh Avoidance Inventory and the Young Compensation Inventory particularly helpful when developing our shared formulations. The Early Signs Scale is useful for initiating relapse plans and monitoring for early signs of relapse. The Personal Beliefs about Illness Questionnaire, Recovery Style Questionnaire and the Hall Engagement Scale are useful for assessing attitude to relapse, recovery style and service engagement respectively. We would add to this list only a good quality-of-life measure such as the Lancashire Quality of Life Profile and the Manchester Short Assessment of Quality of Life. Details of other useful measures are contained in Appendix 1 and in texts such as Tansella & Thornicroft (2001).

If assessment tools are to be used routinely, a rehabilitation team will need training so that, ideally, all team members feel confident to carry out assessment in most of the areas suggested above. Assessment of neuro-cognitive impairment, pharmacological treatment needs and physical health require specialised skills that currently reside in the clinical psychology and psychiatric professions.

Risk assessment

All mental health professionals are now expected to be competent in the assessment of a patient's risk to self or others, a situation highlighted by high-profile incidents in the 1990s. Increasingly, the rehabilitation needs of forensic patients are being recognised, and many individuals referred to rehabilitation services will have had contact with forensic mental health services, which will have conducted very detailed risk assessments. Despite this, rehabilitation services tend to use home-grown risk assessment tools that are often just checklists of known risk factors for harm to self or others and have no proven reliability and validity.

Risk assessment is an inexact science that collates relevant information from epidemiology, history, current mental state and circumstances in an attempt to predict and therefore alter possible outcomes. Although it is important for staff to adhere to their local risk assessment policies and procedures, we must be aware that identifying that a risk exists is of little practical use on its own. What is useful is to formulate the risk issues and identify factors that can be modified to decrease the probability that adverse events will occur. Each behaviour must be clearly defined and assessed individually, as each is likely to involve different factors. Both the probability (likelihood) of the behaviour and its cost (potentially serious consequences) need to be considered (Kapur, 2000). Macpherson et al (2002) describe a system using care programme approach (CPA) documentation to inform multidisciplinary discussion and clinical decisions in their rehabilitation service. In their conclusions they highlight the risks of false positives, especially for a rare event such as homicide. They suggest that an assessment of a more common event, for example violence, is more valid. They also mention the importance of therapeutic risk-taking in people's progress and recovery.

Physical health needs

The physical health of people with schizophrenia and other types of severe mental illness is frequently poor (Phelan *et al*, 2001). Tobacco smoking, physical inactivity, poor diet and nutrition are all contributory factors and there may have been difficulties accessing care. It has long been known that people with long-term mental health problems have higher morbidity and mortality than the general population (Harris & Barraclough, 1998), particularly for diseases of the circulatory, respiratory, digestive, endocrine and nervous systems. Cormac *et al* (2004) have produced a comprehensive review of physical health assessments and possible interventions for long-stay psychiatric in-patients. These assessments should be transferable to other settings and offer opportunities for shared interventions with primary care.

Even before the introduction of antipsychotic medication, schizophrenia was associated with a higher risk of diabetes. Now antipsychotics are themselves associated with the development of diabetes. Fifty years ago Thonnard-Neumann (1956) reported 'phenothiazine diabetes'. More recently, type 2 diabetes (non-insulin-dependent) has received particular attention as one of a number of cardiovascular risk factors known as metabolic syndrome (Holt, 2004). Other assessments are of blood pressure, weight and blood lipids. Current UK guidelines suggest that fasting blood glucose should be measured on starting an antipsychotic drug and then at 6-month intervals. This is especially relevant in those with risk factors such as family history, belonging to a Black or minority ethnic group, obesity, hypertension, dyslipidaemia, lack of physical activity, polycystic ovary syndrome or a history of gestational diabetes or impaired glucose tolerance (Luna & Feinglos, 2001). Medication may have an impact on physical health by direct (e.g. prolongation of QTc interval) or indirect pharmacological action (e.g. hyperprolactinaemia). Antipsychotic-induced hyperprolactinaemia causes menstrual irregularities and galactorrhoea in women and sexual dysfunction in both genders (Cormac *et al*, 2004). In premenopausal women there is also an association of hyperprolactinaemia with premature bone loss and osteoporosis (Wieck & Haddad, 2003).

Assessment of physical health, usually in collaboration with primary care, is mandatory and is strongly emphasised in the NICE schizophrenia guidelines.

The side-effects of medication must be monitored, as they not only contribute to health problems but also influence adherence to treatment regimens. Rehabilitation teams and local primary care services should decide between them who will take responsibility for on-going assessment of such side-effects and potential physical health complications such as diabetes. Care coordinators should arrange an annual physical health check at their client's general practice surgery and make it easy for the client to attend. This check should pay particular attention to endocrine disorders (e.g. diabetes, hyperprolactinaemia), cardiovascular risk factors (e.g. blood pressure, lipids), side-effects of medication, lifestyle factors (e.g. smoking, obesity) and cancer.

The process of assessment

The assessment process involves the conceptualisation of multiple variables and results in a judgement of needs, which in turn informs which services are to be offered and the planning and recording of specific therapeutic interventions. Outcomes (e.g. increased performance or decreased diffi-culties) are measured and these influence the ongoing process of treatment and care.

Enough jargon: how to do it

Case notes are an important source of factual information and will often include detailed descriptions of critical incidents such as relapses that have required acute intervention. Notes are less useful in giving us a picture of change over time. The involvement of many professionals and professions may have led to a variety of attitudes and approaches, to the detriment of a clear and objective history, and to disagreement about diagnosis and treatment. Direct contact with professionals involved in the client's care is preferred when carrying out assessment.

We must also actively involve and engage the client and their carers in the assessment process. Increasing the number of sources of information leads to greater reliability. Meetings are best held in the client's own environment – in their home if this is acceptable (although many people are not used to this and can find the experience threatening and intrusive). The client, carers or family members may be working or have fixed commitments, so professionals need to be flexible in terms of timing. Initial meetings can be lengthy. Multiple meetings are often necessary for an adequate assessment.

Assessment must make use of the attitudes, skills and knowledge of each profession in the multidisciplinary team. All members of the rehabilitation team should agree on the assessment process and value both the process and the information it yields. An initial assessment conference, with presentations to the wider team, should reach a consensus on key issues (e.g. fulfilment of service criteria, risk and initial treatment options) and indicate lines of further assessment and investigation needed to reach a shared formulation. Rating scales may be part of routine practice, in addition to interviews and accurate observations. They may also be suggested when specialist assessment is indicated and are often used in quantifying treatment response and wider outcomes.

Assessments need to be tailored to the individual. Someone with poor attention and concentration (e.g. as part of a psychotic illness) may benefit from a series of short meetings. Those who are socially withdrawn may require a slower pace and greater time to reply. Open questions are important if the person is suggestible and might passively conform to leading questions. People with social anxieties may prefer the involvement of fewer professionals and a less formal approach. If engagement is an issue, practical support and social activities may provide an appropriate forum for assessment.

Specialist advice should be sought if the individual has sensory impairment. Interpreters with knowledge of mental health issues may be useful when asking about difficult situations or symptoms if the client and/or their carers have a limited understanding of English. Family members and friends may sometimes fulfil this role, although the complexities of family dynamics need to be borne in mind.

Rehabilitation can be a slow process and assessment needs to be ongoing. People with long-term mental health problems often show fluctuations even in the absence of relapse or clear exacerbation of symptoms. Longitudinal assessments are preferable, although repeated snapshots may suffice, at an interval determined by the nature and frequency of problems. Assessments should acknowledge the individual's strengths and weaknesses. The information gathered from an assessment should be transferable to other relevant situations and should lead to a client-centred approach that involves realistic, relevant and valued interventions and has a social context. This is discussed further in the next section.

Drawing it all together: the importance of formulation in care planning and treatment

A now widely accepted way of conceptualising the difficulties presented by those who experience psychosis is the biopsychosocial perspective (usually within a stress–vulnerability model). This recognises the importance of biological, psychological and social factors in the onset and maintenance of psychotic symptoms and their associated difficulties. The model provides a valuable perspective when developing a formulation.

Formulation should promote a shared view of the client's difficulties. This is particularly important when attempting to address and manage complex and multiple problems. Developing a shared understanding can have great therapeutic value and has become a cornerstone of some services (Alanen, 1997). It guides therapy and provides the opportunity for dialogue with the individual, carers and the treatment team. It is also likely to reduce the likelihood of competing treatment approaches, promote psychological

> **Box 5.2**   Key elements of the formulation
>
> - Early experiences
> - Vulnerabilities and stressors (past and present)
> - Core beliefs (regarding self and other people)
> - Psychotic experiences (past and present)
> - Emotional and behavioural consequences
> - Coping strategies (past and present)
> - Maintenance factors
> - Social relationships
> - Risk issues

understanding and engage the empathy of staff if negative attitudes towards the individual have developed. Key elements that should be included within the formulation are shown in Box 5.2.

These elements may be linked together diagrammatically or serve as useful headings for summarising key information. One clinician may take the lead in developing a formulation by gathering the relevant information. This can then be progressively shared with team members and, ideally (at some point), with the client and others involved in providing care and support. This could take the form of an assessment conference or a 'case bust', initially consisting of the most involved clinicians and eventually expanding to include all of those concerned in the individual's care. The formulation should be used to plan interventions and develop clear and realistic goals and itself be subject to regular review and revision. We have used such formulations to good effect in promoting team understanding and planning the way forward. The fictional formulation shown in Fig. 5.1 highlights the key information in a functionally useful way.

Population needs assessment

Mental health services should be planned and operated to meet the needs of the population that they serve. Thornicroft & Tansella (2001) provide an accessible general account of the process of undertaking an assessment of need for mental health services at the population level. They emphasise the importance of setting out general service principles that offer an ethical grounding to what is provided and the establishment of 'boundary conditions', the definition of what falls within and outside the remit of the service. This is particularly pertinent to rehabilitation services, which will employ explicit inclusion and exclusion criteria. At present there is no agreed model of rehabilitation service that would help in service planning. In contrast, the Department of Health has produced a very clear set of

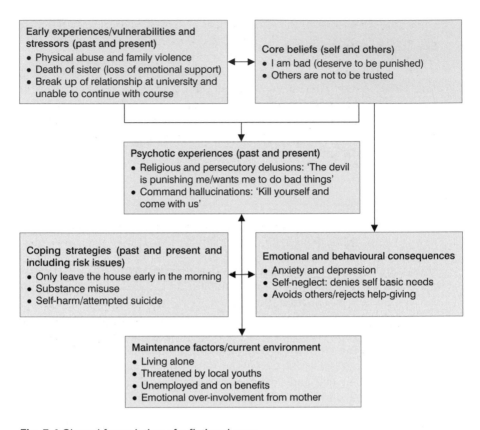

Fig. 5.1 Shared formulation of a fictional case.

specifications for other elements of a comprehensive mental health service in England, such as early intervention, home treatment and assertive outreach (Department of Health, 2001).

The assessment of population needs for mental health services also requires a clear definition of the term 'need', as well as some understanding of the local epidemiology of mental illness. The incidence and prevalence of psychosis varies markedly between catchment areas in a manner correlated with the local demography. Psychosis has been found to be associated with inner-city areas that have high levels of social deprivation, social mobility and substance misuse and high numbers of people belonging to minority ethnic groups. To a lesser extent, the disabilities and consequent service demands associated with psychosis vary according to local conditions.

Thornicroft & Tansella (2001) recommend a pathway for service planning. This begins with the collection of epidemiologically based data (the characteristics of the population being served, who requires treatment and who receives it), considers what is provided by local services (service components, beds, service integration) and identifies what outputs the services achieve (throughput and outcomes). These data together can inform a planning process that identifies gaps in provision and, using comparative data from other services, areas of inefficiency and poor performance.

There are specific issues of needs assessment relevant to rehabilitation services in an era of deinstitutionalisation, when most mental health services expect short in-patient stays and rapid throughput. These include the accumulation of 'new long-stay' patients on acute in-patient wards and the capacity of the service to provide a comprehensive range of accommodation locally for people with long-term severe mental illnesses.

Conclusions

Assessment is a crucial element in the provision of good-quality mental healthcare within rehabilitation, recovery and continuing-care services. In this chapter we have outlined a comprehensive process of assessment and highlighted the importance of promoting meaningful and appropriate outcomes for service users, carers and clinical staff. The service context in which mental health professionals work clearly influences the extent to which comprehensive assessment occurs. Appropriate training and on-going support to enable staff to engage more actively in this process is vitally important.

References

Alanen, Y. O. (1997) *Schizophrenia: Its Origins and Need-adapted Treatment.* London: Karnac Books.

Cormac, I., Martin, D. & Ferriter, M. (2004) Improving the physical health of long-stay psychiatric in-patients. *Advances in Psychiatric Treatment*, **10**, 107–115.

Department of Health (2001) *The Mental Health Policy Implementation Guide.* London: Department of Health.

Derksen, J. (1995) *Personality Disorders: Clinical and Social Perspectives.* Chichester: John Wiley & Sons.

Drake, R. E. & Mueser, K. T. (2001) Substance abuse comorbidity. In *Comprehensive Care of Schizophrenia: A Textbook of Clinical Management* (eds J. A. Lieberman & R. M. Murray), pp. 243–255. London: Taylor & Francis.

Fitzgerald, M. & Corvin, A. (2001) Diagnosis and differential diagnosis of Asperger syndrome. *Advances in Psychiatric Treatment*, **7**, 310–318.

Fowler, D., Garety, P. & Kuipers, E. (1995) *Cognitive Behaviour Therapy for Psychosis: Theory and Practice.* Chichester: John Wiley & Sons.

Gold, J., Queern, C., Iannone, V., *et al* (1999) Repeatable battery for the assessment of neuropsychological status as a screening test in schizophrenia. I: Sensitivity, reliability and validity. *American Journal of Psychiatry*, **156**, 1944–1950.

Haddock, G. & Tarrier, N. (1998) Assessment and formulation in the cognitive behavioural treatment of psychosis. In *Treating Complex Cases: The cognitive behavioural therapy approach* (eds N. Tarrier & A. Wells), pp. 155–175. Chichester: John Wiley & Sons.

Harris, E. C. & Barraclough, B. (1998) Excess mortality of mental disorder. *British Journal of Psychiatry*, **173**, 11–53.

Holt, R. I. G. (2004) Diagnosis, epidemiology and pathogenesis of diabetes mellitus: an update for psychiatrists. *British Journal of Psychiatry*, **184** (suppl. 47), s55–s63.

77

Kapur, N. (2000) Evaluating risks. *Advances in Psychiatric Treatment*, **6**, 399–406.

Lukoff, D., Nuechterlein, K. & Ventura, J. (1986) Manual for expanded Brief Psychiatric Rating Scale (BPRS). *Schizophrenia Bulletin*, **4**, 594–602.

Luna, B. & Feinglos, M. N. (2001) Drug-induced hyperglycemia. *JAMA*, **286**, 1945–1958.

Macpherson, R., Cornelius, F., Kilpatrick, D., *et al* (2002) Outcome of clinical risk management in the Gloucester rehabilitation service. *Psychiatric Bulletin*, **26**, 449–452.

National Institute for Clinical Excellence (2002) *Clinical Guideline 1. Schizophrenia: Core Interventions in the Treatment and Management of Schizophrenia in Primary and Secondary Care.* London: NICE.

Nuechterlein, K. H. & Subotnik, K. L. (1998) The cognitive origins of schizophrenia and prospects for intervention. In *Outcome and Innovation in Psychological Treatment of Schizophrenia* (eds T. Wykes, N. Tarrier & S. Lewis), pp. 17–43. Chichester: John Wiley & Sons.

Phelan, M., Stradins, L. & Morrison, S. (2001) Physical health of people with severe mental illness. *BMJ*, **322**, 443–444.

Roberts, G. & Wolfson, P. (2004) The rediscovery of recovery: open to all. *Advances in Psychiatric Treatment*, **10**, 37–48.

Tansella, M. & Thornicroft, G. (2001) *Mental Health Outcome Measures* (2nd edn). London: Gaskell.

Thonnard-Neumann E. (1956) Phenothiazines and diabetes in hospitalized women. *American Journal of Psychiatry*, **29**, 827–828.

Thornicroft, G. & Tansella, M. (2001) The planning process for mental health services. In *Textbook of Community Psychiatry* (eds G. Thornicroft & G. Szmukler), pp. 179–192. Oxford: Oxford University Press.

Wieck, A. & Haddad, P. M. (2003) Antipsychotic-induced hyperprolactinaemia in women: pathophysiology, severity and consequences. Selective literature review. *British Journal of Psychiatry*, **182**, 199–204.

Wing, J. K., Cooper, J. E. & Sartorius, N. (1974) *Measurement and Classification of Psychiatric Symptoms*. Cambridge: Cambridge University Press.

Wing, J. K., Curtis, R. H. & Beevor, A. (1996) *The Health of The Nation Outcome Scales: Report on Research and Development July 1993–December 1995*. London: Royal College of Psychiatrists' Research Unit.

Wykes, T. & Holloway, F. (2000) Community rehabilitation: past failures and future prospects. *International Review of Psychiatry*, **12**, 197–205.

CHAPTER 6

Mapping and classifying rehabilitation services

Geoff Shepherd

Bennett (1978) defines rehabilitation as a process in which people with physical or psychiatric disabilities are enabled to make best use of residual abilities in order to function optimally in as normal a social situation as possible. This definition highlights the central importance of the 'process' of rehabilitation – the need to provide good-quality care, over long periods of time, with active monitoring of progress and good continuity of support. It also explicitly acknowledges the existence of 'disabilities' – i.e. enduring symptoms or problems in functioning that have to be managed, rather than treated. Finally, it identifies the aim of helping the person find their optimum level in as normal a social context as possible. This places social functioning at the heart of outcomes, whether in hospital or in the community.

To map rehabilitation services, we need first to agree their essential components. Concepts of psychiatric rehabilitation have changed as the organisation of mental health services has moved from one based on hospitals to one based on specialist community teams, with minimal use of in-patient beds. The National Service Framework for Mental Health (Department of Health, 1999) sets out a clear vision for the future of mental health services, based on the operation of specialist teams – assertive outreach, crisis resolution and home treatment, and early intervention. The challenge now is to understand how rehabilitation ideas fit into these new service structures.

Of course, some may claim that there is no need for specialist rehabilitation services when the process of discharging people from long-stay hospitals is more or less complete. But this is to confuse 'rehabilitation' with 'resettlement'. In this chapter I will argue that rehabilitation ideas are just as relevant in these new service structures as they were 50 years ago in mental hospitals. People with problems that are severe and difficult to treat continue to present to mental health services and continue to need long-term, high-quality care with good continuity over time. The principles of rehabilitation offer a way of understanding their needs and formulating treatment and management plans which will effectively address them.

Whether this means that we need separate rehabilitation services, or whether such care can be delivered through mainstream services is open to debate. I will also consider how rehabilitation ideas fit into new models about 'recovery' and 'social inclusion'. Let us begin by trying to spell out an evidence-based set of standards for the provision of high-quality specialist rehabilitation services, located within the current National Service Framework for Mental Health.

Standards for rehabilitation services

A set of evidence-based standards for rehabilitation services was produced by the Health Advisory Service (now the Health and Social Care Advisory Service: HASCAS) in 1999 (Health Advisory Service, 1999). These were used in a series of projects to assess the content of local rehabilitation services and to provide information to guide local service developments. They are set out in Box 1.

Locally agreed definitions

The standards begin with questions of definition. As with any other intervention, rehabilitation services must begin by defining who they are there to serve and how boundaries will be drawn in relation to other services. The client groups that might benefit from a rehabilitation approach are diverse and where the boundaries are drawn may be different in different localities. For example, the kinds of people who are looked after in specialist assertive outreach teams in one locality may be included in specialist rehabilitation services in another. The definition of who is 'suitable' for rehabilitation must therefore take into account these local variations. Agreement on local definitions between all the agencies involved will then form the basis of estimating needs and targeting resources.

In most places, the definitions will cover: (a) 'old long-stay' in-patients (whether still in hospital or resettled in the community); (b) 'new long-stay' in-patients (usually accumulating on acute admission wards, or in the 'revolving door' of brief admission, followed by brief follow-up and frequent readmission); and (c) patients with multiple and long-term needs in the community (who may have significant overlap with the assertive outreach group). Other groups that may be included are those with a dual diagnosis of severe mental illness and substance misuse and people with mental illness and a non-forensic personality disorder. Whatever definitions are used, they should be multidimensional and based on diagnosis, disability and patterns of service use (Powell & Slade, 1996).

Staffing and management

Next, there are questions of staffing and management. Staff in rehabilitation services need an unusual combination of technical skills and human

Box 6.1 Standards for specialist rehabilitation services

1 Shared operational definitions of client groups
- Clear definitions agreed with local agencies, covering 'old long-stay', 'new long-stay' and long-term patients
- Clear definitions agreed with local agencies

2 Staffing and management arrangements
- Dedicated psychiatric consultant medical time (minimum 0.1 sessions/ 30 000 population).
- Dedicated clinical psychology time (minimum 0.2 sessions/100 000 population).
- Identified single manager for specialist teams (or staff) with clearly specified management responsibilities regarding all staff
- Evidence of shared philosophy of care
- Good multidisciplinary team work
- Good communication between the various elements (e.g. in-patient/ community team) *within* specialist service
- Good communication between the various elements (e.g. community team/housing) *between* major statutory agencies

3 Range and quality of in-patient/residential facilities
- Dedicated acute beds
- 24-hour nursed accommodation (transitional and long term)
- Respite beds
- Good-quality individual care planning and review
- Access to appropriate range of psychological and physical treatments
- Access to educational/social/vocational programmes

4 Range of quality of non-hospital residential care
- 24-hour staffed/high-dependency places
- Flexible support for people in their own homes
- Good partnership working between statutory agencies (e.g. community mental health teams) and independent-sector housing providers
- Effective monitoring of individual care planning for residents in independent-sector housing

5 Specialist community teams/dedicated mental health staff
- Coverage 7 days a week
- Out-of-hours access
- Protected case-loads (10–15 cases per worker)
- Integrated social work input
- Appropriate skills mix (including specialists in housing, vocational support, welfare benefits and drug/alcohol misuse
- Integrated medical input
- Care programme approach and care management effectively merged (single paperwork system)
- Pooled budgets (e.g. capacity for 'spot purchasing' at a team level)
- Team-based case management approach (i.e. shared case-loads)
- Access to in-patient beds
- Effective links with primary care teams

continued

Box 6.1 *continued*

6 Training, work and employment opportunities
- Joint planning, commissioning (and funding)
- Clear evidence of vocational component in care planning
- Availability of realistic pre-vocational training
- Vocational guidance, job search and links to employers
- Availability of good-quality sheltered work (social enterprises, etc.)
- Opportunities for supported placements in open employment
- Good links to voluntary work
- Good links to further education

7 User involvement
- Individual peer advocacy services available, specifically targeted to users of 'rehab' services
- Support from within statutory services for development of user involvement (administration, etc.)
- Financial support from statutory services for user involvement initiatives
- User involvement in monitoring service quality at a unit/facility level
- User input into service planning and strategic direction
- Routine consultation on architectural considerations in new projects

8 Range of treatments and interventions (individuals)
- 'Atypical' neuroleptics
- Psychological treatments of known effectiveness (e.g. early-signs monitoring; psychoeducation/self-management techniques; motivational interviewing; individual crisis planning; cognitive–behavioural therapy for psychosis; dialectical behaviour therapy)

9 Range of treatments and interventions (families and carers)
- Expressed emotion-based family interventions
- General family support
- Routine consultation with families and carers during care planning
- Mechanisms for families and carers to comment on service quality

10 Staff training
- Systematic skills audit
- Clear identification of training priorities within a joint training strategy
- Reasonable access to training opportunities
- Examples of joint training initiatives
- Effective mechanisms of clinical supervision for individual cases (including case-load management supervision)

11 Equality issues (age, gender, ethnicity)
- Evidence of attention being paid to these issues in different services (access, representation, monitoring, special programmes, etc.)
- Action plans linked to service monitoring information

12 Use of systematic and targeted audit
- Clear identification of shared audit priorities (e.g. case-mix/targeting; individual care planning; risk assessment and management)
- Evidence that audits of priorities are taking place
- Evidence that interventions based on audit information are being implemented to improve services (closing the audit loop)

(Based on Health Advisory Service, 1999)

qualities. I will discuss therapeutic skills in 'Staff training' (p. 87) but, in human terms, staff need to be able to empathise accurately with users' situation and to be in tune with their priorities. A mixture of ages, backgrounds and experience is important, so that service users can be offered some choice of keyworkers or care coordinators. Some users prefer workers who themselves have had direct experience of receiving mental health services. The advent of the new 'support, time and recovery' (STR) workers may therefore offer important opportunities for expanding the range of staff and skills in rehabilitation teams (Department of Health, 2003a). In terms of general personality, the concept of low expressed emotion (EE) provides a useful framework for identifying and recruiting suitable staff (Ball et al, 1992). The evidence from research on family carers suggests that staff who are able to minimise 'blame attributions' will be most effective. Low-EE staff – like low-EE relatives – also need to have clear and realistic expectations for change. These will be encouraged through good support and supervision.

Regarding the management of rehabilitation teams, as with other specialist teams it is important that there is a single manager with a clear job description and clear authorities regarding operational (general) management responsibilities of staff within the team. The management of community teams has been a consistent area of weakness in mental health services and this has been partly attributed to a lack of clarity regarding the managerial authority of team leaders. There is often a tension between 'professional' and 'operational' management structures and this can lead to a confusion regarding accountabilities. Since rehabilitation teams are, by definition, likely to be multidisciplinary these difficulties need to be addressed. Team leaders should have clear authority over all operational matters (i.e. the day-to-day running of the team, adhering to agreed procedures, local rules and regulations), while professional managers retain responsibility for the maintenance of professional standards. This implies some weakening of traditional professional line-management structures. Staff may therefore have to live with dual accountabilities, with a 'solid line' to general management and a 'dotted line' signifying professional accountability.

Range and quality of hospital beds

Patients receiving care from specialist rehabilitation services will, from time to time, also need access to acute in-patient beds. Traditionally, medical (consultant) cover for these beds has come from the clinician who is responsible for these patients in the community. However, the relatively new crisis resolution/home treatment teams may cut across these arrangements. These teams of mobile community mental health staff, with the back-up of a single consultant, assess individuals in psychiatric crises and provide intensive treatment and care at home. Local services will need to balance the importance of preserving continuity of care with the advantages of being able to call on such specialist acute/crisis resolution services. This same dilemma, of course, arises with other new services, for example early-intervention teams.

To deal with the need for long-term care in a hospital setting (or something very like it) the Department of Health recommends the establishment of specialist long-term residential facilities in the form of 24-hour nursed beds (NHS Executive, 1996). The need for such facilities is also acknowledged in the National Service Framework for Mental Health (Department of Health, 1999: p. 51, para. 4). These units are designed for 'new long-stay' in-patients, who would otherwise have to remain on acute admission wards. Their aim is to combine high levels of professional supervision with a low degree of institutionalisation, in small, domestic-scale environments.

In a review of the evidence, Shepherd (1995) reported that this model of residential care seems to be effective in improving the functioning of up to 40% of those referred sufficient for them to be resettled into less highly supervised accommodation in the community after an average of 2–3 years. Residents generally made more progress regarding their social functioning than matched controls, they showed increased contact with the community and reported higher levels of satisfaction with the residential environment. This greater satisfaction seemed directly related to the increased privacy and choice offered by domestic-scale living arrangements and the more 'normal' atmosphere. For those who are not resettled, the units maintain their functioning more effectively than does remaining in acute beds. Costs are higher than for traditional long-stay wards, but lower than for acute wards.

Despite these encouraging results, such options may not be attractive to all the people they are designed to serve. For some, the advantages of life outside hospital is outweighed by the disadvantages of 'group living' and the stigma of association with others who have severe mental health problems. Specialist residential options such as the 'ward-in-a-house' therefore need to be complemented by a range of ordinary housing options, combined with intensive support from specialised teams, as discussed next.

Non-hospital residential options

Effective care in the community depends on the availability of a good range of high-quality residential accommodation outside of the hospitals (Shepherd & Murray, 2001). The more comprehensive the range of alternatives, the more effectively they can substitute for long-stay in-patient beds. Service users are likely to prefer models of care in which staff are deployed to meet fluctuating levels of need ('floating support'), rather than traditional hostels and group homes where staffing levels are fixed and patients have to move around the system if their needs change. As with 'old long-stay' patients resettled in the community, housing that offers privacy and independence and a minimum of rules and regulations is likely to be most popular with 'new long-stay' patients (Shepherd *et al*, 1996). In practice, a combination of group living and independent living with flexible support is probably needed in each locality. Some people will reject the stigma of traditional hostels and group homes, but without them others will feel lonely and miss the company of group living.

Specialist community teams

As indicated above, there may be considerable overlap between traditional community rehabilitation teams and new assertive outreach services. Choosing whether to establish separate teams or to combine assertive outreach and rehabilitation in a single team therefore needs to take into account local circumstances. In most urban areas, the concentration of people with severe and enduring mental health problems is sufficient to warrant the establishment of specialist teams. However, in rural areas it may be more appropriate to deploy specialist assertive outreach staff within community rehabilitation teams or general community mental health teams (CMHTs). Whatever the local arrangements, it is important to ensure that these workers use effective models of assertive outreach as described in the policy implementation guide (PIG) for assertive outreach (Department of Health, 2001).

Outcome evidence for assertive outreach teams has been well summarised by Mueser *et al* (1998). The most consistent benefits compared with standard aftercare are reduction in the time spent in hospital, improvement in housing stability and increased patient satisfaction with services. There is weaker evidence for the superiority of assertive outreach models regarding reduction in symptoms, improved adherence to medication regimens, reduced substance misuse, and better vocational and social outcomes. To achieve significant improvements in these areas it is necessary to build in more specific and targeted interventions (e.g. motivational interviewing to improve medication adherence; social skills training to enhance social functioning; and access to placement-and-support programmes to improve vocational outcomes).

Work, employment and further educational opportunities

The value of work in hospital-based rehabilitation programmes has long been recognised. However, the range and availability of good-quality work programmes in the community is often very limited. In terms of placing and supporting people in open employment, it now seems clear that 'place-and-train' models such as 'individual placement and support (IPS; Becker & Drake, 1994) are more effective than the traditional 'train-and-place' approaches (Boardman *et al*, 2003). These authors also emphasise the need to integrate clinical and vocational supports. The evidence in favour of the effectiveness of social firms and cooperatives is less strong, although most show some superiority over traditional day care in terms of satisfaction and costs (Grove *et al*, 1997). Most also produce some degree of change in non-vocational outcomes, for example improved self-esteem, wider social networks and less reliance on formal mental health services.

An evidence-based approach to the provision of work and employment opportunities for people with severe and enduring mental health problems should therefore aim to provide access to a range of options, with opportunities for individuals to find whatever suits them best and the chance to move on or stay according to individual preference and circumstances. This is how the rest of us manage our work lives and there is no reason that it should be different for people with mental health problems. To achieve this means establishing effective partnerships between a variety of statutory and independent sectors and having access to good care coordination 'on the ground' (hence the importance of vocational specialists in every community team). They should also link to voluntary work, further education, training and mainstream community social and leisure opportunities.

User involvement

The desire to involve service users (and their carers) more fully in the process of service planning and delivery is now central to Department of Health policy (Department of Health, 2003*b*). This can be particularly difficult in rehabilitation services, where users may need help to express their views or where their wishes seem unrealistic – even self-defeating. There is therefore a need to develop and support advocacy models ('peer' or 'citizen') to ensure that those who are most disabled are given the opportunity to have their voices heard. User involvement should also be sought in the direct monitoring of quality of services at the unit or facility level (e.g. the ward, day centre or residential home). This may be achieved, for example, through user councils or local forums, although these too may require considerable support to be sustained. User involvement is now almost a cliché in mental health services, but involving service users is not just important in terms of civil rights and humanitarian objectives; it is also crucial if we are to successfully engage and maintain contact with those who are at greatest risk if they drop out of services.

Treatments and interventions for service users

The process of rehabilitation has always included the application of treatment interventions, both physical and psychosocial. In recent years, we have seen the accumulation of considerable evidence in favour of the effectiveness of a range of psychosocial interventions for people with severe and enduring mental health problems. Meta-analytic reviews suggest that the strongest evidence exists in relation to EE-based family interventions and cognitive–behavioural therapy for psychosis (Pilling *et al*, 2002*a*,*b*). Evidence for the effectiveness of social skills training and cognitive remediation is weaker, mainly because of problems in successfully generalising treatment effects. Motivational interviewing may also be helpful in improving medication compliance (Kemp *et al*, 1996). Psychoeducational approaches together with early-signs monitoring may be useful in planning and managing symptomatic relapse more effectively (Birchwood & Tarrier, 1992). Of course, the shortage of staff trained to deliver these interventions is a considerable problem (see 'Staff training' below), but the advent of Thorn nurses (http://www.thorn-initiative.org. uk/), combined with the wider availability of good-quality commercial training courses, is beginning to narrow this gap.

Interventions involving families and carers

As indicated above, the evidence for the effectiveness of EE-based family interventions in preventing – or at least postponing – relapse in schizophrenia is very strong. This is particularly true when used in combination with medication and other psychosocial interventions. Given the central role played by family carers in looking after people with severe and enduring mental health problems in the community, all rehabilitation services should have a strong family orientation, involving families as genuine 'partners in care'.

Staff training

Effective staff training is obviously key to effective services. There needs to be a strategic approach to training, with systematic audits of staff skills to identify training priorities and develop programmes to address training needs. The report *Pulling Together* (Sainsbury Centre for Mental Health, 1997) provides a useful list of core competencies for specialist staff working with people with severe mental illness. These include:

- assessment skills – the ability to develop a treatment and care plan based on thorough and comprehensive assessment of the client, family and social system and a psychosocial formulation of the patient's problems;
- treatment and care management skills – knowledge and skills in the provision of assertive outreach and long-term continuing care, awareness of user perspectives;
- collaborative working – the ability to work effectively as a member of a multidisciplinary team, with carers and other agencies;
- management and administration – knowledge of current systems of care, understanding of the roles of various disciplines and the contribution of other agencies.

Training interventions need to be multifaceted and to operate at a number of different levels – individual, practitioner, team and service system. There must also be opportunities to use the skills in practice.

It is of little value to teach staff new skills if they are to be returned to a setting that does not support their use. Services must therefore change at a number of different levels simultaneously for training to have a significant impact and to avoid rapid loss of newly acquired skills because of lack of opportunities to practise.

Sensitivity to special needs

Rehabilitation services are often required to deal with a range of 'special needs' groups (e.g. women, younger people, individuals from Black or minority ethnic groups). They must therefore monitor access and levels of engagement for these groups and use this information to develop specific plans of action, linked to service developments. In relation to people from Black and minority ethnic groups, these are helpfully described in the publication *Inside Outside* (National Institute for Mental Health in England, 2003). The principles of working with excluded minorities – the need to 'reach out' and make contact through community groups, to understand cultural attitudes and norms regarding the expression and management of mental health difficulties, and to offer culturally sensitive interventions (e.g. Khoranic counselling) – are, of course, just as relevant when working with 'mainstream' cultural groups. Specific recruitment policies to target staff from minority groups are also important.

Audit

Finally, we come to the question of audit. Multidisciplinary peer audit is central to clinical governance and attempts to drive up standards and quality. Rehabilitation services therefore need to develop a systematic programme of audit activities (e.g. case-mix issues for teams, quality of individual care planning, quality of care in non-hospital residential facilities, range and quality of vocational provisions, user/carer involvement and support for families) within a clear framework of local priorities. The information obtained needs to be collated and used to improve local services, closing the audit loop. User and carers should play a central role in these activities, giving their opinions, even helping to collect and interpret the data.

Using mapping information to improve services

The standards discussed in the previous section and outlined in Box 6.1 provide a framework for assessing local rehabilitation services. How can we use this information most effectively to improve services? The traditional approach of organisations such as the former Health Advisory Service has been to develop a system whereby the local services would conduct a standards-based self-assessment of performance, which could be discussed with a visiting team of peer experts (selected from our rehabilitation networks). This team would then either confirm or reject the self-assessment, helping with a reformulation of the problem if necessary. The same team would also assist with prioritisation and the formulation of an action plan to remedy deficits. Thus, self-assessment can be a powerful driver for change provided that there is local 'ownership' of the assessment process and it is followed up with the application of real expertise to solve the problems identified.

However, self-assessment on its own is rarely sufficient. It seldom produces new information, but simply serves to confirm – and further define – problems that are already known. Why have these problems not been dealt with? Clearly, local services lack the expertise, perhaps the confidence, imagination or sometimes simply the time, to take the issues forward. External experts can provide this kind of support, but for the process to be effective the sense of local ownership must be retained. Imposed change is unlikely to be effective and seldom lasts (Iles & Sutherland, 2001). Modern approaches to quality improvement stress the importance of formal and informal 'communities of practice', where peers can get together to review what they do, discuss problems and share solutions. This takes time, some expertise (and resources) to organise.

'Separate' or 'mainstream'?

In the present context of mental health service organisation, it is worth asking whether separate rehabilitation services are worth preserving, or whether rehabilitation concepts should simply be integrated into main-stream provisions. The answer, as before, depends on local circumstances. A separate rehabilitation service clearly provides a focus for the maintenance of a rehabilitation 'philosophy'. It helps preserve the unique blend of staff skills and attitudes mentioned earlier and should ensure that patients with the most complex and enduring problems take priority. On the other hand, the concepts of rehabilitation are applicable way beyond traditional rehabilitation services (e.g. in early-intervention, personality disorder and eating disorder services). Segregated rehabilitation services may therefore impede the spread of these ideas, confining them to narrow, segregated services. Separate services also introduce yet more boundaries in the complicated array of specialist teams that now comprise general adult services. It can be difficult for service users to find their way forwards (and backwards) across these boundaries. In some areas (e.g. in a rural area with no history of mental hospital provision) there may be insufficient numbers of people with very complex long-term problems to justify a separate rehabilitation service. Here it may be more sensible to concentrate on the development of the new National Service Framework services – assertive outreach, crisis resolution/home treatment and early intervention – and try to ensure that they take on board the principles of continuity of care, social management, family involvement and so on.

Rehabilitation and recovery

In conclusion, let us examine the relationship between rehabilitation and the concepts of recovery (Repper & Perkins, 2003) and social inclusion (Social Exclusion Unit, 2004). As indicated already, rehabilitation provides a profoundly 'social' model for psychiatry. It reminds us that for many service users their contact with mental health services is much more like a journey than an episode of care. In addition, it places the process of helping people function in social roles (social inclusion) at the heart of reintegration and therefore of long-term outcomes. In all these respects, rehabilitation is very like current recovery models.

Recovery is also not about cure (Roberts & Wolfson, 2004): it is about *hope*, about building a life, trying to find some meaning in the chaos and distress of serious mental illness. This will be a unique and personal journey. Mental health professionals can assist with this journey, although more often – wittingly or unwittingly – they may actually interfere with it. Other individuals – friends, family, neighbours – may be just as important, and other agencies – housing, employment, education – may have just as profound an influence on long-term outcomes as any intervention delivered by mental health services. However, the individual must be 'in charge' of their own recovery, they must set the goals and (mostly) set the pace. This represents a profound challenge for mental health professionals – and policy makers. Are we really ready to serve our clients, to be 'on tap' not 'on top'? It is radically different to think of service users being helped to choose and shape their own treatment and management plans, rather than have well-meaning professionals do it for them. As Rachel Perkins has put it,

'Any services, or treatments, or interventions, or supports must be judged in these terms – how much do they allow us to lead the lives we wish to lead?' (Repper & Perkins, 2003: p. 27).

Perhaps this is the greatest challenge of the recovery model.

Conclusions

The concept of rehabilitation still contains some profoundly important ideas that are highly relevant to modern practice. The importance of a long-term orientation to care – 'journeys' as opposed to 'episodes' – a social model based on individual needs, where reintegration into key social roles is seen as the primary vehicle for rebuilding identity, improving status and facilitating positive long-term outcomes: these are its key elements. Evidence-based reviews of local rehabilitation services can be useful to identify gaps and help improve quality, although the information obtained from self-assessments needs to be combined with the advice of expert peer reviewers to provide development plans that are locally owned. So, how can we keep these important ideas alive in a service environment in which rehabilitation may seem like an outmoded concept? Paradoxically, the answer may lie not in not trying to keep separate rehabilitation services alive. It may be better to incorporate modern ideas of recovery, which add the dimension of personal meaning and direction, into traditional rehabilitation services. Maybe 'rehabilitation' is indeed dead; but if it is, combined 'rehabilitation and recovery' will give an exciting new direction in which to support and develop these fundamentally important ideas.

References

Ball, R. A., Moore, E. & Kuipers, L. (1992) Expressed emotion in community care staff. A comparison of patient outcomes in a nine month follow-up of two hostels. *Social Psychiatry and Psychiatric Epidemiology*, **27**, 35–39.

Becker, D. R. & Drake, R. E. (1994) Individual placement and support: a community mental health centre approach to vocational rehabilitation. *Community Mental Health Journal*, **30**, 193–206.

Bennett, D. H. (1978) Social forms of psychiatric treatment. In *Schizophrenia: Towards a New Synthesis* (ed. J. K. Wing). London: Academic Press.

Birchwood, M. & Tarrier, N. (1992) *Innovations in the Psychological Management of Schizophrenia*. Chichester: John Wiley & Sons.

Boardman, J., Grove, B., Perkins, R., *et al* (2003) Work and employment for people with psychiatric disabilities. *British Journal of Psychiatry*, **182**, 467–468.

Department of Health (1999) *National Service Framework for Mental Health: Modern Standards and Service Models*. London: Department of Health.

Department of Health (2001) *The Mental Health Policy Implementation Guide*. London: Department of Health.

Department of Health (2003a) *Support, Time and Recovery (STR) Workers*. London: Department of Health.

Department of Health (2003b) *Choice, Responsiveness and Equity in the NHS and Social Care: A National Consultation*. London: Department of Health.

Grove, R., Freudenberg, M., Harding, A., *et al* (1997) *The Social Firm Handbook: New Directions in the Employment, Rehabilitation and Integration of People with Mental Health Problems*. Brighton: Pavilion Publishing.

Health Advisory Service (1999) *Avon and West Wiltshire Mental Health Trust: Review of Specialist Mental Health Rehabilitation Services*. London: HAS.

Iles, V. & Sutherland, K. (2001) *Organisational Change: A Review for Health Care Managers, Professionals and Researchers*. London: NCCSDO London School of Hygiene and Tropical Medicine.

Kemp, R., Hayward, P., Applewhaite, G., *et al* (1996) Compliance therapy in psychotic patients: a randomised controlled trial. *BMJ*, **312**, 345–349.

Mueser, K. T., Bond, G. R., Drake, R. E., *et al* (1998) Models of community care for severe mental illness: a review of research on case management. *Schizophrenia Bulletin*, **24**, 37–74.

National Institute for Mental Health in England (2003) *Inside Outside: Improving Mental Health Services for Black and Minority Ethnic Communities*. London: NIMHE.

NHS Executive (1996) *24-Hour Nursed Care for People with Severe and Enduring Mental Illness*. Leeds: NHS Executive.

Pilling, S., Bebbington, P., Kuipers, E., *et al* (2002a) Psychological treatments in schizophrenia. I: Meta-analysis of family intervention and cognitive behaviour therapy, *Psychological Medicine*, **32**, 763–782.

Pilling, S., Bebbington, P., Kuipers, E., (2002b) Psychological treatments in schizophrenia II. Meta-analysis of social skills training and cognitive remediation, *Psychological Medicine*, **32**, 783 – 791.

Powell, R. & Slade, M. (1996) Defining severe mental illness. In *Commissioning Mental Health Services* (eds G. Thornicroft and G. Strathdee). London: TSO (The Stationery Office).

Repper, J. & Perkins, R. (2003) *Social Inclusion and Recovery*. Ballière Tindall: London.

Roberts, G. & Wolfson, P. (2004) The rediscovery of recovery: open to all. *Advances in Psychiatric Treatment*, **10**, 37–48.

Sainsbury Centre for Mental Health (1997) *Pulling Together: The Future Roles and Training of Mental Health Staff*. London: Sainsbury Centre for Mental Health.

Shepherd, G. (1995) The 'ward-in-a-house: residential care for the severely disabled. *Journal of Mental Health*, **31**, 53–69.

Shepherd, G. & Murray, A. (2001) Residential care. In *Textbook of Community Psychiatry* (eds G. Thornicroft & G. Szmukler). Oxford: Oxford University Press.

Shepherd, G., Muijen, M., Dean, R., *et al* (1996) Residential care in hospital and in the community: quality of care and quality of life. *British Journal of Psychiatry*, **168**, 448–456.

Social Exclusion Unit (2004) *Mental Health and Social Exclusion. Social Exclusion Unit Report*. London: Office of the Deputy Prime Minister.

CHAPTER 7

Understanding madness

Glenn Roberts

'The physician knows madness in one way; he collects the symptoms of it, the causes and cure; but the madman in his way knows it far better. The terror and the glory of the illusion, which after all, are the madness itself, are open only to the madman or to some sympathetic spirit as prone to madness as he is.'

Santayana (1925)

'Towards the end of an acute episode of schizophrenia, service users should be offered help to better understand the period of illness, and given the opportunity to write their account in their notes.'

National Institute for Clinical Excellence (2002: p. 12)

From our first encounter with madness we are confronted with the problem of understanding and meaning. The above quotations mark out our boundaries. They suggest the possibility of finding straightforward patterns of understanding alongside the inevitability of mystery. They also suggest that sympathetically listening to the stories of those who experience madness may provide more meaningful guidance to the inner world than can statisticians and diagnosticians. There are many obstacles too, the greatest of which is in believing that in madness we have reached the limits of understanding, that by definition it is impossible to understand, and therefore we do not even try to make sense of psychosis.

Madness and meaninglessness have long been companion concepts, an association that may powerfully contribute to stigma, alienation and discrimination. As Jaspers (1963, p. 310) noted, 'Everything understandable has a constituent potentiality of worth. In contrast we do not value the un-understandable'. Those suffering from persisting psychotic states, often regarded as some of the least understandable, have also been some of the least valued. Emily Dickinson's (1924) observation that 'Much madness is divinest sense to a discerning eye' at first appears to simply fly in the face of all this, and is readily dismissed as the romantic notions of a mad poet, for she was both, but seldom at the same time. Nowadays she may be more politely regarded as an expert by experience.

This chapter is about exploring the role of understanding madness in recovery-oriented rehabilitation. It considers the potential for understanding to be potently antipsychotic, and explores some of what it takes to develop a 'discerning eye'. I hope to demonstrate that there are many possible interrelationships between meaning and madness. Finding specific and concrete meanings may be of direct therapeutic significance such that understanding what the person is talking about can be taken as an invitation to look for non-psychotic ways of engaging with these meanings. Understanding metaphoric or thematic associations similarly offers a means of seeing through the madness and engaging with the person struggling with their life and experience. Gaining some understanding of the purpose and significance of an individual's elaboration of their psychosis may shed light on how, and sometimes why, they have reconstructed their 'perspectival world' (Cox & Theilgaard, 1987) within madness. Each of these may in turn serve to highlight some of the complex implications in recovery from psychosis and the significance of leaving behind delusional and hallucinatory constructions.

Terms of engagement

The pejorative connotations of 'madness' have been overturned in recent years by service users (e.g. Curtis *et al*, 2000) and non-medical authors (e.g. Read *et al*, 2004), who have preferred 'madness' over more technical diagnostic terms such as bipolar disorder or schizophrenia. These resonate with the views of Seymour Krim, who, in his exotically titled autobiography *Views of a Nearsighted Cannoneer* (in Kaplan, 1964), expressed a clear preference for the term, choosing '"madness" for its human sound, over the legalistic, "insanity", or the antiseptically cold and clinical "psychosis"'. In this chapter I have used the terms madness and psychosis interchangeably, with the aim of linking clinical and societal discourse.

The purpose of understanding

We shall be mostly looking to understand current psychotic symptoms in the context of people's life experience and there is a perennial risk that this backwards search for meanings can become endless, and a problem in its own right. Any gardener knows that digging up the roots is not a good way to promote growth. Within rehabilitation the purpose of understanding is not in seeking to 'crack the code', but always in the service of supporting the individual's journey in recovery and getting on with life. However, like everywhere in psychiatry, rehabilitation practice is dependent on forming relationships in which there is hope and trust, and it may be hard if not impossible to develop a meaningful relationship with someone you cannot understand. The search for meaning and understanding is fundamentally a search for relationship and relatedness, a means of de-alienation and a bridge to reintegration. It is not a question of trying to understand everything so much as trying to understand something, for a little understanding goes a long way. It can be like a Rosetta Stone, offering some translatable meanings which support confidence in meaningfulness rather than assumptions of meaninglessness. In this sense the search for understanding is powerfully antipsychotic, and a significant contribution to recovery-based rehabilitation.

Where have all the meanings gone?

At present the overall impression of clinical services is that they give little emphasis to understanding madness in terms of people's life experience. The recovery and service user movements (see Roberts & Wolfson, Chapter 2, and Perkins, Chapter 8, this volume) have documented a strong interest from people who want to understand their experiences in terms of social and cultural contexts, and as Thomas & Bracken (2004) have noted, 'many of them find biomedical interpretations limited – at best unhelpful, and at worst harmful'. Other obstacles to understanding include the progressive de-emphasising of case history and personal stories (Hauerwas, 1993) and quantitatively driven models of evidence-based medicine (Watson, 2005). The sort of trust that supports understanding is hard won and it is common for patients to withhold descriptions of their inner life out of fear, based on experience, that disclosure will result in pressure to take additional medication or accept admission to hospital. The problem is compounded by patterns of professional training that fail to support in-depth relationships between clinicians and patients (Conran, 1999). From this critical perspective traditional psychiatry is seen as inhospitable to understanding and an impediment to recovery (Thomas & Bracken, 2004).

It may not always have been like this. At the inception of the schizophrenia concept, and based on an unusually close relationship with his patients, we find Bleuler (1951) observing that:

'At first all this may appear sheer nonsense, [but] on closer scrutiny we find understandable connections in every one of these cases ... the delusions of the paranoiac form a logical structure with only a few false premises and inferences in its foundation, or amongst its building stones; the delusions of the schizophrenic are not as systematic, yet they are not the chance heap of unruly chaos which they seem on superficial observation' (p. 403).

Jung (1914), working alongside Bleuler, also saw continuity with ordinary mental life as well as discontinuity:

'when we penetrate into the human secrets of our patients, the madness discloses the system upon which it is based, and we recognise insanity to be simply an unusual reaction to emotional problems which are in no wise foreign to ourselves'.

In searching for the boundaries between the possibility and limits of understanding, these 'few false premises' and the origins of these 'unusual reactions' to ordinary problems must be accounted for. But if there was once a more balanced view of understanding and incomprehension, it begs the question 'Where did all the meanings go?'

Kathleen Jones (2004), like many others, has attributed this to the uncoupling of psychotherapeutic approaches from mainstream psychiatry from the 1950s onwards, and with it the splitting off of clinical approaches based on narrative, context and personal meaning, from those focused on biological dysfunctions and drug treatments. Ciompi (1989) has described this as a 'disastrous splitting' into either biological or psychosocial reductionism, often caricatured as the difference between mindlessness and brainlessness.

There are signs that bridges are at last being built across this historical divide. In Murray's (2004) authoritative review of recent advances in understanding psychosis (Box 7.1) we can see a simultaneous awareness of dysregulation of naturally occurring chemicals in the brain in a person

---

Box 7.1 Recent advances in understanding psychosis

- *Genetics*   Identification of specific 'susceptibility genes'
- *Neurodevelopmental models*   These have limited application and 60% of people with psychosis show no early dysfunction, emphasising that there are many pathways to psychosis
- *Environmental factors*   Highly significant factors include: drug misuse, urbanicity, social isolation and being of African–Caribbean descent
- *Understanding symptoms – process*   Single-photon emission computed tomography has demonstrated that 'inner speech' is processed by systems usually involved in external speech, leading to misattribution. In acute psychosis, dysregulation of mesolimbic dopamine transmission leads to the excessive assignment of salience to external and internal stimuli, and the making of aberrant or unusual meaningful connections
- *Understanding symptoms - contents*   Hallucinatory voices are linked to inner speech, so that what the person is saying through their symptoms may be meaningfully related to significant life experiences
- *Relief from acute symptoms*   This may depend on the attenuation of the underlying dopaminergic drive achieved with medication, which then reduces abnormal attribution of salience
- *Effective treatment for psychosis*   This is recognised to depend on far more than treatment of symptoms: it needs to embrace the person in their social and biographical context
- *Recovery from psychosis*   Recovery is seen to be a complex process, including recognition that delusions may have arisen as convincing explanations of altered experience which are subsequently remembered as real. Such beliefs can be integrated into persisting explanatory systems of personal belief, and come to constitute a world view that may be highly resistant to change

who lives within a social and societal context and who struggles between adaptation to disorder and hope of recovery, is hampered by isolation, stigma and discrimination, and mobilises whatever human resources are available with which to make sense of such a predicament.

Understanding is clearly a concept with many usages. In this chapter we are particularly concerned with seeking to understand the individual's psychotic experiences in the context of their accounts of their lives. To do this we first need to be clear concerning what we mean by 'understanding'.

The difference between explaining and understanding

Jaspers (1913) began his exploration of meaningful connections between psychosis and life history with the critical distinction between understanding (*verstehen*) and causal explanation (*erklaren*). This is also one of the key principles guiding his monumental *General Psychopathology*, which remains one of the foundations of contemporary psychiatric thought and practice (Sims, 1988; Fulford *et al*, 2003).

Jaspers was interested in inner experience and what might be the natural boundaries of different mental phenomena. He sought to describe them without recourse to theory or interpretation, and thereby established an atheoretical descriptive psychopathology on the basis of phenomenology.

For Jaspers, understanding proceeds by way of empathy, and the process of establishing meaningful connections is based on an intuitive identification with the experience of another, in effect 'I see what you mean'. This contrasts with explaining as a process of building causal theory on the findings of experimentation and measurement. Many of the disputes and difficulties in understanding madness have arisen from a failure to adequately grasp the distinction between understanding meaningful connections and explaining causes.

For example, it is common to find sexual and other abuse in the early histories of people presenting with psychosis as adults. This has understandably led to the strongly held, but disputed, view that psychosis has traumatic origins. The only large prospective study to date (Spataro *et al*, 2004) to follow up children who have been unequivocally subject to penetrative sexual abuse in a large community sample (500 000) found no significant association between childhood sexual abuse (at an average age of 9.4 years) and subsequent psychosis (at average age 27.1 years). Like any such experimental finding, the evidence is both valued and disputed, and awaits attempts at replication to achieve verification. Such causal explanation is in search of general rules and is amenable to objective and standardised evaluation, supported by rigorous analysis and replication.

The process of understanding meaningful connections is different and dependent on empathy rather than experimentation. A young man hears a voice threatening 'I'm going to desecrate your daughter's grave'. Prior to a recurrence of his psychotic illness he heard indirectly that his daughter, living far away with his estranged wife, had died some months earlier and he had missed the funeral. He did not even know where she was buried. There seemed a meaningful connection between his life experience and his current symptoms. We could understand that he felt guilty and bereaved, that this news of loss had rekindled a deep sense of failure and loneliness, that his self-critical and self-punishing feelings had some relationship with the threatening voice – but how could this ever be proven? What kind of experimental method comparing people who had experienced either bereavement or psychosis would give sound evidence of a causal connection? Understanding these meaningful connections was very helpful in his care and treatment and unlocked many other meanings besides, but they clearly did not explain why he was presenting with a psychotic illness.

How and where might we look for understanding in madness?

If understanding is desirable but difficult, it may be useful to be reminded that 'understanding proceeds primarily by way of story' (Romanshyn, in Cox & Theilgaard, 1987). To be clinically useful we need a simple method which is readily accessible to patients and staff alike; it is always possible to make it more complex later (see Davidson, 2003). If we are seeking to build meaningful connections we can begin by asking what we are trying to connect and how. The only essential prerequisite for developing understanding is a trusting relationship. This is the means through which it becomes possible to gain a deepening sense of what is happening to someone in their life and their mind and what may be the links between the two. Moreover, this is a circular and self-reinforcing process, for developing a sense of understanding with someone significantly supports a deepening relationship with them. Such understanding can be developed in a sit-down process of sessional enquiry, but is more likely if the clinician and the team talk together frequently, compare notes and keep the following questions alive in all their interactions:

- What is your inner world like? – Build up a detailed description of symptoms, unusual beliefs and altered experience of reality
- What has your life been like? – Construct a comprehensive biographical picture with the patient and from all available sources
- How can one be understood in the context of the other? – A collaborative enquiry into meaningful connections.

These rather simple questions are easily forgotten in the confusing and apparent bizarreness of psychosis, but can act as guiding principles that need to be kept constantly in mind.

The results of searching for meaning and understanding emerge at many different levels, and each carries different implications for care and treatment. I have found it useful to map them out as follows:

- understanding the meaning *of* madness: how does it arise?
- understanding meaning *in* madness: the search for specific, metaphorical and thematic associations
- understanding meaning *through* madness: existential considerations.

What follows are some examples derived from living with these questions over time in rehabilitation settings and considering people's responses under these three categories of meaning. Like Jaspers, I shall aspire to be 'atheoretical' and be guided by empathic affirmation (Davidson, 2003), but this is of course nonsense, as every word or phrase we use carries the semantic detritus of its origins and the numerous discarded theories it has been acquainted with. There are no theory-free facts or observations. But we can at least seek to avoid refracting observations through whole complex interpretive theories which, for example, colour and risk prejudicing our perspectives as Kleinian, Jungian or even the medical model.

Understanding the meaning of madness – how does it arise?

Madness does not arrive fully formed, although our current tendency to first meet people in crisis, after lengthy periods of untreated psychosis, gives exactly that impression. The ambition to reduce the duration of untreated psychosis and work progressively closer to onset ('up-stream'), has re-emphasised that early psychosis presents as subtle shifts of gestalt perception, affect and associated behavioural changes, and that these fluctuating or progressive changes often appear months, and sometimes years, before unequivocal psychotic symptoms emerge (Box 7.2; Power *et al*, Chapter 9, this volume). The inception of this psychotic process has not yet been convincingly explained as a meaningful reaction to adverse life experiences, like grief following bereavement, in that there are no psychosocial conditions that would reliably predict the occurrence of madness in the majority of those who develop it. The onset of psychosis appears much more as a manifestation of a psychophysiological process arising from a toxic interaction between stressful life circumstances and still-mysterious pre-psychotic vulnerabilities, the product of which exceeds a critical threshold for inception. This stress–vulnerability model continues to be hotly debated (Read *et al*, 2004), but underpins most current rehabilitative approaches.

There is then a temporal succession from these rather non-specific early signs, which overlap with normal adolescence, to the prodromal state of emerging psychosis, which in turn is followed by the first delusions and hallucinations and, if unchecked, various more complex states of elaboration or deterioration. The development of a psychotic disorder often

Box 7.2 Early signs of psychosis

- Withdrawal from activities and social contacts
- Irrational, angry or fearful responses to friends
- Sleep disturbance
- Deterioration in studies or work
- Inappropriate use of language – words do not make sense
- Sudden excesses, such as extreme religiousness, extreme activity
- Deterioration in personal hygiene
- Difficulty controlling thoughts, difficulty concentrating
- Hearing voices or sounds others do not hear
- Seeing people or things others do not see
- A constant feeling of being watched
- Inability to turn off the imagination, delusions, bizarre ideas
- Mood swings
- Increasing anxiety
- Bodily symptoms: weakness, pains, odd inexplicable sensations

(British Columbia Schizophrenia Society, 2003. Adapted with permission.)

goes through discernible steps and stages, and the characteristic symptoms develop gradually over time, sometimes many years, as secondary features based on these primary alterations. Some of the most familiar features of madness – delusions and hallucinations – can therefore be understood as coping mechanisms, acts of creative intelligence, whereby an individual defuses the occult potential of these initial disturbing and disruptive experiences, through the attribution and elaboration of meaning (Roberts, 1999). The meanings appropriated in the process of a developing psychosis arise from the memory and imagination of the individual and, although the underlying psychotic process may not be amenable to understanding, the content of these subsequent symptoms may be.

Understanding meaning in madness: every symptom tells a story

The style of personal, biographical and phenomenological studies that supports an exploration of meaning and understanding has been out of favour in scientific psychiatry for some time. However, much of the growing volume of user-led research is more personal, narrative-based work, which upholds the significance of what is specific, individual and unique rather than boiling everything down to meaningless generalisations (Strauss, 1994; Leibrich, 1999).

The clinician seeking understanding may require a different approach from 'taking a history' in order to 'make a diagnosis'. It is a matter of gaining sufficient trust to be welcomed in and shown around the person's subjective world. This may be helped by adopting a posture of curious uncertainty and avoiding 'beating the drums of logic' (Huszonek, 1987). It may help to freely express your confusion or uncertainty and to ask the person to help you make (their) sense. It is also important to remain aware that you are a guest within this inner world, and know how to avoid overstaying your welcome.

Specific connections: truth in non-sense

Sartre criticised psychiatry for being 'too quickly satisfied when it throws light on the general structures of delusions and does not seek to comprehend the individual, concrete content of the psychosis' (cited in Sims, 1988). This is an attitude perhaps typified by the depiction of delusions as 'empty speech acts, whose informational content refers to neither world nor self' (Berrios, 1991). And yet if we look, it is sometimes possible to find unequivocal personal and biographical associations. Kaffman's study (1984) of 34 families in which at least one member had developed a delusional system concluded that there was always a basis in historical reality for the contents and that this may support the incorrigibility of these 'false beliefs', for in a transformed and distorted way the individual is telling some truth about their lives (see Boxes 7.3 and 7.4 for examples).

Working both to understand the life story and its relationship with delusional phenomena then becomes the means of connecting with the person within the psychosis:

'the crux of therapy becomes the task of empathising with the schizophrenic's perspective and attempting to understand its essential plausibility and validity ... the therapist in searching for kernels of truth is better able to construct an empathic appreciation of the patient's experience than by focusing on what appears distorted and unrealistic' (Josephs & Josephs, 1986).

Box 7.3 A tale of a pig

A late-middle-aged man had spent 20 years in the back wards of a hospital and continued to be troubled by a voice that said 'He buggered a pig'. It said other derogatory and critical remarks, but mostly repeated this offensive accusation. It did not seem to have occurred to anyone to wonder whether this was true. On being asked more details he clearly recognised the voice as that of his old headmaster. With his permission my colleagues and I were able to track down this elderly gent, who remembered our patient and that there had indeed been an embarrassing incident with a pig on the school farm. It had resulted in punishment, but ever after the boy had been taunted by the other children and regarded with suspicion by the staff. It was possible to gently introduce this into conversation, and although the experiences persisted, there was a greater sense of compassion for his life experience, opening a greater sense of connection and relationship.

Box 7.4   Sand for brains

Billy, a young man with psychosis, described his life as including successive educational failures and shaming. Throughout his childhood he had been repeatedly told that he 'had no brains', and at some stage he had decided that they had been replaced by sand. He said that he could hear it when he moved his head. When Billy demonstrated this, the interviewer also heard a grating swishing noise, but attributed it to osteoarthritis in the cervical spine rather than sand in his head.

In these two examples, discovering what appeared to be a factual basis, or kernel of truth, for these 'auditory hallucinations' and 'delusional beliefs' by following methods similar to those of Romme & Escher (2000) did not change them, or at least not quickly, but it did create a climate of understanding for these isolated men who continued to be taunted and haunted by their past and gave staff caring for them something more tangible and meaningful to work with. Recovering a biographical perspective reinstated an awareness of the person of the patient and fostered respect.

The search for understanding is not always about trying to make sense of something that is initially obscure. Sometimes complex but specific meanings are concealed behind the obvious. It is not uncommon in madness for there to be meanings within meanings – hence the value of maintaining an attitude of curious uncertainty. It is always possible for new information to emerge as long as we have not already prematurely closed the door against it (Box 7.5).

Box 7.5   'I want to change my medication'

This is such a common request that it is taken for granted, but within madness it is always worth asking why. Sometimes there are surprising answers.

Emily explained that she wanted to change her medication 'because I don't want to kill anyone'. After this baffling response Emily was asked how this was related to taking her medication. She replied that she had looked it up. Unfortunately Emily had looked up her medication not in the *BNF* but in an old dictionary in the ward office. At that time she was prescribed Seroquell (quetiapine) but had limited herself to looking up the meaning of -quell. Among other usages the dictionary had informed her that quell came from the old English cwellen – to kill. A discussion of etymology and shifting meanings over time was sufficient to persuade her that her tablets had more to do with the modern usage of quell as to soothe, and she continued with her prescribed medication.

Metaphorical links and purposeful dis-association

Bateson's (1973) definition of delusions as 'unlabeled metaphors' implies that understanding may be found through looking for symbolic or metaphorical associations (Cox & Theilgaard, 1987). This process of reattaching detached meanings requires an imaginative jump, but the sureness of landing is greatly enhanced by making the gap as narrow as possible. The more that is known of a person's life and the intricacies of their delusional systems, the closer the two come together. We may also seek to understand why it is that the labels have come off, how is it that the person cannot easily see the links themselves and what it means that they 'lack insight'. It may be that the labels did not just fall off in some haphazard way: sometimes they appear to have been peeled off for good reasons. For example, a detained patient struggling to get a tune out of the ward piano states that 'they' must have broken his fingers when he was 'in captivity' and complains that as a consequence he can no longer reach the keys – rather than recognising that he is hopelessly out of practice, anxious and distracted, and was still feeling traumatised by his sojourn in the police station prior to admission. This and other examples (Box 7.6) may illustrate that a denial of meaningful connections can itself be meaningful and purposeful.

Box 7.6 Who is Osmicron?

Over a considerable time of building trust, Mary grew more interested and willing to engage in trying to make sense of her unusual experiences. She was persecuted by a magical creature that she called Osmicron, who was a malicious male that taunted her and sought to disrupt her and relationships. From knowing something about her life it appeared potentially meaningful to ask her to compare the characteristics of Osmicron with those of her father. She was able to list both, in adjacent columns on a single sheet of paper. The lists were strikingly similar and raised the obvious possibility that she was 'haunted' by past experience of a traumatic relationship with her father, manifest as Osmicron. Remarkably, she could not see the similarities at all. When her attention was drawn to the parallels that she had recorded in almost the same words, instead of drawing the obvious conclusions she wondered instead whether Osmicron had made her father like that. Furthermore, in response to gentle questioning she could say that despite all her experience, she still longed for her father to love her. Thus, her lack of insight appeared understandable and also purposeful.

These discoveries, tentatively held, created a strong sense of understanding Mary and something of what her life had been about and her continuing needs. Without requiring her to agree with the clinician's view of what her symptoms meant, it became more possible to draw alongside and successfully support her as she worked towards recovery, which was achieved without either medication or agreement concerning diagnosis.

Two-thirds of young people experiencing psychosis do not recognise it for themselves – they have 'impaired insight' and believe that they really are being poisoned, persecuted, brainwashed, etc. This greatly complicates seeking and offering help in an acceptable way. Lack of insight is so common as to almost be the defining feature of madness, and given the strange and altered view of reality that people commonly hold, this not-knowing is quite extraordinary. It is clearly a complex phenomenon and amenable to a host of causal theories (Amador & David, 2004), but to speculate on whether this dis-association, this characteristic 'lack of insight', is an affliction (a disability that is part of 'the illness'), whether it represents some complex attributional bias or whether unconscious psychological defences of denial, splitting and projection are at work is to stray into the domain of causal explanation. However, from an empathic perspective, it is not difficult to see many meaningful connections, and the intractability of some delusions may be less puzzling if their explanatory power is acknowledged. As coping mechanisms they are understandably protected from challenge. Engagement may be assisted by a form of therapeutic collusion, not in offering any false or superficial agreement, but through respecting these belief structures as meaningful and valuable to the person, and seeking to build trust on whatever common ground can be won.

Taken in context, it can be understandable that someone would wish to preserve their delusional perspective in preference to awakening to the reality of their lives, which would include an acceptance of having been mad (Roberts, 2000a). There are many contradictory and paradoxical processes at work in recovery. For some, it is simply a relief when psychotic processes diminish; others appear reluctant to let them go. Unless the complex interweaving of illness and coping are understood, it is easy to mistake them (Davidson & Strauss, 1995) and be similarly confused when planning treatment and making sense of resistance.

Thematic associations: listening to the tune rather than the words

The Vienna group under Berner *et al* (1986) presented a multiaxial classification of delusional states including an axis recording exact contents, and concluded that the specific circumstances in the personal history are frequently of great importance in choice of delusional theme. Moreover, recognition of the meaningfulness of these delusional themes in supportive relationships can correspondingly provide a basis for empathic connection and communication. The link here is more diffuse than any kind of one-to-one decoding. It is more a resonance between psychotic and ordinary life experience that implies a meaningful connection (Box 7.7).

In looking for understanding through specific, metaphoric and thematic associations, our aim is not trying to understand everything so much as to understand something, as a step towards increasing confidence that understanding is possible and more so than is commonly recognised.

Box 7.7 In pursuit of the FBI

'A friend called me when he was having a tough time. He was clearly panicked and said that the FBI has bugged his apartment. He was also worried that if he left, they would follow him. That experience was very real for him. I knew it wouldn't be useful or respectful to tell him not to worry, that it was not really happening. Instead I asked him what we could do together to help him feel less afraid. I shared a story about a fear I'd often had of people reading my mind. I told him that this fear had gotten easier to deal with after remembering someone reading my diary and then being hospitalised. He said that his father had been a judge and that he'd felt like every move he made was being scrutinised. Slowly but surely he sounded sad rather than panicked. We talked about helping each other with old feelings and responses.'

(From Copeland & Mead, 2004: p. 39 with permission)

One problem is in how we set our depth of focus when looking into psychosis. On the one hand, we are familiar with the 'shallow' discipline of diagnosis which gives the same name to very different constellations of experience. On the other, we have the bewilderingly complex and richly kaleidoscopic transformations described in biographies and autobiographies (North, 1987; Jamison, 1995; Nasar, 1998; Bottoms, 2001) and gathered in collections of personal experience (Leibrich, 1999). Both are needed and each serves very different purposes. We need succinct and thin descriptions to do any comparative research in the search for valid generalisations, but if we are unaware of these 'thick' descriptions, we are badly misinformed concerning what madness is like, and the multitude of factors that are significant to different individuals. In practice, many different types of meaningful association coexist (Roberts, 1999) (Box 7.8).

Meaning through madness – existential considerations

Laing's comment that 'the mad things said and done by people with schizophrenia will remain a closed book until we can see them in their existential context' (Laing, 1990: p. 17) finds resonance with Jaspers' view that 'Extreme psychotic states offer a human parable' and that 'in psychotic reality we find an abundance of content representing fundamental problems in philosophy' (Jaspers, 1963: p. 309). They both point towards the significance of some extraordinary shifts of belief and understanding that characterise madness.

This complex and contradictory perspective appears to be supported by a study of 17 individuals with long-standing delusional belief systems, who were found to have less self-rated depression and a greatly enhanced sense of meaning and purpose in life than a group of patients who had recovered

Box 7.8 It is better…

A young man had been detained in hospital for treatment of his schizophrenia; he had a range of hallucinatory experiences and delusional beliefs, and at times was additionally depressed to the point of despair at his predicament in life with an insightful awareness of all he had lost. Clozapine 'worked' in terms of diminishing his hallucinations, but was unacceptably sedating for him and he adamantly refused it. He had become a Christian in a desperate search for faith and freedom, but found only intermittent solace and relief, in the context of persisting symptoms.

His hallucinations included two sets of oppositional voices, the 'little ones' which said nice things, and the 'big ones' which were nasty. One day he absconded from the ward, took a motor bike and drove to the coast, where he removed one of the wheels, tied himself to it, walked to the edge of a small cliff and threw himself into the sea, intending to end his life. To his surprise the still-inflated tyre on the wheel caused it to float and a dog walker raised the alarm, which resulted in his return to the ward. For some weeks he denied that this had been a suicide attempt, but that he had been in some way doing what his voices told him. He said he was disappointed not to have died, but seemed to lack any real feeling and was mildly amused by all the fuss, including the air-sea rescue. He specifically appeared detached from understandable despair and conflict over the limitations of both his faith and our treatment.

Over the next few weeks he was gradually willing to piece together the story of what had happened. He had been feeling more unhappy and trapped on the unit, the disturbance between his voices had grown and it had reached the point where the big ones had told him forcibly that he would harm the little ones, which caused him more distress. From his Bible readings he had found that 'if anyone causes one of these little ones who believe in me to sin, it would be better for him to have a large millstone hung around his neck and to be drowned in the depths of the sea' (Matthew 18:6, New International Version). In his own way he had set off to do exactly that.

His hallucinations appeared to hold for him both hope and despair in conflictual dialogue; he was metaphorically in two minds. His concrete interpretation of Biblical text seemed related to his deep desire to find healing and release through religious observance and simultaneously an ambivalent wish simply to end his life.

from severe psychotic illness and those treating them (Roberts, 1991). This touches on the paradoxical possibility that there are comforts in madness (Sayers, 1989), even if the individual remains exquisitely uncomfortable and finds meaning and purpose at the cost of isolation.

Looking for issues of meaning and purpose accompanying the elaborations of madness may shed light on some aspects that are otherwise perverse and inexplicable. For example, it was hard to understand why a patient in our rehabilitation unit seemed to actively resist almost all favourable experiences that we believed could support his recovery – until the nurse working with him asked 'What are you most afraid of?' We were surprised but enlightened when he replied 'Happiness'. It then became possible to understand much of his 'negativism' as an active resistance to the threat of recovery and all that it implied, including the risk of hope, which had so often in the past been raised only to collapse again. There are clear therapeutic implications in discovering that the otherwise straightforward hope of recovery may be accompanied by profound ambivalence:

'There are days when I wonder if it might not be more humane to leave the schizophrenic patient to his world of unreality, not to make him go through the pain that it takes to become part of humanity. These are the days when the pain

---

Box 7.9   The story of Jimmy 'JC'

Jimmy came for treatment after attempting to walk across a local river and realising something was wrong when he was waist deep. He had been 'ill' for some years but was something of a local tourist attraction because of his flamboyant dress and continuous good mood. He had established a reciprocal and collusive relationship with 'the public' such that people would have their photographs taken with him and he would grant them wishes, 'I was Jimmy the Healer, JC'. Until the incident with the river his only reason for visiting the psychiatry unit was to offer his services in healing patients. But he had frightened himself through acting on the strength of his beliefs, which then seemed false and vulnerable. He accepted regular medication, which cured him of his grandiosity and messianic identifications. Initially, he felt completely lost but gradually he became an appreciated and integrated member of a day centre and was able to re-establish relationships with his children which had been lost for many years. He sometimes looks back on his madness with nostalgia: 'They were happy times, but I was ill, I was like a Martian, somebody nobody had seen before who had come back to Earth'. And despite having lived very poorly he spoke of being in charge of his own world: 'I could do what I liked … I used to be Jimmy the boring, then I became Jimmy the saviour. I used to be an ordinary person, them I became a super-person'.

Jimmy managed a successful re-entry into a shared and social world, one in which he acknowledged the benefits of medication, which he is now afraid not to take lest he 'cross over and go back again'. He fears that he would lose contact with his children again: 'they didn't speak to me for years, I used to embarrass them … the medication brings me back to the real world, I'm stable now, the kids say "dad is better"'. His pattern of recovery also contains and retains something of his previous life, in that other members of the resource centre affectionately refer to him as 'JC' after he had signed the attendance register as Jimmy 'JC'.

The apostrophes that he is now able to put around JC appear to represent the integration of his two stories and the fact that he has achieved a warm acceptance within a community with both. This appears to have helped him achieve the transition into sanity without shame or humiliation concerning his previous beliefs and behaviour, and with a balanced acknowledgement of the continuing tension between the losses and gains implied in his symptomatic and personal recovery.

is so great, I think I might prefer the craziness until I remember the immobilising terror and the distance and isolation that keep the world so far away and out of focus. It is not an easily resolved dilemma' (Anonymous, 1986).

A critical issue may be to find satisfactory answers to the question of what else the patient has in life apart from his madness (Box 7.9). This goes to the heartland of recovery-oriented rehabilitation.

Conclusions

Greg Bottoms' distressing and confusing experience of coping with his brother's psychosis led him to conclude that 'with sympathy the early stages of schizophrenia are a massive burden; without sympathy and understanding, without love and care even in the face of the strangest behaviours, schizophrenia is a wrecking ball' (Bottoms, 2001).

As psychiatrists, we face limitations both in our discipline and in ourselves. In a complementary pair of cautionary notes we find Kleinman (1988) worrying that modern medicine (not just psychiatry) unintentionally 'does just about everything to drive the practitioner's attention away from the experience of illness' and Fulford *et al* (2003: p. 30) warning against jumping to the conclusion that 'our incomprehension is a product of another's incomprehensibility'.

There are many dimensions to understanding, including understanding that someone has an illness. This chapter has particularly emphasised the possibility and benefit of recontextualising symptoms within the life experiences of the person as a more secure foundation for making and sustaining therapeutic relationships. I began with Jaspers' observations that we give little value to that which we cannot understand, and have explored a number of ways by which understanding in some measure can restore a sense of value and significance. There is much to support the development of narrative skills – story making and breaking, listening and telling, sharing and critically evaluating – as basic tools within recovery-based practice.

The various experiences of madness that commonly bring people to rehabilitation services are still regarded by some as inherently meaningless and un-understandable. In this and so many other ways, madness is about detachment and alienation; it follows that the mad will cease to be so when they find the means to re-associate themselves with the realities of their past and present lives, which may include the painful awareness of having been mad. I have suggested that in this sense the experience of understanding can be potently antipsychotic for both patients and staff.

I have attempted to convincingly illustrate meaningful connections, specifically, metaphorically, thematically and existentially, between the symptoms of psychosis and the life experience of the individual. These are not proven links so much as highly suggestive associations, and in using a method that relies on our empathy and imagination there is a need to hold our findings tentatively and with caution. We have seen that understanding madness is more like the resolution of a koan than the cracking of a riddle. Comprehension emerges although mystery remains. But we will surely find our patients less incomprehensible if we actively look for meaning and are better trained in the possibilities of understanding.

The clinician looking for meaningful connections may not find the patient a ready customer for these discoveries and may have to hold them in trust, sometimes for long periods. But a team approach can be built up around seeking understanding and valuing meaningful connection, whether or not these discoveries find immediate application with the individual. A clinical climate of meaningfulness will be very different from a climate of meaninglessness.

Elizabeth Baxter, a psychiatrist who survived a severe psychosis and went on to win an award for helping people with schizophrenia reintegrate into their communities, speaks for many in her reported observation that 'one crucial reason people with serious mental illnesses recover is because they find someone who believes in them and their recovery' (Kupersanin, 2002). This key process, of seeing through the madness to the person struggling with their altered experience of reality, will be powerfully supported by developing skills and confidence in understanding. It may be hard to imagine an element in our training that values understanding the dynamics of story making and breaking and creative speculation over meaning as much as power calculations underpinning statistical confidence. However, such approaches offer complementary and interweaving dimensions to the more traditional clinical (medical) disciplines which are of particular relevance to the practice of recovery-based rehabilitation (Roberts, 2000b).

A note on confidentiality

Andrew Solomon (2002: p. 11), in setting out his method for writing a richly evocative book on the experience of depression, writes that he asked his patients to allow him to use their actual names 'because real names lend authority to real stories'. He goes on to state that if one is aiming to remove the burden of stigma from mental illness, it is important not to play to that stigma by hiding the identities of those affected. His logic and aspirations are shared by this chapter, but at present the stigma and complex social implications associated with madness are much greater than with depression, and I have therefore followed the current convention (Draper & Rogers, 2005) of disguising the identity of those whose experience is described or offering descriptions that have been previously reported with consent.

References

Amador, X. & David, A (2004) *Insight and Psychosis: Awareness of Illness in Schizophrenia and Related Disorders* (2nd edn). Oxford: Oxford University Press.

Anonymous (1986) 'Can we talk?' The schizophrenic patient in psychotherapy. *American Journal of Psychiatry*, **143**, 68–70.

Bateson, G. (1973) *Steps to an Ecology of Mind*. St Albans: Paladin.

Berner, P., Gabriel, E., Kieffer, S. (1986) Paranoid psychosis: new aspects of classification and prognosis coming from the Vienna research group. *Psychopathology*, **19**, 16–29.

Berrios, G. E. (1991) Delusions as 'wrong beliefs': a conceptual history. *British Journal of Psychiatry*, **159** (suppl. 14), 6–13.

Bleuler, E. (1951) Autistic thinking. In *Organisation and Pathology of Thought* (ed. D. Rapaport). New York: Columbia University Press.

Bottoms, G. (2001) *Angelhead: My Brother's Descent into Madness*. London: Headline Book Publishing.

British Columbia Schizophrenia Society (2003) *Early Psychosis: What Friends and Family Need to Know*. Richmond, BC: BCSS. http://www.bcss.org/Get_Information/Schizophrenia/early_psychosis.html

Ciompi, L. (1989) The dynamics of complex biological–psychosocial systems. Four fundamental psycho-biological mediators in the long-term evolution of schizophrenia. *British Journal of Psychiatry*, **155** (suppl. 5), 15–21.

Conran, M. (1999) Sorrow, vulnerability and madness. In *Psychosis (Madness)* (ed. P. Williams), chapter 2. London: Institute of Psychoanalysis.

Copeland, M. E. & Mead, S. (2004) *Wellness Recovery Action Plan and Peer Support*. Dummerston, VT: Peach Press.

Cox, M. & Theilgaard, A. (1987) *Mutative Metaphors in Psychotherapy: The Aeolian Mode*. London: Tavistock Press.

Curtis, T., Dellar, R. & Leslie, E. (2000) *Mad Pride: A Celebration of Mad Culture*. London: Chipmunka Publishing.

Davidson, L. (2003) *Living Outside Mental Illness: Qualitative Studies in Recovery in Schizophrenia*. New York: New York University Press.

Davidson, L. & Strauss, J. (1995) Beyond the biopsychosocial model: integrating disorder, health and recovery. *Psychiatry*, **58**, 44–55.

Dickinson, E. (1924) Life: XI. In *The Complete Poems of Emily Dickinson*. Boston, MA: Little, Brown,

Draper, H. & Rogers, W. (2005) Re-evaluating confidentiality: using patient information in teaching and publications. *Advances in Psychiatric Treatment*, **11**, 115–124.

Fulford, W., Morris, K., Sadler, J., et al (2003) Past improbable, future possible: the renaissance in philosophy and psychiatry. In *Nature and Narrative: An Introduction to the New Philosophy of Psychiatry* (eds B. Fulford, K. Morris, J. Sadler, et al), chapter 1. Oxford: Oxford University Press.

Hauerwas, S. (1993) *Naming the Silences: God, Medicine and the Problem of Suffering*. Edinburgh: T&T Clark.

Huszonek, J. J. (1987) Establishing therapeutic contact with schizophrenics: a supervisory approach. *American Journal of Psychotherapy*, **XLI**, 185–193.

Jamison, K. R. (1995) *An Unquiet Mind: A Memoir of Moods and Madness*. New York: Alfred A. Knopf.

Jaspers, K. (1913) Causal and 'meaningful' connections between life history and psychosis. Reprinted (1974) in *Themes and Variations in European Psychiatry* (eds S. Hirsch & M. Shepherd; trans. J. Hoenig). Bristol: John Wright and Sons.

Jaspers, K. (1963) *General Psychopathology* (trans. J. Hoenig & J. W. Hamilton), Manchester: Manchester University Press. Reprinted (1998) by John Hopkins University Press, Baltimore, MD.

Jones, K. (2004) The historical context of therapeutic environments. In *From Toxic Institutions to Therapeutic Environments: Residential Settings in Mental Health Services* (eds P. Campling, S. Davies & G. Farquharson), chapter 1. London: Gaskell.

Josephs, L. & Josephs, L. (1986) Pursuing the kernel of truth in the psychotherapy of schizophrenia. *Psychoanalytic Psychology*, **3**, 105–119.

Jung, C. G. (1914) The content of the psychoses. Reprinted (1960) in *The Collected Works of C. G. Jung* (eds H. Read, M. Fordbam, G. Adler, *et al*; trans. R. F. C. Hull), vol 3. Princeton, NJ: Princeton University Press.

Kaffman, M. (1984) Paranoid disorders: the core of truth behind the delusional system. *International Journal of Family Therapy*, **6**, 220–232.

Kaplan, B. (1964) *The Inner World of Mental Illness: A Series of First-Person Accounts of What it is Like*. New York: Harper and Row

Kleinman, A. (1988) *The Illness Narratives: Suffering, Healing and the Human Condition*. New York: Basic Books.

Kupersanin, E. (2002) Psychosis fails to block psychiatrist's career path. *Psychiatric News*, **37**, 5.

Laing, R. D. (1990) *The Divided Self*. London: Penguin.

Leibrich, J. (1999) *A Gift of Stories: Discovering How to Deal with Mental Illness*. Dunedin: University of Otago Press.

Murray, R. (2004) New ways of thinking about and treating psychosis. *Progress in Neurology and Psychiatry*, **8**, 20–26.

Nasar, S. (1998) *A Beautiful Mind*. London: Faber and Faber.

National Institute for Clinical Excellence (2002) *Clinical Guideline 1. Schizophrenia: Core Interventions in the Treatment and Management of Schizophrenia in Primary and Secondary Care.* London: NICE.

North, C (1987) *Welcome Silence: My Triumph over Schizophrenia*. New York: Simon and Schuster.

Read, J., Mosher, L. R. & Bentall, R. P. (2004) *Models of Madness: Psychological, Social and Biological Approaches to Schizophrenia*. Hove: Brunner-Routledge.

Roberts, G. (1991) Delusional belief systems and meaning in life: a preferred reality? *British Journal of Psychiatry*, **159** (suppl. 14), 19–28.

Roberts, G. A. (1999) The rehabilitation of rehabilitation: a narrative approach to psychosis. In *Healing Stories: Narrative in Psychiatry and Psychotherapy* (eds G. Roberts & J. Holmes), chapter 8. Oxford: Oxford University Press.

Roberts, G. A. (2000*a*) Awakening: the complexity of recovery. *Clozaril Newsletter*, issue 23 (Winter), 8–9.

Roberts, G. A. (2000*b*) Narrative and severe mental illness: what place do stories have in an evidence-based world? *Advances in Psychiatric Treatment*, **6**, 432–441.

Romme, M. & Escher, S. (2000) *Making Sense of Voices: A Guide for Mental Health Professionals Working with Voice-Hearers*. London: Mind Publications.

Santayana, G. (1925) *Dialogues in Limbo*. London: Constable and Co.

Sayers, P. (1989) *The Comforts of Madness*. London: Sceptre.

Sims, A. (1988) *Symptoms in the Mind: An Introduction to Descriptive Psychopathology*. London: Elsevier.

Solomon, A. (2002) *The Noonday Demon: An Anatomy of Depression*. London: Vintage.

Spataro, J., Mullen, P. E., Burgess, P. M., *et al* (2004) Impact of child sexual abuse on mental health. Prospective study in males and females. *British Journal of Psychiatry*, **184**, 416–421.

Strauss, J. S. (1994) The person with schizophrenia as a person. II: Approaches to the subjective and complex. *British Journal of Psychiatry*, **164** (suppl. 23), 103–107.

Thomas, P. & Bracken, P. (2004) Critical psychiatry in practice. *Advances in Psychiatric Treatment*, **10**, 361–370.

Watson, C. (2005) The P value of empathy. Personal view. *BMJ*, **330**, 101.

CHAPTER 8

First person: 'you need hope to cope'†

Rachel Perkins

'When I was diagnosed I felt this is the end of my life. It was a thing to isolate me from other human beings. I felt I was not viable unless they found a cure... I felt flawed. Defective.'

Cited in Sayce (2000)

If you have serious mental health problems you face a multifaceted catastrophe. You feel all the unfamiliar and often frightening experiences on which your diagnosis is based – experiences profoundly different from those of other people. You may be unable to organise your thoughts; the ordinary things of everyday life – getting up, dressing, shopping, talking to friends – may become impossibly difficult; you may experience altered sensations and perceptions that no one else appears to share; you may know that strange – and dangerous – things are happening. The isolation and distress of unshared experiences are compounded by the disbelief that lurks on the faces of those around you. Things you know to be true they dismiss as ludicrous, imagined, unreal:

'Not believing that I really feel, see or hear the things that trouble me – that's what makes me really lonely. People say things like "Don't worry", "It's in your imagination", "Of course no one is talking in your head" ... "It's just not happening"' (cited in Perkins & Repper, 1999).

You become the images that the media paint of you. Basically you have two choices. On the one hand, you are the dangerous, unpredictable 'mad axe murderer' of tabloid media fame: two-thirds of all British press and television coverage on mental health includes an association with violence (Health Education Authority, 1998). On the other hand, you are seen as incompetent, unable and unfit to participate in society – in need of others to look after you and make decisions for you. The prejudice and discrimination arising from popular beliefs of danger and incompetence mean that too

---

†This was written on a 'graffiti wall' at a consultation event for Black service users – 'Canerows and Plaits' – held at Sound Minds in Wandsworth, London, in May 2004.

often you are ostracised. Sometimes the discrimination and exclusion are quite subtle:

'Friends, family, people you meet everyday – people treat you differently. Like they are treading on eggshells ... they think that if they say the wrong thing you're going to flare up or whatever' (cited in Repper *et al*, 1998).

But sometimes rejection takes more frightening forms: Read & Baker (1996) provide accounts of people who have been attacked, had eggs thrown at them, dog faeces pushed through the front door, simply because they were known to have mental health problems.

Social networks contract as former friends and social contacts drift away – or as you avoid former contacts for fear of what they might think – leaving you more alone. This day-to-day rejection is compounded by exclusion from a range of opportunities and services. Negative attitudes pervade all areas of society: the police, housing and benefit agencies, businesses, insurance companies, community organisations, churches, clubs, physical health services (see Read & Baker, 1996; Rose, 1996; Dunn, 1999; Sayce, 2000), and within mental health services themselves:

'even the briefest perusal of the current literature on schizophrenia will immediately reveal to the uninitiated that this collection of problems is viewed by practitioners almost exclusively in terms of dysfunction and deficit. A positive or charitable phrase or sentence rarely meets the eye ... Deficit obsessed research can only produce theories and attitudes which are disrespectful of clients and are also likely to induce behaviour in clinicians such that service users are not properly listened to, not believed, not fairly assessed, are likely treated as inadequate and are not expected to be able to become independent and competent individuals in managing life's tasks' (Chadwick, 1997).

If even the experts believe that you will never amount to very much, what hope is there?

Employment is central to social inclusion and to the lives of most people. Work offers more than a source of income; it provides social contacts and social support, social status and identity, activity and involvement, a means of structuring and occupying time, and a sense of personal achievement (Rowland & Perkins, 1988; Royal College of Psychiatrists, 2003).

For people who are already excluded as a consequence of their mental health problems, work takes on an even greater significance (Rogers, 1995). Yet they experience greater discrimination within, and exclusion from, the labour market than any other disabled people (Burchardt, 2000). Repeated surveys of employers demonstrate a reluctance to even think of taking on people with mental health problems for jobs (see Department of Work and Pensions, 2001), ensuring that almost 76% of people with such difficulties are unemployed (Office for National Statistics, 2003).

The belief that people with mental health problems are not capable of working is not restricted to employers: many mental health professionals share this perception (Rinaldi & Hill, 2000). Yet a increasing body of

113

research demonstrates that, with the right sort of help and support, as many as 60% of people with serious mental health problems can gain and sustain employment (Crowther *et al*, 2001; Bond, 2004).

And unemployment results in poverty, which further exacerbates isolation and reduces opportunity:

'Out of the blue your job has gone and with it any financial security you may have had. At a stroke, you have no purpose in life and no contact with other people. You find yourself totally isolated from the rest of the world. No one telephones you. Much less writes. No one seems to care if you are alive or dead' (cited in Bird, 2001) …

'Because of my low income … I go for foods with cheaper prices and those with special offers, I have not bought new clothes for years and have not been out for a meal, cinema or a holiday for more than 10 years' (cited in Bird, 2001).

The possibility of recovery

Serious mental health problems are a life-changing experience. There is no way back to the way things were before your problems started, but they do not have to be the end of life (Repper & Perkins, 2003). Many people with such difficulties have shown us that recovery is possible.

Recovery is not the same as cure (Deegan, 1993): it does not mean that all symptoms have been removed or that functioning has been fully restored. It is about recovering meaning, purpose and identity – about pursuing your interests and ambitions, and discovering new ones, in the presence of ongoing or recurring problems:

'Recovery refers to the lived or real life experience of people as they accept and overcome the challenge of the disability … they experience themselves as recovering a new sense of self and of purpose within and beyond the limits of the disability' (Deegan, 1988).

Recovery is not something that services do, it is the journey of the individual who experiences mental health problems: the process of finding a new meaning and identity. Mental health professionals and services cannot do recovery – but they can help people to make the best of their abilities and resources and find new purpose and value in life.

Serious mental health problems: a bereavement

If mental health professionals are to help people to recover a meaningful and valued life they need to understand the nature of the challenges these individuals face and what they wish to achieve in life. Too often, the focus is only on problems associated with the 'illness' itself – the recurring, fluctuating or ever-present cognitive and emotional problems that the person experiences – with scant attention to the other sources of trauma with which the person must contend, such as:

- the treatment of their difficulties, including the side-effects of medication and stigma associated with using mental health services;
- the negative attitudes and prognoses of professionals whose primary concern is symptom relief and who may lack the skills necessary to help individuals to rebuild their lives;
- devaluing and disempowering services – housing in depressing, shabby buildings – that encourage passivity and where 'them and us' attitudes are rampant;
- the multiple manifestations of prejudice in a society where people with mental health problems are seen as dangerous, incompetent or both;
- the discrimination and social exclusion – lack of opportunity to engage in valued roles and activities – that result from these stereotypes.

It is the multiple interlocking traumas, which create a compound experience, that have such a devastating impact on people's lives and leave them feeling disconnected from the themselves, from family and friends and from the communities in which they live (Repper & Perkins, 2003).

Being diagnosed with serious mental health problems is a bereavement. It involves loss of the privileges of sanity: loss of the life you had or expected to lead and loss of the person you were or thought you would become. Like any bereavement, the experience of serious mental health problems is associated with a range of emotions, from denial to despair (Box 8.1).

Emotions such as these are ordinary responses to devastating life events. Yet, in someone who has serious mental health problems, they are too often pathologised – seen as symptoms to be treated: denial becomes a 'lack of insight' that is supposed to be inherent in the disorder, not an ordinary response to catastrophic life events. Hopelessness, apathy, withdrawal are understood as the 'negative symptoms' and 'lack of motivation' that characterise the disorder. Anger is seen as 'acting out' or 'attention-seeking'.

Box 8.1 The emotional effect of diagnosis

Diagnosis of mental illness can evoke a range of emotions

- Denial: 'It must be a mistake', 'Everything will be back to normal soon'
- Anger: 'Why me?', 'It's not fair'
- Terror: 'Now what will happen to me?'
- Guilt: 'I must have done something wrong'
- Grief: 'My life is over', 'Everything is hopeless'
- Shame: 'I hope no one finds out'
- Isolation: 'Now no one will want to have anything to do with me'
- Worthlessness: 'I'm useless', 'Everyone else copes, I'm just not good enough'

(O'Donoghue, 1994; Repper & Perkins, 2003)

This attitude can leave people with mental illnesses feeling devalued and ignored and cause them to mistrust and become alienated from mental health services (Spaniol *et al*, 1997).

Unless mental health professionals can understand the ordinary human responses to the bereavement associated with serious mental health problems, they may inadvertently impede recovery by alienating people from those very services that are supposed to assist them.

Recovery is about whole lives, not just symptoms

There are many pharmacological, psychological and social interventions that can help people to gain symptomatic relief. But symptoms do not define a person or their life. The problems that impede recovery extend well beyond the relief of cognitive and emotional problems: housing, money, relationships, employment/education, social and leisure activities are central to recovery. But expertise in these areas falls outside the traditional competencies of mental health professionals.

Rehabilitation services need to ensure that individuals have the opportunity to explore all facets of themselves with people who have a range of skills and experiences. And this must include access to the expertise of personal experience. Who better to help someone face the challenge of life with serious mental health problems than someone who had faced the same challenge themselves?

Recovery is about growth

'Schizophrenia is an "I am" illness, one which may take over and redefine the identity of the person.'

Estroff (1989)

It is very easy for people who experience serious mental health problems to become nothing other than the array of symptoms that characterises their illness: 'a schizophrenic', 'a manic–depressive', 'a nutter'. Recovery involves redefining identity in a way that includes these difficulties but is not defined by them. It is very easy for a person's interests, talents and dreams to be eclipsed by their problems. People are always more than their illness. Lives cannot be rebuilt on problems and deficits – they are rebuilt on the foundation of abilities and ambitions. It is these that enable us to grow, develop and move beyond our problems.

It is not uncommon for mental health professionals to believe that they must always protect those they serve from further failure in a hostile and unwelcoming world. But growth necessarily involves the risk of failure. Every time a person enters a relationship they risk rejection. Every time a person applies for a job they risk not getting it. Without taking risks we can never pursue our dreams.

Recovery is a continuing journey

'Recovery is a process, not an end point or destination. Recovery is an attitude, a way of approaching the day and the challenges I face. ... I know I have certain limitations and things I can't do. But rather than letting these limitations be occasions for despair and giving up, I have learned that in knowing what I can't do, I also open up the possibilities of all I can do.'

Deegan (1993)

Too often mental health professionals judge the effectiveness of an intervention – helping a person to go to college, get a job, live in the community – in terms of whether the individual is able to do things when support is withdrawn. They judge the effectiveness of services in terms of the extent to which they enable a person to become 'independent' – move on, cease to need their support. If recovery is a continuing journey, then rehabilitation must be a continuing process. The critical yardstick of success is not whether the person can become independent of support and services, but what they are able to achieve in the presence of that support.

To take a parallel with physical impairment. The effectiveness of a wheelchair in helping someone with a broken spine is never judged in terms of whether it enables the person to walk again. We judge the effectiveness of the wheelchairs, hearing loops, lifts and personal assistants that a person with mobility or sensory impairments may need in terms of the extent to which they enable the person to do the things they want to do.

Rehabilitation services might usefully move away from models of 'illness/ cure' to a 'disability/access' perspective (Sayce, 2000; Repper & Perkins, 2003; Royal College of Psychiatrists, 2003). If people are viewed as 'ill', then efforts are directed towards making them better, finding a cure, and there is the assumption that they should be relieved of responsibilities – 'tucked up in bed' – their lives suspended, until they get better. Rehabilitation services are replete with people whose lives have been suspended for many years, and while they are waiting to 'get better' and the patient role eclipses all others they become nothing but their illness. If people are viewed as disabled rather than ill – emotional and cognitive problems are approached in the same way as mobility and sensory impairments – then the agenda changes. Attention is directed towards access – the supports and adaptations that may be necessary to help the person to do the things they want to do.

Throughput models are inappropriate in the context of ongoing problems, and recovery is not a linear process: there will be problems and setbacks along the way. Mental health problems typically fluctuate, and relapse is not 'failure' but part of the recovery process – part of the impairments with which individuals have to contend in rebuilding their lives. Setbacks can be dispiriting and it can be tempting to give up. At such times people need someone who can hold onto hope – continue to believe in their possibilities when they are not able to believe in them themselves. If professionals cannot be such holders of hope then they cannot promote recovery.

Recovery is not dependent on professional intervention

Mental health professionals can facilitate recovery, but they do not hold the key: a person's own resources and those available to them outside mental health services are central (Anthony, 1993; Deegan, 1993; Young & Ensing, 1999). The sources of meaning and purpose in people's lives do not lie in mental health services; they lie in our work, our homes, our relationships, our leisure pursuits, our spiritual beliefs... If people with mental illnesses are not able to access the range of ordinary opportunities that their non-disabled peers take for granted, then it is unlikely that they will be able to rebuild a satisfying and meaningful life.

The expertise of personal experience is also central: many people have described the enormous support and hope they have gained from others who have faced similar challenges. Therefore services need to maximise opportunities for people to support and learn from each other.

Visions of recovery

Just as professionals have developed a range of organic, psychological and interpersonal models for understanding mental distress and impairment, so people who experience such problems have adopted different ways of understanding their predicament: from biological, to environmental, social, spiritual and political explanations (Jacobson, 1993).

A recovery vision does not commit one to a particular understanding of distress and disability (Anthony, 1993; Repper & Perkins, 2003). People need to find ways of understanding their situation, but whichever framework they choose, the process of recovery – rebuilding a satisfying and meaningful life – is equally important. If a person's explanatory framework is to facilitate recovery it must make sense to them and offer them hope for the future. If services insist that everyone adopt a single understanding of their difficulties, this is likely to alienate those who prefer alternative explanations and thus impede the recovery process.

Recovery is possible for everyone

Some people may never be free of their cognitive and emotional problems, but no matter how severe the impairment, they can still develop sources of meaning and value in their lives. Rehabilitation is not about selecting people who are 'motivated' and can be 'rehabilitated into the community'. It is about enabling everyone to make the most of their lives. The challenge for professionals is to discover people's ambitions and abilities, especially when these are overshadowed by their problems. And some people will need a high level of support on an indefinite basis if they are to make the most of their talents.

There are no rules of recovery – no one formula for success. Each person must find their own way. But it remains common for services to develop sets of rules about how people must use them – like 'You can only have lunch at the day centre if you go to a group first' – or to adopt a 'ladder' approach, for example, 'You start in the rehabilitation ward and move on to a hostel before progressing to a flat of your own'. Rules like these impede recovery. They inevitably mean that services cannot be tailored to individual needs, preferences and aspirations. They can also serve to prevent people from using their abilities to the full and/or alienate by offering a service that they find unacceptable.

Although everyone's recovery journey is different, two factors repeatedly emerge as central: hope and opportunity (Deegan, 1988, 1993; Spaniol & Koehler, 1994; Young & Ensing, 1999; Kirkpatrick *et al*, 2001; Repper & Perkins, 2003). It is not possible to rebuild your life if you do not believe that a better future is possible or if everywhere you turn you are debarred from doing the things that give your life meaning and value. If services are to promote recovery they must foster hope and promote opportunity.

Fostering hope

Hope has been identified as important in coping with physical illnesses (e.g. Hickey, 1986), in the success of psychotherapy (e.g. Frank, 1968), in successful outcome in first-episode psychosis (Aguilar *et al* 1997) and in psychiatric rehabilitation (e.g. Kirkpatrick *et al*, 1995). Conversely, a number of studies have demonstrated a link between hopelessness and suicide (e.g. Drake & Cotton, 1986; Beck *et al*, 1990).

Hope – the belief that things can be better – lies at the heart of an individual's ability and willingness to take on the challenge of rebuilding their life:

'For those of us who have been diagnosed with mental illness and who have lived in the sometimes desolate wastelands of mental health programs and institutions, hope is not a nice sounding euphemism. It is a matter of life and death' (Deegan, 1996).

But hope does not exist in a vacuum. It occurs in the context of relationships (Byrne *et al*, 1994). It is not possible to believe in your own possibilities if everyone around you believes you will never amount to very much. And in this context, mental health professionals are particularly powerful – for good or ill. If those experts who are supposed to be helping you cannot believe in your potential, what hope is there? It unfortunately remains the case that many people continue to report that contacts with mental health services have left them discouraged and dispirited.

A number of skills appear to be important in developing hope-inspiring relationships that can enable people to gain the confidence and self-belief that is necessary if they are to rebuild their lives (Russinova, 1999; Repper & Perkins, 2003). These include:

- valuing the person for who he or she is
- believing in the person's worth
- seeing, and having confidence in, the person's skills, abilities and potential
- listening to and heeding what the person says
- believing in the authenticity of the person's experience
- accepting, and actively exploring, the person's experiences
- tolerating uncertainty about the future
- seeing problems and setbacks as part of the recovery process: helping the person to learn from, and build on, them.

If these are some of the necessary skills it begs the question of how to promote and propagate these in clinical settings. Clearly, these capacities can be sought during the complex process of staff selection, but can they also be taught, and cultivated through subsequent staff and team development? And what should be done if any kind of audit finds these qualities lacking?

However, relationships between practitioners and clients are only a small part of the story. Such relationships are neither elective nor reciprocal. The professional does not elect to enter the relationship with a particular client – they are paid to do so – and the purpose of the relationship is to benefit the client rather than the practitioner (except indirectly via the salary paid or job satisfaction gained). Therefore the role of such relationships in enabling patients or clients to gain a sense of their own value and worth is limited. Perhaps the quality of a relationship between client and practitioner should be judged in terms of the extent to which it supports or enables people to develop their own relationships with friends and family? For it is these elective, reciprocal relationships on which we all rely so heavily that provide us with our social context and personal identity.

The restoration of hope in those whose self-confidence and self-belief have been shattered by serious mental health problems can be a time-consuming affair and may involve a number of components (Repper & Perkins, 2003):

- helping people to grieve what they have lost
- challenging the myths associated with serious mental health problems ('I will never be able to get married, have a home of my own, get a job…')
- understanding what has happened – not simply at the level of neuro-transmitters, but in relation to those broader, philosophical questions: 'Why me?', 'What's the point in life?'
- taking back control:

    'I have more control over my illness than I ever realised … Knowing that gives me more hope because I know the next time when I start to get ill I can turn it around. You don't have to let your illness run your life' (client cited in Kirkpatrick *et al*, 2001)

- learning from others who have been there themselves – either in person or by their writing:

  'My suggestion is to get as many success stories as possible from those who have schizophrenia to give a sense of hope to those just beginning their journey' (client cited in Kirkpatrick *et al*, 2001).

However, it is not possible to sustain hope in the absence of opportunity.

Promoting opportunity

It is very easy for mental health professionals to look at the extent of a person's problems and the discrimination that exists and give up – decide that there is nothing that they can do to change things. This is a mistake and is not consistent with the evidence base.

Broadly, there are two ways in which professionals can help people to access the opportunities they seek. They can either change the person so that they fit in, or they can change the world so that it can accommodate the person. Traditional approaches have focused on the former by reducing symptoms – via pharmacological or psychological means – and developing the person's skills. Although such endeavours are undoubtedly valuable, there are two major problems.

First, many people have ongoing symptoms that cannot be removed by treatment, and skills training does not always enable people to use the competencies they have developed unaided because of their continuing cognitive and emotional difficulties. Access and inclusion cannot be contingent on a person ceasing to have problems. Professionals in the mental health field need to think about the psychiatric equivalent of the wheelchairs, ramps and personal assistants that facilitate access for people with impaired mobility.

Second, in the time it takes for symptoms to abate, it is likely that the person will have lost many or all of their former roles, and no matter how much symptoms can be reduced or skills developed, discrimination exists and a history of mental health problems can be as much of a barrier to participation as their continued presence (Sayce, 2000). Promoting opportunity must involve actively reducing these barriers.

There is much that can be learnt from the physical disability arena. At least as important as the treatment of symptoms are the ways in which mental health services can help people to gain access to the opportunities they desire (Repper & Perkins, 2003).

For example, they can provide support and assistance: the psychiatric equivalent of the wheelchair and the personal assistant. This might involve, for example, having someone (not necessarily a mental health professional) do things with the person, practical help and relief from some responsibilities to enable the individual to take on others: how many of us have someone to clean our home, or buy take-away meals so that we can get on

121

with the things we really want to do? There is now considerable evidence of the effectiveness of this sort of approach in helping people to access employment and education (Crowther *et al*, 2001) and of assertive outreach approaches in helping people to live independently (Mueser *et al*, 1998).

They can also adjust what is expected of the person, so that he or she is able to meet those expectations: the psychiatric equivalent of ramps and lifts. It is important to remember that roles are relational – negotiated between the different parties involved (Shepherd, 1984). This means that they can be renegotiated. Negotiations about hours, duties and supervision requirements have helped many people to gain access to employment and college courses. Negotiations around expectations within families have helped people to participate in family life.

A most important function for people working within mental health services is to break down discrimination and prejudice. There is now considerable evidence that the best way of reducing prejudice is to enable a devalued group to participate on equal terms (Hewstone, 2003). There is a great deal that can be done to facilitate this via advocacy and support: extolling a person's skills and assets, explaining any adjustments they may need and dispelling the fears of employers, colleges, or the local church, leisure centre or football club that the person may be dangerous or incompetent. It might also involve providing support to an employer (or college tutor, or religious leader…) – perhaps something as simple as a number they can call if they have problems – and understanding and promoting people's rights.

The Disability Discrimination Act 1995 includes people with mental health problems. It goes further than rendering illegal discrimination in employment, education and the provision of goods and services, by requiring that employers, educators and the purveyors of goods and services make 'reasonable adjustments' to accommodate people with such difficulties. Mental health professionals have a major role to play in enabling people to understand their rights and helping clients, employers, educators and service providers to think about what adjustments might be needed.

Images of possibility

If psychiatric rehabilitation services are to promote recovery – enable people to rebuild their lives within and beyond the limitations of serious mental health problems – images and stories of possibility are essential. If a person is to rebuild their life with mental health problems they must believe in the possibility of a positive future. If mental health professionals are to facilitate recovery, then they must be able to see beyond deficit and dysfunction and envision a positive future for those whom they serve. If people with mental health problems are to access the opportunities they seek, then those outside mental health services – employers and educators, social and leisure facilities, friends and relatives – must be able to see what those with mental health problems have to offer. Mental health professionals can help them to do this and offer the support they need to accommodate and integrate those with mental health problems.

There are a great many theories and speculations about the nature and origins of mental health problems, but in relation to recovery, it is a person's talents, opportunities and ambitions – and helping them to make the most of these – that become paramount in enabling them to live the lives they wish to lead and do the things they want to do. This may involve a wide range of interventions, services and supports, but these will be helpful only in as much as they foster hope and promote opportunity. Recovery is about helping people to rebuild satisfying, meaningful and valued lives, but it is important to remember that sources of meaning, satisfaction and value are different for different people. Recognition of the expertise of personal experience, and a willingness to learn from and with those whom we serve, are of the essence. Those we serve will always be our most important teachers.

References

Aguilar, E. J., Haas, G., Manzanera, F. J., et al (1997) Hopelessness and first episode psychosis: a longitudinal study. Acta Psychiatrica Scandinavica, **96**, 25–30.

Anthony, W. A. (1993) Recovery from mental illness. The guiding vision of the mental health system in the 1990s. Innovations and Research, **2**(3), 17–24.

Beck, A. T., Brown, G., Berchick, J., et al (1990) Relationship between hopelessness and ultimate suicide. A replication with psychiatric outpatients. American Journal of Psychiatry, **147**, 190–195.

Bird, L. (2001) Poverty, social exclusion and mental health. A survey of people's personal experiences. A Life in the Day, **5**, 3.

Bond, G. R. (2004) Supported employment. Evidence for an evidence-based practice. Psychiatric Rehabilitation Journal, **27**, 345–359.

Burchardt, T. (2000) Enduring Economic Exclusion: Disabled People, Income and Work. York: Joseph Rowntree Foundation.

Byrne, C., Woodside, H, Landeen, J., et al (1994) The importance of relationships in fostering hope. Journal of Psychosocial Nursing, **32**, 31–34.

Chadwick, P. K. (1997) Schizophrenia: The Positive Perspective. In Search of Dignity for Schizophrenic People. London: Routledge.

Crowther, R. E., Marshall, M., Bond, G. R., et al (2001) Helping people with severe mental illness to obtain work. Systematic review. BMJ, **322**, 204–208.

Deegan, P. (1988) Recovery. The lived experience of rehabilitation. Psychosocial Rehabilitation Journal, **11**(4), 11–19.

Deegan, P. E. (1993) Recovering our sense of value after being labeled mentally ill. Psychosocial Nursing and Mental Health Services, **31**(4), 7–11.

Deegan, P. (1996) Recovery as a journey of the heart. Psychiatric Rehabilitation Journal, **19**, 91–97.

Department of Work and Pensions (2001) Recruiting Benefits Claimants: Quantitative Research with Employers in ONE Pilot Areas (Research series paper no. 150). London: Department of Work and Pensions.

Drake, R. E. & Cotton, P. G. (1986) Depression, hopelessness and suicide in chronic schizophrenia. British Journal of Psychiatry, **148**, 554–559.

Dunn, S. (1999) Creating Accepting Communities. Report of the Mind Inquiry into Social Exclusion and Mental Health Problems. London: Mind Publications.

Estroff, S. E. (1989) Self, identity, and subjective experiences of schizophrenia. In search of the subject. *Schizophrenia Bulletin*, **15**, 189–196.

Frank, J. (1968) The role of hope in psychotherapy. *International Journal of Psychiatry*, **5**, 383–395.

Health Education Authority (1998) *Discrimination Hurts* (press release 5th October). London: Health Education Authority.

Hewstone, M. (2003) Intergroup contact: panacea for prejudice? *The Psychologist*, **16**, 352–355.

Hickey, S. S. (1986) Enabling hope. *Journal of Cancer Nursing*, **9**,133–137.

Jacobson, N. (1993) Experiencing recovery: a dimensional analysis of recovery narratives. *Psychiatric Rehabilitation Journal*, **24**, 248–255.

Kirkpatrick, H., Landeen, J., Byrne, C., *et al* (1995) Hope and schizophrenia. Clinicians identify hope-instilling strategies. *Journal of Psychosocial Nursing and Mental Health Services*, **33**, 15–19.

Kirkpatrick, H., Landeen, J., Woodside, H., *et al* (2001) How people with schizophrenia build their hope. *Journal of Psychosocial Nursing and Mental Health Services*, **39**, 46–53.

Mueser, K. T., Bond, G. R., Drake, R. E., *et al* (1998) Models of community care for severe mental illness. A review of research on case management. *Schizophrenia Bulletin*, **24**, 37–74.

O'Donoghue, D. (1994) *Breaking Down the Barriers. The Stigma of Mental Illness: A User's Point of View*. Aberystwyth: US, The All Wales User Network.

Office for National Statistics (2003) *Labour Force Survey 2003*. London: Office for National Statistics.

Perkins, R. E. & Repper, J. M. (1999) *Working Alongside People with Long Term Mental Health Problems*. London: Stanley Thornes.

Read, J. & Baker, S. (1996) *Not Just Sticks and Stones. A Survey of the Stigma, Taboos and Discrimination Experienced by People with Mental Health Problems*. London: Mind Publications.

Repper, J. & Perkins, R. (2003) *Social Inclusion and Recovery. A Model for Mental Health Practice*. London: Ballière Tindall.

Repper, J., Perkins, R. & Owen, S. (1998) 'I wanted to be a nurse ... but I didn't get that far': women with serious ongoing mental health problems speak about their lives. *Journal of Psychiatric and Mental Health Nursing*, **5**, 505–513.

Rinaldi, M. & Hill, R. (2000) *Insufficient Concern – The Experience, Attitudes and Perceptions of Disabled People towards Open Employment in One London Borough*. London: Merton Mind.

Rogers, J. (1995) Work is key to recovery. *Psychosocial Rehabilitation Journal*, **18**, 5–10.

Rose, D. (1996) *Living in the Community*. London: Sainsbury Centre for Mental Health.

Rowland, L. A. & Perkins, R. E. (1988) You can't eat, drink or make love eight hours a day: the value of work in psychiatry. *Health Trends*, **20**, 75–79.

Royal College of Psychiatrists (2003) *Employment Opportunities and Psychiatric Disability* (Council Report CR111). London: Royal College of Psychiatrists.

Russinova, Z. (1999) Providers' hope-inspiring competence as a factor optimizing psychiatric rehabilitation outcomes. *Journal of Rehabilitation*, **65**(4), 50–57.

Sayce, L. (2000) *From Psychiatric Patient to Citizen. Overcoming Discrimination and Social Exclusion*. London: Macmillan.

Shepherd, G. (1984) *Institutional Care and Rehabilitation*. London: Longman.

Spaniol, L. & Koehler, M. (1994) (eds) *The Experience of Recovery*. Boston, MA: Center for Psychiatric Rehabilitation.

Spaniol, L., Gagne, C. & Koehler, M. (1997) Recovery from serious mental illness. What it is and how to assist people in their recovery. *Continuum*, **4**(4), 3–15.

Young, S. L. & Ensing, D. S. (1999) Exploring recovery from the perspective of people with psychiatric disabilities. *Psychiatric Rehabilitation Journal*, **22**, 219–231.

Part 2

Therapeutic practices

Early intervention in first-episode psychosis and its relevance to rehabilitation psychiatry

Paddy Power, Jo Smith, David Shiers and Glenn Roberts

'The experience of the Retreat has already proved the great importance of placing the insane under proper care in an early stage of the disorder ... experience has this year abundantly convinced us, of the advantage to be derived from an early attention to persons afflicted with disorders of the mind ... and that of the six cases of 'recent instance', four had recovered and been discharged within three months and the other two were clearly recovering.'

Samuel Tuke, forefather of rehabilitation psychiatry (1813)

The current emphasis in the UK on early intervention for young people in their first episode of psychosis grew out of dissatisfaction with our 'one size fits all' approach, regardless of the age of the patient or stage of illness. Early intervention emphasises that individuals who develop psychosis when young require phase-specific interventions tailored to the particular needs and aspirations they have as young people. This chapter describes both the development of early-intervention services and their potential relationship with rehabilitation as essential components of a wider family of psychosis services built round the changing needs of the individual and their family over time.

Early-intervention services are built on the observation that long-term outcome is strongly determined by what happens during the initial phase (Harrison *et al*, 2001). In the great majority of cases, psychosis begins in adolescence and young adulthood, at a crucial time for intellectual development, social functioning and emerging personal autonomy. The first 3 years of illness have been described as the critical period (Birchwood *et al*, 1998) during which therapeutic, illness and life experiences are likely to have important long-term consequences (Box 9.1). It is the time when the neuropathological process of psychosis is at its most active (Lieberman, 1999), but it is also when treatments can achieve their best response. Early-intervention services are based on the belief that effective and sustained intervention over this critical period maximises the potential for recovery, protects against relapse and improves the individual's long-term trajectory and outcome.

Box 9.1 The critical period

- Outcomes at 3 years strongly predict those at 20 years (Harrison *et al,* 2001)
- Most of those who take their own lives (66%) do so in the first 5 years of illness (Mortensen & Juel, 1993)
- Two-thirds of patients relapse in the first 3 years (Robinson *et al*, 1999)
- Early-stage relapse predicts the risk of future relapse (Wiersma *et al*, 1998)
- Delay or difficulty in gaining employment predicts longer-term difficulty
- Patterns of disability, persisting symptoms and poor engagement are established
- Losses with longer-term consequences set in – social networks, education, self-image and self-esteem
- Persisting psychosis during adolescent neurodevelopment is 'neurotoxic'

The wider view: 'prevention is better than cure'

Early intervention in psychosis follows trends seen in other areas of healthcare. Conditions such as diabetes and coronary artery disease provide useful models where health professionals and the public's perspective have shifted significantly towards health promotion, early intervention and collaborative management. Although the search continues for the key factors that mediate occurrence, renewed optimism has come through securing quick access to high-quality treatment to reduce the risk of serious long-term morbidity.

In most areas of psychiatry, the pessimistic Kraepelinian view of schizophrenia as a dementia praecox (Kraepelin, 1896) whose treatment could be best characterised as 'the orderly management of decline' (Birchwood, 2002) has given way to a more optimistic and proactive view. The seeds of this revised view can be seen in the writings of Sullivan (1927), Cameron (1938) and Meares (1959). Following the advent of antipsychotic drugs, outcome studies from the early 1980s (Ciompi, 1980) showed that even the most severely affected could achieve partial or even complete recovery, particularly if supported by comprehensive psychosocial rehabilitation (Harding *et al*, 1987). The value of being treated in an atmosphere of optimism and hope, as a precondition for all other aspects of treatment, has been emphasised in recent guidance (National Institute for Clinical Excellence, 2002: section 1.1.1.1) and personal testimony of recovery (May, 2004).

Early-intervention services are part of a wider reform movement to modernise mental health services in the UK. Some clinicians and academics remain sceptical, believing that developments in early intervention have moved beyond the evidence base; service managers range from enthusiastic to dismissive. However, early intervention offers a face validity and intuitive logic to service users, families and healthcare providers, and consumer-led organisations such as the Initiative to Reduce the Impact of Schizophrenia (IRIS) and Rethink have given powerful impetus to these political reforms (Box 9.2).

Box 9.2 Development of policy and commitment to early-intervention services in the UK

1998 *Modernising Mental Health Services* (Department of Health, 1998) A clear statement of intent to review and revise the content, process and organisation of mental health services – modernisation.

1999 *National Service Framework for Mental Health* (Department of Health, 1999) This first NSF provided a blueprint for a modernised mental health service to be developed over 10 years and included the target of local early-intervention services throughout England responding to the needs of the 7500 young people who develop a psychosis each year.

2000 *The National Health Service Plan* (Department of Health, 2000) A wide-ranging document describing the modernisation agenda for the entire NHS, including commitment to developing 50 early-intervention teams, each covering about I million of the general population (by April 2004) so that 'all young people who experience a first episode of psychosis, such as schizophrenia, will receive the early and intensive support they need'. Commitment to reduce the duration of untreated psychosis to a service average of 3 months (maximum for one individual: 6 months) and continuous service support for the first 3 years.

2001–2002 *Task Force and Policy Implementation Guide* (Department of Health, 2001) Described the aims, objectives and service configuration for each of the new functional services specified in the NSFs and NHS Plan – including early-intervention services. It offered a detailed description of an ideal service and the expectation that services develop with high fidelity to the prescribed model. It specified a service for people aged 14–35 for the first 3 years of illness.

2002 *NICE schizophrenia guidelines* (National Institute for Clinical Excellence, 2002) Recommendations for early intervention as a phased response – part of the total care pathway.

2002 *Improvement, Expansion and Reform – The Next 3 Years* (Department of Health, 2002) Document distilling the multitude of targets in the NHS Plan and NSFs into the top priorities – which preserved early-intervention services as a leading goal in mental health.

2002 *Child and Adolescent Mental Health Target* (Department of Health, 2002: Appendix 5B) Resetting of national targets to establish comprehensive early-intervention services by 2006.

2004 *NSF for Children, Young People and Maternity Services* (Department of Health, 2004) Reiterates the need for early-intervention services for young people that effectively integrate child, adolescent and adult mental health services through joint commissioning and collaborative working.

2004 *Early Psychosis Declaration* (World Health Organization & International Early Psychosis Association, 2004) Developed by IRIS and the International Early Psychosis Association, an international consensus about service targets to meet the needs of young people with psychosis and their families.

2004 *NIMHE/RETHINK Early Intervention Development Programme* A 3-year programme to support and guide the implementation of early-intervention services and put into action the Early Psychosis Declaration (D.S. and J.S. are the national co-leads of this programme). See Box 9.7 for website and details.

In the vanguard of the reform movement, early intervention has needed to navigate between aspirations and criticisms, idealism and realism, and innovation and cost-saving diversion of existing resources into redevelopments. Anyone who lived through the era of deinstitutionalisation can recount important benefits but remember many difficulties inadvertently created, and most clinicians acknowledge that it will be a hollow achievement if current resources are stretched to cover early intervention only for significant holes to open up elsewhere. Early-intervention reform needs to proceed carefully (Edwards & McGorry, 2002) and learn to integrate itself effectively and sensitively with the range of constituencies, including continuing care and rehabilitation, making the most of its pivotal location on the interface between traditional and innovative services.

Is there really a need to change existing practice?

'Services just seemed to passively wait until he was really ill ... the service oozed pessimism, lack of investment and lack of imagination.'

A carer's view of service provision in 1998

Johannessen (2004: p. 319) writes 'If we ask, "For how long is it decent to let a young person suffering from psychosis go undiagnosed and untreated in our society?" – the answer would be obvious to most people'. Current services have been summarised as 'too little, too late' (Box 9.3) – and it has been estimated that up to 17% of those who develop schizophrenia never actually receive treatment or mental health services (Link & Dohrenwend, 1980).

Box 9.3 Treatment as usual

Every 3 days about 100 young people in the UK develop first-episode psychosis
After 12 months:
- 80% have dropped out of education or work
- 1–2% have died by suicide
- 50% have received no specialist help – although 1:3 tried to get help but were turned away
- Of those who got help:
  - 50% were sectioned, often with police involvement
  - 80% were admitted to adult wards
  - 60% were lost to follow-up
  - 45% suffered post-traumatic stress disorder – partly attributable to treatment
  - 10% received psychological therapy
  - Few (possibly only one) received optimal treatment, voluntarily in a suitable location

(C. Prior, Rethink, personal communication, 2005)

For those who do manage to gain access to treatment for their emerging illness, the delay between symptoms emerging and treatment being sought is lengthy: during the prodromal period before frank psychosis develops it is typically 2–3 years in schizophrenia (shorter in bipolar disorder) (Jackson *et al*, 2003) and during the phase of frank psychosis it is typically 1–2 years (Johannessen, 2004). There is compelling evidence that this excessive delay is a significant contributor to poor response to treatment, recovery and relapse rates.

Once in services, the quality of the treatment and care provided has considerable shortcomings (Garety & Rigg, 2001). Most young people are initially hospitalised, in crisis, commonly with traumatic police involvement and use of the Mental Health Act 1983, lengthy hospital stays and coercive in-patient practices (Yung *et al*, 2003). Levels of psychosocial treatment provision are unacceptably low. Clients and carers too frequently complain of how little practical help and education about psychosis is offered. Clinicians' attention tends to focus on treatment, while personal adaptation, functional recovery, relapse prevention and carer needs tend to be neglected. Not surprisingly, drop-out rates are depressingly high: the majority are lost to follow-up within 6 months and more than half have relapsed by 18 months (Craig *et al*, 2004). Relapse is most likely to occur between the end of the first and the third year of follow-up (Robinson *et al*, 1999), causing further disruption to educational, vocational, family and social functioning and increased risk of secondary depression, anxiety and substance misuse (Jager *et al*, 2003). With each relapse, the speed and quality of remission are progressively impaired, the risk of further relapse and persisting symptoms increases (Fig. 9.1) and service costs rise (Almond *et al*, 2004). By 5 years, the majority (55%) of patients will have failed to achieved remission from episodes of psychosis (Robinson *et al*, 1999) and most of the suicides will have occurred (Mortensen & Juel, 1993).

There are many and complex reasons for these delays and the poor quality of services provided. Current community services are characterised as overstretched and under-resourced, unable to engage in prevention, early detection or assertive follow-up for young people with psychosis, and the prospect of additional cases are a disincentive for beleaguered services to reduce thresholds for referral or engagement. Similarly, those with comorbid presentations such as drug problems or learning disability have additional needs and risk being treated conservatively or, in some cases, actively excluded from services as somebody else's problem. These scenarios combine to result in assessment services setting high thresholds for referral or engagement, which prioritises only the most severely ill and perversely colludes with the progressive deterioration of individuals to a point when crisis and legal detention in hospital becomes inevitable.

Follow-up case management services focus mainly on 'revolving-door' patients with long histories and multiple admissions. In-patient units are populated with a high and, to a young person, demoralising proportion of middle-aged patients with chronic disabling illnesses in relapse. Standard

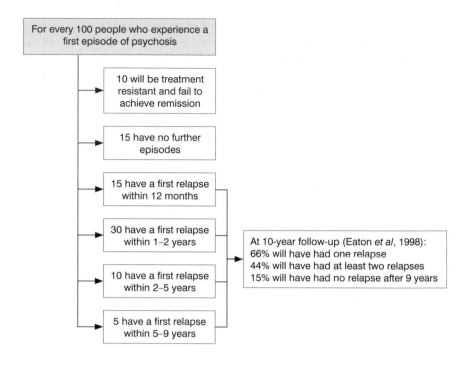

Fig. 9.1 An algorithm based on known recovery and relapse rates. Data from Wiersma *et al* (1998).

pharmacological and psychosocial interventions cannot necessarily be applied successfully without adaptation to young people in their first episode (Linszen *et al*, 2001; Gaebel *et al*, 2002). Rehabilitation is often reserved for those with the most serious and established forms of illness, and young people may be excluded from some settings on the basis of age. This can result in a catch-22 whereby adult services 'don't do young people' and child and adolescent mental health services (CAMHS) 'don't do psychosis' – so what becomes of a 16-year-old presenting with ambiguous signs of a possible first episode? At present, they risk sitting outside services until they are over 17 and they develop an unambiguous and severe illness that grants them access to acute admission to hospital under the Mental Health Act.

The result of services failing to regard young people merely at high risk of psychosis as 'core business' results in referrals being returned to general practitioners and others with little advice about appropriate support and treatment options. This demotivates referrers from seeking help or advice for similar patients. For young people and their families, these obstacles can be extremely stressful and demoralising, bringing about the risk that they will lose hope in accessing effective help and the possibility of recovery.

These observations, criticisms and consequences have generated deeply felt concerns which have driven the inception of early-intervention services. Furthermore, the introduction of these new services is in turn beginning to prompt a revision of standard services in the direction of early-intervention practices such as the use of low-dose atypical antipsychotic regimens ('start low, go slow') and the routine use of psychosocial interventions, including cognitive–behavioural therapy (CBT). Early research publications and more recent educational meetings on first-episode psychosis have gradually gained a higher profile, and attendance at the International Early Psychosis Association has multiplied tenfold since its first meeting about a decade ago. There is still a long way to go, but there are encouraging signs that the major reform is beginning to reach routine practice, and the benchmarks set by the National Institute for Clinical Excellence (NICE) (2002) (now the National Institute for Health and Clinical Excellence) and the Early Psychosis Declaration (World Health Organization & International Early Psychosis Association, 2004) are beginning to be implemented.

Aims and activities of early-intervention services

The broad aims and activities of early-intervention services can be clustered under six main headings: prevention, detection, early intervention, improved treatment, relapse prevention, and onwards care-pathway connections (Box 9.4). Current services and international models vary considerably in their level of activity across these categories.

Is early intervention successful?

'Our overwhelming feeling was of an opportunity missed for someone so young and at such an important stage of her life – to what extent she was needlessly disabled by those first four years of care we'll never know.'
Mother commenting on her daughter's prospects (1998)

The need for dedicated early-intervention services depends on how well current services respond to early psychosis. There is no doubt that standard services can provide high-quality care and treatment, but the extent to which this alone can address the aims of early intervention remains very unclear. However, when good-quality standard mental health services are compared with early-intervention services, the latter show shorter duration of untreated psychosis (Larsen et al, 2000), less use of legal detention, reduced hospital admissions (Yung et al, 2003), lower relapse rates (Craig et al, 2004), better recovery (Garety et al, 2006), better service engagement and client and carer satisfaction, lower suicide rates (Power, 2004) and better cost-effectiveness (Mihalopolous et al, 1999).

An important group of patients with first-episode psychosis (about 14–20%) become treatment refractory within the first year (Lieberman et al, 1993). Within an early-intervention service such as the Early Psychosis

Box 9.4 Aims and activities of early-intervention services

1 Reduce the risk of developing psychosis by:
- public health policies that reduce general risk factors for psychosis (universal prevention)
- strategies in asymptomatic high-risk groups (selective prevention)
- interventions in symptomatic high-risk groups (indicated prevention)

2 Improve detection by:
- promoting public health education
- promoting professional education and opening referral and care pathways
- low-threshold responsiveness to help-seeking by individuals, carers or referrers
- early detection and outreach assessment services, to maximise early collaborative engagement in the community
- comprehensive integrated biopsychosocial assessments by clinicians skilled in the assessment of young people with first-episode psychosis

3 Reduce delays in accessing treatment for patients with psychosis by:
- public health education, increasing understanding, reducing stigma and promoting help-seeking
- improved access and availability of services
- building bridges between primary and secondary care
- structuring services across the inception age span (14–35 years)

4 Maximise symptomatic and functional recovery of people with psychosis by:
- making a better start, reducing the trauma of initial contacts with services by offering early home-based or in-patient treatment in high-quality youth-sensitive settings
- providing integrated treatments with low-dose atypical antipsychotics and phase-specific cognitive–behavioural treatments
- focusing on functional recovery and adaptation through psychosocial recovery programmes
- addressing comorbidity (e.g. cannabis dependence, depression, suicidality) early through specific cognitive–behavioural interventions
- addressing treatment refractoriness early through graded treatment protocols and cognitive–behavioural interventions for positive symptoms
- ensuring that carers are offered a range of services early, including psycho-education about psychosis, carer support groups, family intervention and access to services for unwell family members

5 Prevent relapse after the first episode of psychosis by:
- ensuring assertive follow-up and psychoeducation during the critical period (the first 3 years)
- providing relapse-prevention counselling and advice about long-term management

6 Plan for continuing needs and onwards care pathways by:
- recommending appropriate follow-up services, depending on need and risk
- brokering collaborative arrangements with clinically adjacent services to open care pathways before needed
- ensuring smooth transition of care and communication between early-intervention services and appropriate follow-on services, with co-working in the overlap

(Initiative to Reduce the Impact of Schizophrenia, 2000)

Prevention and Intervention Centre (EPPIC) this group can be limited to just 6% (Edwards *et al*, 1998). This may in part be due to the early identification of those at highest risk and targeting them with specific interventions such as psychosis-focused CBT and clozapine to improve treatment response (Edwards *et al*, 2004). This is possible as early as 3 months into treatment, when at least 19% of individuals in their first episode will still be experiencing positive symptoms (Edwards *et al*, 2002). Individuals with treatment-refractory psychosis commonly have complex needs with particularly difficult histories of poor premorbid functioning and educational achievement, social exclusion, early substance use, violence, long duration of untreated psychosis, contact with police and probation services, and established patterns of disengagement from help. Clinical experience suggests that they are at especially high risk of drop-out and relapse, and rapidly develop chronic treatment resistance, cognitive deficits and social disability. It is a major challenge for services to reverse this deteriorating course and successfully engage this group of young adults early (particularly in deprived inner-city areas) in youth-sensitive psychosocial programmes promoting well-being and independent functioning as well as targeting treatment-refractory symptoms. Whether an early-intervention service can better address this group's needs remains untested. It is possible that involvement in intensive rehabilitation services may prove the best option for some.

Putting the principles into practice

Types of early-intervention service

No two early-intervention services look the same. Over the past two decades a rich variety of early-intervention service models have emerged (Box 9.5; Edwards & McGorry, 2002; Johannessen, 2004), which between them carry an international consensus of the clinical and organisational processes involved in achieving a fully functioning early-intervention service (Box 9.6). Most early-intervention programmes have arisen out of adult services stretching down into the older-adolescent group. A smaller minority are youth-based, with upper age limits reaching up into the younger-adult age-group. Which of these many configurations (Box 9.6) is more effective remains unclear and is the focus of several UK national research projects: Evaluating the Development and Impact of Early Intervention Services (EDEN) in the West Midlands, the First Episode Research Network (FERN) and the London Development Centre's Early Intervention Research Network's MiData study. In the meantime, it is important that service commissioners and providers resist the temptation to choose the cheapest early-intervention option as a way of fulfilling NHS targets. There is no clarity concerning the necessary 'dose effect' for early intervention, but choosing the lowest will almost certainly fail to have any real impact.

Box 9.5 Principles guiding the development of early-intervention practice

1 *Early detection and assessment of frank psychosis*
   This will require auditing pathways to care and collaboration between primary and secondary care and a willingness to work with diagnostic uncertainty

2 *Early and sustained keyworker engagement*
   Allocation of a keyworker as early as possible to develop engagement and rapport and to stay with the individual and their family throughout the critical period, preferably within an assertive outreach model

3 *A comprehensive, collaborative and shared assessment plan*
   An assessment plan should be drawn up that is both comprehensive and collaborative and driven by the needs and preferences of the individual and their family

4 *Dual approach of low-dose pharmacotherapy and psychosocial interventions*
   Management of acute psychosis should include low-dose, atypical antipsychotic medication, cognitive therapy for positive symptoms and family interventions

5 *A family approach*
   Family and friends should be actively involved in the engagement, assessment, treatment and recovery process

6 *Relapse prevention*
   Relapse prevention and treatment resistance strategies should be implemented, embracing vulnerability factors, prophylaxis and early detection of relapse

7 *Access to work and valued occupation*
   A strategy to facilitate pathways to training, work and valued occupation should be developed

8 *Assessment of basic needs of everyday living*
   Care plans should address the basic needs of everyday living, ensuring that housing, money and practical support needs are met and regularly reviewed

9 *Assessment and treatment of comorbid problems*
   Interventions should include the assessment and management of comorbid problems, including substance misuse, depression and suicidal thinking

10 *Public education strategy*
   A local strategy to promote a positive image of psychosis, emphasising its treatability, the production of youth-friendly education materials (e.g. *Getting Back on Your Feet*, Jackson & Reading, 2004) and encourage awareness of how and where to seek help

   (Derived from Initiative to Reduce the Impact of Schizophrenia, 2000)

The state of play

Most early-intervention services focus on the youth age-group (16- to 25-year-olds), providing assertive outreach and psychosocial recovery and relapse prevention programmes via designated early-intervention clinicians with small case-loads (typically 12–15 per full-time case manager) (Edwards & McGorry, 2002; Bywaters *et al*, 2004). Standard mental health

Box 9.6 Models of early-intervention services

Option 1
Services based in:
- the community, hospital services or both
- child and adolescent mental health services
- adult mental health services
- primary care
- youth services
- research institutions

Option 2 Specialist v. generic service model
Specialist early-intervention services:
- stand-alone service
- hub-and-spoke model
- piggy-back supplementary model
- tertiary consultation services/clinic
Generic-based services:
- top up with embedded early-intervention worker/s
- top up with early-intervention training and clinical guidelines
Research-based interventions:
- time-limited trials of interventions/programmes in any of above settings

Option 3: Non-mental health programmes
- Public health promotion campaigns
- Early-intervention initiatives within social services, education, employment, housing, alcohol and drug services, service user agencies

services are usually the first point of contact and assessment for new referrals. Well-developed early-intervention services have unequivocally demonstrated that it is possible to substantially reduce the duration of untreated psychosis, for example from 114 to 17 weeks in the Norwegian TIPS (Early Identification and Treatment of Psychosis) project (Larsen *et al*, 2000). However, in the UK at present, designated in-patient services for people with first-episode psychosis are rare, as are early-detection teams and prodrome services. Even rarer are the major public health education programmes that made TIPS so successful. Consequently, most current early-intervention services have little capacity to effect early detection and reduce duration of untreated psychosis. Their main focus is on recovery and relapse prevention. However, for those services that do genuinely target duration of untreated psychosis the effect will be to gradually bring down the average age of their client population and increase the need for a good working relationship with adolescent services.

Many psychosis early-intervention programmes are selective, recruiting only those with non-affective disorders and excluding certain comorbid conditions such as learning disability. Many more are unintentionally selective because of the manner in which they depend on referrals from standard mental health services (as evidenced by their throughput, which represents only a fraction of people presenting in their first episode of psychosis). The length of follow-up by early-intervention services varies from 18 months (EPPIC) to 5 years (North Birmingham early intervention service). Commonly, new early-intervention services take several years to evolve clear discharge policies, putting them at risk of saturation as case-loads gradually increase and they struggle to liaise effectively with continuing care and rehabilitation services.

By the end of 2004, over half of the NHS trusts in the UK had set up early-intervention teams (Pinfold *et al*, 2006). The Department of Health (2001) presented a model service for which central funding was provided, but in reality not always fully funded or delivered at the local level. Rethink and IRIS have supported these new developments with guidelines and an accompanying toolkit (Initiative to Reduce the Impact of Schizophrenia, 2000), and have set bold health outcome targets for early intervention summarised in the Early Psychosis Declaration (World Health Organization & International Early Psychosis Association, 2004). Regional networks of early-intervention services have emerged across the UK, coordinated through the National Institute for Mental Health in England's (NIMHE's) eight development centres and supported by a NIMHE/Rethink National Early Intervention Programme. There are also expanding first-episode service and research networks such as those of the London Development Centre and FERN. These networks not only provide considerable support for new teams and encourage good practice models, they are also a valuable resource for comparisons between different service models, which in time may give much-needed evidence to guide early-intervention practice. Health education programmes and training materials are better developed in longer-standing overseas services such as EPPIC and the British Columbia Schizophrenia Society, but there is steady growth in very useful UK publications (e.g. Jackson & Reading, 2004), web-based support (Box 9.7) and innovative health education programmes (Warner, 2005). Box 9.7 also shows online addresses for many of the organisations mentioned here.

Steps towards effective prevention of psychosis

In any one individual, the final process in the pathway to psychosis may be highly dependent on the chance accumulation of myriad factors over time. There is considerable interest in understanding and potentially intervening to interrupt this sequence of events and consequences. The supportive research foundations for early intervention include just such pathway analysis and there is hope that better understanding of risk factors for psychosis will open up a major opportunity for public health education and progressively more ambitious preventive strategies. For example, in response to renewed concern over the link between cannabis and psychosis Henquet *et al* (2005) concluded that 'cannabis use moderately increases

---

Box 9.7 Web-based addresses of early-intervention networks, associations and related support organisations

Early-intervention networks and associations
- British Columbia Schizophrenia Society at http://www.bcss.org
- Early Psychosis Prevention and Intervention Centre (EPPIC, Melbourne) at http://www.eppic.org.au
- First Episode Research Network (FERN, England) at http://www.fernonline.org
- International Early Psychosis Association (IEPA) at http://www.iepa.org.au
- London early intervention services and research networks, follow links for mental health at the London Development Centre website: http://www.londondevelopmentcentre.org

UK-related support organisations websites
- Initiative to Reduce the Impact of Schizophrenia (IRIS) at http://www.iris-initiative.org.uk
- National Early Intervention Programme: follow links from http://www.rethink.org/about_mental_illness/early_intervention
- Rethink at http://www.rethink.org
- Support and Training for Elation and Depression in Youth (Steady) at http://www.steady.org.uk
- YoungMinds at http://www.youngminds.org.uk

---

the risk of psychotic symptoms in young people but has a much stronger effect in those with a predisposition to psychosis'. They reported that cannabis use from adolescence into adulthood quadruples the likelihood of psychosis. These findings have been sufficiently concerning to become front-page news, and have prompted the UK government to reconsider drugs legislation (Frean, 2005). An evidence-based public health message might be 'If schizophrenia runs in your family, then don't use cannabis – it's likely trigger the same in you'.

As the markers for those at highest risk become more refined, there is hope that very early detection and intervention could reduce the progression to psychosis. Several studies are currently testing whether CBT and/or low-dose antipsychotic medication offered to individuals at ultra-high risk of psychosis can reduce the risk of subsequent psychosis as well as ameliorate prodromal symptoms. Two such trials have already reported very promising results. The Personal Assessment and Crisis Evaluation (PACE) study in Melbourne (McGorry *et al*, 2002) showed a reduction in the risk of first-episode psychosis from 35% to 10% while in treatment with low-dose atypical antipsychotics and CBT, but the benefits disappeared when the treatment was withdrawn. Morrison *et al* (2004) demonstrated that almost the same lowered conversion rate to psychosis (12%) could be achieved with CBT alone in a similar group of patients.

So far, these studies have been conducted in relatively small selected samples of people at high risk of psychosis, willing to seek help. Whether their findings can be generalised across the broader at-risk group remains to be seen. None the less, the implications of these results are considerable and could significantly change the landscape in which future rehabilitation services will operate. Such targeted public health preventive strategies may reduce the overall local incidence or even the severity of psychosis, thereby reducing subsequent demands on continuing care and rehabilitation services. They may also help de-stigmatise these illnesses and encourage people and families to be better informed from the start and more receptive to earlier rehabilitative interventions.

Implications for rehabilitation services

The recommendation that rehabilitation should begin at first contact contrasts with the reality that referrals to rehabilitation services often happen when individuals have exhausted the therapeutic hope and energy of the service they are in. Early intervention offers a clinical philosophy and approach that is equally applicable to raising standards in psychiatric rehabilitation services, indeed in all mental health services.

Early intervention and rehabilitation hold much in common. They both have a guiding emphasis on recovery, social inclusion, hope and the value of psychosocial therapies. In fact, several flagship early-intervention services, for example EPPIC and the North Birmingham early-intervention services, emerged from in-patient adult rehabilitation and recovery units.

By providing strategies for early detection, early-intervention services inevitably draw in a small number of patients who otherwise might never have attended mental health services. Assertive follow-up by early-intervention services similarly maintains engagement with patients who might otherwise have been lost by standard services. These factors might well increase the throughput of new patients in the first years of treatment. However, countering this increase are the benefits of early-intervention services in reducing initial admission rates (Power et al, 2004), improving recovery rates (Garety et al, 2006) and preventing relapse (Craig et al, 2004). There is hope that these early gains will improve the long-term trajectory and life experience of people with psychosis and reduce demands on continuing care and rehabilitation services.

The shift towards early intervention has other implications. The focus on youth is likely to identify a younger population for whom rehabilitation services are critical to recovery and independence (Lloyd et al, 2000). This may challenge rehabilitation services to become more youth friendly and sensitive to family perspectives. The educational content of rehabilitation programmes may need to be enhanced and vocational programmes attuned to youth culture. Drug use and risk behaviours common in young people present particular challenges, especially for residential and day-programme services attempting to accommodate younger patients with complex needs.

The culture within early-intervention services that adopts the language and style of collaborative decision-making and encourages patients and carers to be better informed about care and treatment options is consistent with recovery-based practice. Assertive outreach, home treatment, CBT and greater carer involvement all place heavy burdens on staff. Furthermore, patients and carers who have experienced such approaches may carry greater expectations with them when they move into established services. Better-informed patients and their carers will present challenges to services but also an opportunity for a richer and more sophisticated exchange of ideas for staff to draw on when designing treatment programmes.

It is similarly important for early-intervention services to avoid an inappropriately optimistic idealism and to acknowledge that a proportion of patients (10%) will need continuing care and rehabilitative support. These individuals should be identified early, and pathways to rehabilitation services negotiated to avoid unhelpful delay. This group will require sustained long-term intervention, family support, supported accommodation and daytime activities, and specialist interventions such as CBT for positive and negative symptoms, cognitive remediation programmes and clozapine. Early intervention is not an single 'injection' that sustains functioning and outcomes throughout life (Linszen *et al*, 2001). It is particularly important to plan carefully how these clients will move from early-intervention to rehabilitation services, so that the focus is maintained on recovery and long-term optimal functioning, the risk of relapse is minimised and healthy relations with carers are sustained. Many of these difficulties can be overcome and services enhanced if there are joint training and staff development opportunities.

Can early-intervention and rehabilitation services work together?

The words of Samuel Tuke that opened this chapter point to the heritage shared by rehabilitation and early-intervention services. Both service models are concerned with integrating a more holistic approach to individuals' care and treatment for psychosis so that their best chances of recovery can be realised. Both services have much to learn from each other's expertise. There could be mutual and creative benefits to patients, carers, staff and services if they were brought into neighbourly relations as part of a family of services for psychosis, mirroring the natural history of the disorder. Without losing their distinctive phase-specific emphasis or altering case-loads, staff could benefit from shared training, joint management, staff rotations, education, supervision, shared resources and effective communication and liaison.

Better integration and dovetailing of early-intervention and rehabilitation services clearly presents challenges. But as with many initial interface issues between services, obstacles quickly evaporate in the context of a common purpose and a focus on the patient's best interests. Leadership is crucial to this end.

A common aim: recovery

'…can't get a job, can't get a girlfriend, can't get a telly, can't get nothing … it's just everything falls down into a big pit and you can't get out.'

(service user, cited in Hirschfeld *et al*, 2005)

Many of the factors that influence the mental well-being of people with emerging psychosis lie outside the traditional remit of health and social care. Respect for the person, everyday interactions, family life, social relationships, leisure, satisfactory accommodation, sufficient finances and meaningful occupation are as important as therapeutic/symptom change. Equally, raising awareness, tackling stigma and discrimination, providing equal access to opportunities and addressing cultural factors are vital in promoting successful community inclusion. These aspirations are embodied in the 2002 Newcastle Declaration and subsequent international Early Psychosis Declaration (World Health Organization & International Early Psychosis Association, 2004) and are strongly represented in user-led recovery literature (see Roberts & Wolfson, Chapter 2, and Perkins, Chapter 8, this volume). Social inclusion, engagement and offering not just an abstract or sentimental hope of recovery but practical means to do so are the cornerstones of both early intervention and rehabilitation. They share Johannessen's (2004: p. 331) perspective that 'The growing understanding of psychosis as something that develops gradually, in phases or stages, and which is therefore possible to prevent, delay, modify and reverse, has serious implications for how we structure our services'.

We are in a process of revitalising old structures and creating new ones. New services cannot prosper in isolation and established ones will wither if cut off from the lifeblood of innovation and challenge. Early intervention in first-episode psychosis is emerging not only as the aim of specific new services but as a quality standard for psychosis services as a whole. Indeed, what criteria would guide us to think 'late intervention' a good idea? Many philosophical, clinical and operational concerns are held in common by early-intervention and rehabilitation services, which implies benefits in cultivating mutually supportive relationships. There is a continuing and shared challenge to develop the partnerships between health, social, educational and employment services needed to realise the goal of offering relevant, accessible and effective programmes for young people with serious mental illness. It is a challenge that both rehabilitation and early-intervention services must work on together if they are truly to effect recovery and improve the lives of all people experiencing psychosis and those caring for them.

References

Almond, S., Knapp, M., Francois, C., *et al* (2004) Relapse in schizophrenia: costs, clinical outcomes and quality of life. *British Journal of Psychiatry*, **184**, 346–351.

Birchwood, M. (2002) *Keynote Address: Development of Comprehensive Early Intervention Services in the UK*. International Early Psychosis Association 3rd International Conference on Early Psychosis, Copenhagen, Denmark. Victoria: IEPA. http://www.iepa.org.au/conference/past.cfm

Birchwood, M., Todd, P. & Jackson, C. (1998) Early intervention in psychosis. The critical period hypothesis. *British Journal of Psychiatry*, **172** (suppl. 33), 53–59.

Bywaters, J., Birchwood, M., Shiers, D., *et al* (2004) Early intervention in psychosis in the UK: a radical plan for nationwide service reform. In *Best Care in Early Psychosis Intervention: Global Perspectives* (eds T. Ehmann, G. W. MacEwan & W. G. Honer), pp. 109–118. London: Taylor & Francis

Cameron, D. E. (1938) Early schizophrenia. *American Journal of Psychiatry*, **95**, 567–578.

Ciompi, L. (1980) Catamnestic long-term outcome studies on the course of life of schizophrenics. *Schizophrenia Bulletin*, **6**, 606–618.

Craig, T., Garety, P., Power, P., *et al* (2004) The Lambeth Early Onset (LEO) team: randomised controlled trial of the effectiveness of specialised care for early psychosis. *BMJ*, **329**, 1067–1070.

Department of Health (1998) *Modernising Mental Health Services: Safe, Sound and Supportive* London: TSO (The Stationery Office).

Department of Health (1999) *National Service Framework for Mental Health: Modern Standards and Service Models*. London: Department of Health.

Department of Health (2000) *The NHS Plan: A Plan for Investment, a Plan for Reform* (Cm 4818–I). London: TSO (The Stationery Office).

Department of Health (2001) *The Mental Health Policy Implementation Guide*. London: Department of Health.

Department of Health (2002) *Improvement, Expansion and Reform – The Next 3 Years: Priorities and Planning Framework 2003–2006*. London: Department of Health.

Department of Health (2004) *The National Services Framework for Children, Young People and Maternity Services: The Mental Health and Psychological Wellbeing of Children and Young People*. London: Department of Health.

Eaton, W., Thara, R., Federman, E., *et al* (1998) Remission and relapse in schizophrenia. The Madras longitudinal study. *Journal of Nervous and Mental Disease*, **186**, 357–363.

Edwards, J. & McGorry, P. (2002) *Implementing Early Psychosis Services in Psychosis: A Guide to Establishing Early Psychosis Services*. London: Martin Dunitz.

Edwards, J., Maude, D., McGorry, P. D., *et al* (1998) Prolonged recovery in first-episode psychosis. *British Journal of Psychiatry*, **172** (suppl. 33), 107–116.

Edwards, J., Maude, D., Herrmann-Doig, T., *et al* (2002) A service response to prolonged recovery in early psychosis. *Psychiatric Services*, **53**, 1067–1069.

Edwards, J., Wade, D., Herrmann-Doig, T., *et al* (2004) Psychological treatment of persistent positive symptoms in young people with first-episode psychosis. In *Psychological Interventions in Early Psychosis: A Practical Treatment Handbook* (eds J. Gleeson & P. D. McGorry), pp. 191–208. London: John Wiley & Sons.

Frean, A. (2005) Cannabis dangers prompt review of 'soft' law. *The Times*, 19 March, p. 1.

Gaebel, W., Jaenner, M., Frommann, N., *et al* (2002) First vs multiple episode schizophrenia: two-year outcome of intermittent and maintenance medication strategies. *Schizophrenia Research*, **53**, 145–159.

Garety, P. & Rigg, A. (2001) Early psychosis in the inner city: a survey to inform service planning. *Social Psychiatry and Psychiatric Epidemiology*, **36**, 537–544.

Garety P. A. Craig, T. K. J., Dunn, G., *et al* (2006) Specialised care for early psychosis: symptoms, social functioning and patient satisfaction. Randomised controlled trial. *British Journal of Psychiatry*, **188**, 37–45.

Harding, C. M., Brooks, G. W., Asolaga, T., *et al* (1987) The Vermont longitudinal study of persons with severe mental illness. 1: Methodological study sample and overall status 32 years later. *American Journal of Psychiatry*, **144**, 718–726.

Harrison, G., Hopper, K., Craig, T., *et al* (2001) Recovery from psychotic illness: a 15- and 25-year international follow-up study. *British Journal of Psychiatry*, **178**, 506–517.

Henquet, C., Krabbendam, L., Spauwen, J., *et al* (2005) Prospective cohort study of cannabis use, predisposition for psychosis, and psychotic symptoms in young people. *BMJ*, **330**, 11–14.

Hirschfeld, R., Smith, J., Trower, P., *et al* (2005) What do psychotic experiences mean for young men? A qualitative investigation. *Psychology and Psychotherapy: Theory, Research and Practice*, **78**, 249–270.

Initiative to Reduce the Impact of Schizophrenia (2000) *Early Intervention in Psychosis: Clinical Guidelines and Service Frameworks*. Birmingham: West Midlands Partnership for Mental Health.

Jackson, A., Cavanagh, J. & Scott, J. (2003) A systematic review of manic and depressive prodromes. *Journal of Affective Disorders*, **74**, 209–217.

Jackson, C. & Reading, B. (2004) *Getting Back on Your Feet: Understanding and Recovering from Psychosis*. Birmingham: Birmingham Early Intervention Service. Available from: BEIS, Harry Watton House, 97 Church Lane, Aston, Birmingham, UK.

Jager, M., Hintermayr, M., Bottlender, R., *et al* (2003) Course and outcome of first admitted patients with acute and transient psychotic disorders (ICD–10: F23). Focuses on relapses and social adjustment. *European Archives of Psychiatry and Clinical Neuroscience*, **253**, 209–215.

Johannessen, J. O. (2004) The development of early intervention services. In *Models of Madness: Psychological, Social and Biological Approaches to Schizophrenia* (eds J. Read, L. Mosher & R. Bentall), pp. 319–334. London: Brunner-Routledge.

Kraepelin, E. (1896) Dementia praecox. Reprinted (1987) in *The Clinical Roots of the Schizophrenia Concept* (eds J. Cutting & M. Shepherd), pp. 13–24. Cambridge: Cambridge University Press.

Larsen, T. K., Johannessen, J. O., McGlashan, T., *et al* (2000) Can duration of untreated psychosis be reduced? In *Early Intervention in Psychosis: A Guide to Concepts, Evidence and Interventions* (eds M. Birchwood, D. Fowler & C. Jackson), pp. 143–165. London: John Wiley & Sons.

Lieberman, J. (1999) Is schizophrenia a neurodegenerative disorder: a clinical and pathophysiological perspective. *Biological Psychiatry*, **46**, 729–739.

Lieberman, J., Jody, D., Geisler, S., *et al* (1993) Time course and biologic correlates of treatment response in first-episode schizophrenia. *Archives of General Psychiatry*, **50**, 369–376.

Link, B. & Dohrenwend, B. P. (1980) Formulation of hypotheses about the ratio of untreated to treated cases in the true prevalence studies of functional psychiatric disorders in adults in the United States. In *Mental Illness in the United States: Epidemiological Estimates* (eds B. Link, B. P. Dohrenwend, B. S. Dohrenwend, *et al*), pp. 13–148). New York: Praeger.

Linszen, D., Dingemans, P. & Lenior, P. (2001) Early intervention and a five year follow-up in young adults with a short duration of untreated psychosis: ethical implications. *Schizophrenia Research*, **51**, 55–61.

Lloyd, C., Bassett, J. & Samra, P. (2000) Rehabilitation programmes for early psychosis. *British Journal of Occupational Therapy*, **63**, 76–82.

May, R. (2004) Making sense of psychotic experience and working towards recovery. In *Psychological Interventions in Early Psychosis: A Treatment Handbook* (eds J. F. Gleeson & P. D. McGorry), pp. 245–260. Chichester: John Wiley & Sons.

McGorry, P. D., Yung, A. R., Phillips, L. J., *et al* (2002) Randomised controlled trial of interventions designed to reduce the risk of progression to first episode psychosis in a clinical sample with sub-threshold symptoms. *Archives of General Psychiatry*, **59**, 921–928.

Meares, A. (1959) The diagnosis of prepsychotic schizophrenia. *Lancet, i* , 55–59.

Mihalopolous, C., McGorry, P. D. & Carter, R. (1999) Is phase-specific community-oriented treatment of early psychosis an economically viable method of improving outcome. *Acta Psychiatrica Scandinavica,* **100**, 47–55.

Morrison, A. P., French, P., Walford, L., *et al* (2004) Cognitive therapy for the prevention of psychosis in people at ultra-high risk. Randomised controlled trial. *British Journal of Psychiatry,* 185, 291–7.

Mortensen, P. B. & Juel, K. (1993) Mortality and causes of death in first admitted schizophrenic patients. *British Journal of Psychiatry,* **163**, 183–189.

National Institute for Clinical Excellence (2002) *Clinical Guideline 1. Schizophrenia: Core Interventions in the Treatment and Management of Schizophrenia in Primary and Secondary Care.* London: NICE.

Pinfold, V., Smith, J. & Shiers, D. (2006) Audit of early intervention in psychosis service development in England in 2005. *Psychiatric Bulletin,* in press.

Power, P. (2004) Suicide prevention in first episode psychosis. In *Psychological Interventions in Early Psychosis* (eds P. McGorry & J. Gleeson), pp. 175–190. Chichester: John Wiley & Sons.

Power, P., Iacoponi, P., Russell, M., *et al* (2004) A randomised controlled trial of an early detection team in first episode psychosis: provisional findings of the LEO CAT study. *Schizophrenia Research,* **70**, 1 (suppl.), 131.

Robinson, D., Woerner, M., Alvir, J., *et al* (1999) Predictors of relapse following response from a first episode of schizophrenia or schizoaffective disorder. *Archives of General Psychiatry,* **56**, 241–247.

Sullivan, H. S. (1927) The onset of schizophrenia. Reprinted (1994) in *American Journal of Psychiatry,* 151 (suppl. 6), 135–139.

Tuke, S. (1813) *Description of the Retreat.* Reprinted (1996) in facsimile edition (foreword by K. Jones). London: Process Press.

Warner, L. (2005) Fringe benefits: a review of the interactive health education drama programme on first episode psychosis 'On the Edge'. *Mental Health Practice,* **8**(6), 22–24.

Wiersma, D., Nienhuis. F., Sloof, C., *et al* (1998) Natural course of schizophrenic disorders: a 15 year follow-up of a Dutch incidence cohort. *Schizophrenia Bulletin,* **24**, 75–85.

World Health Organization & International Early Psychosis Association (2004) *Early Psychosis Declaration: An International Consensus Statement about Early Intervention and Recovery for Young People with Early Psychosis.* Geneva: WHO/IRIS. http://www.iris-initiative.org.uk/irisdeclaration.pdf

Yung, A., Organ, B. & Harris, M. (2003) Management of early psychosis in a generic adult mental health service. *Australian and New Zealand Journal of Psychiatry,* **37**, 429–436.

CHAPTER 10

Management of medication when treatment is failing

Melinda Sweeting

Even though, as this book demonstrates, pharmacological treatment is but one aspect of an array of strategies for the treatment, care and support of people experiencing major mental illnesses, it plays an essential role. In this chapter I discuss how to assess and then optimise medication management for people with schizophrenia and schizoaffective disorder, the most common conditions resulting in referral to psychiatric rehabilitation services, from the perspective of the clinician taking over responsibility for treatment from the 'acute' mental health services. I focus on people who are identified as 'treatment resistant', i.e. remain significantly symptomatic after standard care, and the practicalities of prescribing clozapine. Readers seeking to increase their understanding of the mechanisms of drug action should consult one of the standard textbooks on psychopharmacology. Stahl (2000), for example, provides an excellent introduction. The Maudsley Prescribing Guidelines (Taylor *et al*, 2005) are a regularly updated guide to practical aspects of prescribing. I have constructed this chapter to address five key issues in medication management: optimising medication, drug choice, adherence, side-effects and the NICE schizophrenia guidelines (National Institute for Clinical Excellence, 2002*a*).

Optimising medication

There are a number of tasks that should be carried out when taking over the care of a person with a psychotic illness who remains actively symptomatic. (Box 10.1.) Before one can conclude that an individual is treatment resistant, it is important to review thoroughly key aspects of treatment. Questions should be asked to assess the person's history and current situation, allowing a discussion with the patient and carers about changes to treatment.

Reviewing the patient's history at this stage allows the clinician both to understand them as a person and to evaluate critically the diagnosis. It is important to consider comorbid or primary disorders that might have been missed, such as an organic mental disorder (e.g. temporal lobe epilepsy) or autistic-spectrum disorder. Equally, one should review the current symptomatology to ensure that treatment is effectively targeting the symptoms that are distressing the patient and their carers. Reviewing the medication history is important: what worked in the past might be effective again now. Also assess adherence to treatment. Finally, evaluate side-effects: the akathisia produced by typical antipsychotics, for example, can be mistaken for agitation requiring increased doses of antipsychotic.

At this point one should be in a position to identify the best treatment options, in terms of both medication and psychological and social

---

Box 10.1 Approaches to the assessment of the patient whose symptoms persist

Review the patient's history
- Are there any unaddressed perpetuating factors?
- Is the diagnosis correct?
- Have organic mental illnesses been excluded?
- Have psychosocial difficulties been addressed?
- What do the patient and carer think?

Review patient's current symptomatology
- Are the primary symptoms psychotic?
- Does the patient have affective symptoms and are they being treated?
- Does the patient have anxiety symptoms and are they being treated?
- Does the patient have any other symptoms?

Review medication history, current use and patient's knowledge
- What has been tried before?
- What worked and what didn't (including doses and why not)?
- What do the notes say?
- What does the patient think?
- What do the carers say?
- If there are other family members with the illness, what treatment did they have and was it successful?
- What medication is the patient taking now? And how was it chosen? (By the patient, carer and/or professional?)

Is the patient adhering to the medication regimen?
- Have blood medication levels been assessed? Simple blood tests to determine levels are readily available for clozapine, olanzapine, valproate, lamotrigine, lithium, carbamazepine, phenytoin and some tricyclic antidepressants
- If the patient is not compliant, why not? Do they have insight? Do they have side-effects from existing medications?

Can side-effects be addressed?
- Is the patient taking as few medications as possible? Are minimum effective doses being prescribed?
- Can they be switched to an alternative antipsychotic to alleviate side-effects?

interventions. It is particularly important to remember that medication is only part of the treatment package. Treatment options should be discussed in as much detail as possible with the patient and any involved carer and this discussion recorded in the case notes (National Institute for Clinical Excellence, 2002a). The better the patient and carers understand the illness and the available treatments, including medication, the more informed their choices can be. Being given choice should increase treatment adherence and encourage the patient on their way to recovery (both in the sense of decreased symptoms and, just as importantly, in gaining autonomy in the management of their illness). Active dialogue about treatment options should, of course, continue even when the individual is being treated under the Mental Health Act 1983.

Medication options

Drugs that have a specific effect on the florid symptoms of psychosis (delusions, hallucinations, thought disorder) have been available since the introduction of chlorpromazine over 50 years ago. Although effective, a major drawback of traditional antipsychotic drugs was their propensity to produce extrapyramidal side-effects (pseudo-parkinsonism, akathisia, dystonia and tardive dyskinesia). The subsequent generation of anti-psychotics, the so-called atypicals, are characterised by an absent or lower potential to produce such side-effects (although other definitions of atypicality are also in use (Taylor *et al*, 2005: p. 16)).

Guidelines on the treatment of schizophrenia published in 2002 by the National Institute for Clinical Excellence (now the National Institute for Health and Clinical Excellence; NICE) recommend that atypical anti-psychotics be used as the first-line treatment. At the time of writing, six atypicals are available for use in the UK: clozapine, amisulpride, risperidone, olanzapine, quetiapine and aripiprazole (it is also argued that sulpiride can be considered an atypical). There is growing evidence that some atypicals are more effective than traditional antipsychotics, not only in the treatment of negative symptoms, but also because they have mood-stabilising effects and possibly improve cognition.

Atypicals as a class continue to have significant side-effects, which differ between drugs. Prescribers should be aware of these and the contemporary expectations on monitoring. Weight gain and impaired glucose tolerance are a particular cause of concern with clozapine, olanzapine and, to a lesser extent, risperidone and quetiapine.

Treatment adherence: the use of depot and other preparations

Medication does not work if the patient does not take it or therapeutic levels are not established. Unfortunately, simple blood tests to determine levels of antipsychotic medication are routinely available only for a few agents. Even in supervised settings people may by subterfuge avoid taking prescribed treatment. Depot medication (using long-acting injectable preparations) should be considered if there is evidence that the individual has an established pattern of non-adherence with oral medication. The advantage of depot is that it is clear whether the medication has been taken or not. Note, though, that there is only modest evidence that prescription of depot antipsychotic preparations improves treatment adherence in the long term. Some patients prefer depot since it relieves them of responsibility for taking medication daily (and provides a reason for regular contact with the services). The choice of drug will depend on individual patient variation and side-effect profile, a detailed discussion of which is beyond the scope of this chapter. It is important to note that the pharmacokinetic properties of depot preparations make frequent dosage alteration irrational.

Risperidone is the only atypical depot preparation available at the time of writing. If depot risperidone is planned, the patient should be established on the oral preparation, and the full drug dose should be maintained for 3–4 weeks after the first injection, to ensure therapeutic plasma levels. Alternatively, cross-titration protocols can be used.

Both risperidone and olanzapine are also available in rapidly dispersing oral preparations that generally assure adherence if nurses are supervising while patients take their medication. Unless the patient has a strong preference, there is no obvious reason to continue to prescribe these preparations if supervision ends.

Managing treatment resistance

The NICE schizophrenia guidelines define treatment-resistant schizo-phrenia as a lack of satisfactory clinical improvement despite the sequential use of the recommended doses for 6–8 weeks of at least two antipsychotics, at least one of which is an atypical (National Institute for Clinical Excellence, 2002a). In practice, it is important to have excluded other factors (as described in 'Optimising medication', above) before concluding that the patient has treatment-resistant schizophrenia. Clozapine is the only anti-psychotic that has robustly demonstrated efficacy in treatment resistance (Davis *et al*, 2003). Although not in its product license, clozapine is also a highly effective antimanic. It would have been very widely used following its introduction in the 1970s were it not for the range and potential severity of its side-effects. The most obvious of these side-effects are neutropenia and agranulocytosis, which initially resulted in its withdrawal from most markets in the world and, on its reintroduction, has mandated close haematological monitoring. With haematological monitoring in place, weight gain and its consequences, impaired glucose tolerance and constipation, are in practice more concerning (although patients are understandably distressed and worried by the requirements for haematological monitoring). Early side-effects include sedation, hypersalivation, hypertension, hypotension, tachycardia, fever and nausea. A combination of tachycardia and fever may indicate myocarditis. Nocturnal enuresis is common and distressing, and seizures a risk at high doses. Other rare but serious side-effects include thromboembolism and cardiomyopathy.

General principles for commencing clozapine

The general eligibility criteria for commencing clozapine are that the patient:

(a) if well, is likely to take oral medication and allow blood tests;
(b) is resistant to other antipsychotics;
(c) if possible, gives consent to taking the drug and understands both the risks and potential benefits associated with it.

Although it is possible to commence clozapine on an out-patient or day-patient basis, for people who have a history of non-adherence or substance misuse, who present a risk to themselves or others or have physical health problems treatment should be started in hospital. Before starting clozapine treatment, it is recommended that the clinician review the patient's medical history, checking in particular that there is no history of significant cardiac problems, seizures, agranulocytosis or active liver disease. The Maudsley prescribing guidelines recommend baseline measurement of full blood count, glucose, HbA_{1c} (glycosylated haemoglobin, type 1c), liver function, pulse, blood pressure, temperature, weight and electrocardiogram (ECG). (These measures relate to documented adverse effects of clozapine.) Unless there is a local system for generic prescribing, the patient must be registered with the Clozaril Patient Monitoring Service.

The Maudsely Prescribing Guidelines (Taylor et al, 2005) provide a titration regimen for in-patient and out-patient initiation of prescribing, the latter being significantly slower and cross-tapered with other selected antipsychotics. The standard in-patient titration regimen results in a dose of 300 mg/day in divided doses after 3 weeks. If dose increases are required beyond 300 mg they should be made in increments of 50 mg a week, with the aim of achieving a trough level of 350–500 µg/l. It is recommended that blood serum levels are measured at 300 mg or earlier if the patient is small, elderly, of East Asian decent, female or a non-smoker, or if treatment non-adherence is suspected. Daily amounts of up to 200 mg may be given in a single dose at night. The current average clozapine dose in the UK is 450 mg/day; doses above 600 mg are significantly more likely to result in fits. Doses that result in plasma levels greater than 1000 µg/l should not be given, because of the risk of seizures.

If using the in-patient titration regimen, on initiating clozapine blood pressure and pulse should be monitored hourly for 6 h. Temperature, blood pressure and pulse should then be taken twice daily (as well as before and after the morning dose) for at least 2 weeks, or until there are no unacceptable adverse effects. Monitoring should continue daily or every other day (depending on the rate of titration) until a stable dose is reached. Thereafter, these parameters should be monitored when blood tests are taken. The Maudsley Prescribing Guidelines (Taylor *et al*, 2005) give recommendations on monitoring using the out-patient titration regimen.

With either regimen, staff should inform the prescriber if:

- the patient's temperature rises above 38°C (although it is important to note that elevated temperatures are common and clozapine does not usually need to be stopped in these situations);
- the pulse rate rises to more than 100 bpm (which is also common, but important, as in rare cases it is linked to myocarditis, a severe side-effect of clozapine);
- there is a postural blood pressure drop of greater than 30 mmHg;
- the patient is clearly oversedated or otherwise distressed by side-effects.

As with a number of other atypical antipsychotics, weight gain is a major problem with clozapine and weight should be regularly monitored. The Maudsley Prescribing Guidelines provide additional recommendations for monitoring the metabolic and cardiac effects of clozapine, and these are regularly updated as the evidence base expands. Much of the skill in using clozapine is in effectively managing its side-effects, which includes supporting the patient who is experiencing them. One of the disadvantages of clozapine is that if there is a break in treatment of over 48 h it must be re-titrated, albeit at a faster rate than for drug-naïve patients. There is also some evidence that a rebound psychosis may occur on abrupt discontinuation of clozapine.

Augmentation strategies: suggestions and what is known

Full benefit from clozapine may take many months to emerge. If a patient continues to have distressing symptoms, even though clozapine is improving their illness, augmenting clozapine with other medications should be considered. When deciding on augmentation options, first consider whether the individual has symptoms that would suggest particular options. For example, for symptoms of mania consider adding a mood stabiliser, and for depression consider an antidepressant. When considering the use of multiple medications, it is important to also to consider the possibility of additional side-effects, pharmacological interactions, compliance and cost-effectiveness.

The literature on augmentation of clozapine is sparse. Options include sulpiride (Shiloh *et al*, 1997), amisulpride (Munro *et al*, 2004) and risperidone (Josiassen *et al*, 2005; Yagcioglu *et al*, 2005). Limited data on aripiprazole indicate that this may also be an augmentation option. There are reasons to avoid olanzapine (which may increase the risk of agranulocytosis) and agents that have a documented effect on QTc interval, for example pimozide, quetiapine and ziprasidone (the last of which is not licensed

151

in the UK). Co-prescription of clozapine and typical antipsychotics is frowned upon except during periods of cross-titration, and data are lacking.

Many people with treatment-resistant psychosis have affective features, and there is some evidence that sodium valproate can be useful as an adjunctive treatment for these (Kando *et al*, 1994). It also has the advantage of being prophylactic against clozapine-induced seizures used at the same doses and therapeutic range as usual. Results on its effect on clozapine levels, however, are conflicting (Taylor, 1997), and there have been reports of acute liver failure (Wirshing *et al*, 1997), sedation and confusion (Costello & Suppes, 1995).

Lithium has been reported to be effective augmentation of clozapine (Small *et al*, 2003) at plasma levels ≥ 0.5 mmol/l, but it should be used with caution. It is important to note that, although lithium increases neutrophil and total white blood cell counts, it does not protect against clozapine-induced agranulocytosis. One case of fatal agranulocytosis and one of treatment resistance to granulocyte/macrophage colony-stimulating factor (GMCSF) have been reported with lithium and clozapine. Lithium has been used to boost white blood cell counts in people with benign ethnic neutropenia (a normal ethnic variation on white blood cell count range), but the Clozaril Patient Monitoring Service provided by Novartis recently devised a lowered blood scale for this group, reducing the need for artificially increasing white blood cells. If using this combination watch for symptoms of lithium toxicity, which can occur with therapeutic lithium levels.

Lamotrigine has also been reported as a useful augmenting agent (Tiihonen *et al*, 2003) at doses of 200 mg/day. Reported side-effects included hypersalivation, asthenia, rash, constipation, ejaculatory dysfunction and failing memory. There has been one case of lamotrigine-associated agranulocytosis reported.

Carbamazepine is not recommended for clozapine augmentation, owing to the reported risk of agranulocytosis, neuroleptic malignant syndrome and lowered clozapine serum levels. Phenytoin should not be used because of the risk of agranulocytosis.

Trials of augmentation with antidepressants are sparse and conflicting. Selective serotonin reuptake inhibitors tend to increase clozapine serum levels and should therefore be used with caution because side-effects may be exacerbated (the exception is citalopram, which is probably therefore the drug of choice in treating comorbid depression).

To date there have been three double-blind randomised trails of the use of fish-oil preparations as augmentation agents. On balance, although doubts remain about the extent of efficacy, it appears that fish oils may be a worthwhile augmentation option (particularly as they are cheap and well tolerated) (Taylor *et al*, 2005). There are some case reports of the safe use of electroconvulsive therapy as an adjunctive agent, although a lengthening of seizures has been noted.

What if clozapine cannot be used?

Some patients are unable to tolerate clozapine or do not show symptomatic improvement after a reasonable trial. Pharmacological options for these individuals are very limited. It is doubtful that atypical antipsychotics in standard doses would be effective alone in treatment-resistant schizophrenia and the practice of 'mega-dosage' therapy using typicals is now discredited. High-dose olanzapine (30–60 mg/day) may be effective, but its use at such doses is off licence and risks cardiac difficulties. Electroconvulsive therapy is the only well-used option, but its effects may be short lived.

Using a combination of non-clozapine atypical antipsychotics to treat patients with treatment-resistant illness intolerant to clozapine is common, despite a very sparse evidence base. Chan & Sweeting (2006) report that combinations using (a) olanzapine with either amisulpride or risperidone or (b) quetiapine with risperidone, which act in theory on different receptor profiles, show improvement in symptoms in the limited data available, have been used frequently and on balance have more data on safety. Initial case reports suggest that aripiprazole combined with non-clozapine atypicals may worsen psychosis. Owing to the lack of data on safety, caution is recommended when combining non-clozapine atypicals.

Adherence issues

Ongoing symptoms may reflect non-adherence to medication regimens rather than true treatment resistance. Adherence is likely to be greater if patients are in control of choices and are aware of the likely benefits and potential side-effects of their medication and treatment options for side-effects. Dolder et al (2003) reviewed the literature on interventions to improve antipsychotic medication adherence. Combinations of educational, behavioural and affective strategies appear to be the most successful in terms of adherence and secondary outcomes (such as symptoms, relapse and admissions).

A meta-analysis by Nosé et al (2003) looking at clinical interventions for treatment non-adherence in psychosis suggests that, at a median follow-up of 6-months, these had more than doubled the likelihood of adherence to psychotropic medications and attendance at scheduled appointments. The interventions included educational sessions, psychotherapeutic approaches and telephone prompts. One well-structured approach is compliance therapy (Kemp et al, 1998), which uses a combination of motivational interviewing and cognitive techniques to encourage individuals to reflect on their illness and the role that psychotropic treatment might play in its management (Box 10.2). (Not all studies of compliance therapy have shown it to be better than non-specific counselling (O'Donnell et al, 2003).)

As stated above, adherence can be monitored by testing blood levels of medication; prescription should aim to minimise side-effects; and depot administration is recommended if non-adherence is a serious concern.

Box 10.2 Principles of compliance therapy

- Symptoms or problems reported by the patient are used as treatment targets
- The therapist openly predicts common misgivings about treatment, e.g. fears of addiction, loss of control, loss of personality. If the patient has any untoward fears, a cognitive approach is used to address them
- Confusion between illness symptoms and side-effects is discussed
- Any other meanings attached to medication are explored
- The natural tendency to stop medication if feeling well is discussed, in combination with an exploration of the patient's views of the consequences
- Indirect benefits of medication are highlighted, e.g. getting on better with other people
- The therapist tries to instil a feeling that poor adherence works against the patient's long-term goals, e.g. sustaining work, avoiding hospital, looking after their children
- Certain metaphors are introduced, e.g. 'medication offers a protective layer', 'medication is an insurance policy'

(After Kemp *et al*, 1998)

Management of side-effects

Side-effects may create a significant burden for patients and affect their attitudes towards their illness, medication adherence, their relationship with staff and carers, and subsequently their prognosis. In the past, inadequate attention was paid to the burden of adverse effects of treatment, and some side-effects were ignored completely (e.g. the effects of antipsychotics and antidepressants on sexual functioning). One obvious and important strategy when prescribing antipsychotics is to use the minimum effective dose. Standard psychopharmacology textbooks such as Stahl (2000) and Taylor *et al* (2005) provide accounts of the side-effect profiles of medications in common use; the latter also contains an extended discussion of side-effect management. The greatest concerns used to relate to the extrapyramidal effects of typical antipsychotics and the rare but potentially fatal neuroleptic malignant syndrome. However, now that atypicals dominate the market, concern has shifted to the health impact of weight gain, impaired glucose tolerance and the rare occurrences of sudden death on antipsychotics, which is generally thought to be related to ventricular arrhythmia.

People with schizophrenia have an increased risk of dying from cardio-vascular disorders, which is significantly contributed to by smoking and obesity. Weight gain is particularly associated with clozapine and olanzapine and less likely with amisulpride, ziprasidone and aripiprazole. A small volume of literature examining behavioural interventions to reduce weight gain has shown some positive results. It is important that patients are warned about the risks when started on antipsychotics, that weight is monitored and that dietetic advice is available.

Owing to worries about potential cardiac and metabolic side-effects, clinical practice is moving towards routine monitoring of ECGs (particularly when dosages are high) and glucose metabolism in patients taking anti-psychotics over the long term. More immediately relevant to the prescriber of clozapine are the array of common annoying effects associated with its complex pharmacology, such as constipation (often requiring treatment with laxatives), sialorrhoea (treated with hyoscine) and enuresis (which responds to desmopressin). Sedation is distressing and may be managed by careful adjustment of the timing of doses.

The NICE schizophrenia guidelines

The National Institute for Health and Clinical Excellence is responsible for making recommendations about the treatments to be provided within the National Health Service in England. It has published a number of documents on psychosis and its treatment, including clinical guidelines on the treatment of schizophrenia and a technology appraisal on the use of atypical antipsychotics (respectively National Institute for Clinical Excellence, 2002a,b). All practitioners in England need to be aware of NICE recommendations and should deviate from them only if they have a good reason.

The NICE schizophrenia guidelines (National Institute for Clinical Excellence, 2002a) make recommendations for social, psychological and pharmacological management. In terms of drug treatment two sets of recommendations are pertinent. First, what should be prescribed. There is a strong preference for use of atypicals, a steer towards the early use of clozapine if other medications have failed and the suggestion that depot medication be considered where adherence is an issue. It is highly likely that as the evidence base expands these recommendations will require modification. Second, the guidelines set out how prescribing should be undertaken. Here the emphasis is on offering the patient and carers a say in prescribing decisions, with the aim that decisions are made by the patient as an informed choice. Discussions with patients and carers are to be documented in case notes, information is to be provided and advance directives should be encouraged and followed. This represents a major and probably irreversible paradigm shift in the treatment of psychosis. It is fully in line with the overall theme of this book, which focuses on the individual with a major mental illness as an active participant in the management of their illness and their individual process of recovery rather than the passive recipient of treatment.

Conclusions

People coming into psychiatric rehabilitation services have generally responded poorly or incompletely to pharmacological treatments for their psychotic illnesses and may experience a significant burden of side-effects. Careful attention to detail, including assessment of adherence to treatment, optimising standard treatments and judicious use of adjunctive strategies, can result in marked symptomatic improvement. It is important for rehabilitation practitioners to remain aware of advances in pharmacological treatment and take an evidence-based approach. It is recommended that prescribers venturing into prescribing where there is a poor evidence base should seek a second opinion.

References

Chan, J. & Sweeting, M. (2006) Combination therapy with non-clozapine atypical antipsychotic medication: a review of current evidence. *Journal of Psychopharmacology*, in press.

Costello, L. E. & Suppes, T. (1995) A clinically significant interaction between clozapine and valproate. *Journal of Clinical Psychopharmacology*, **15**, 139–141.

Davis, J. M., Chen, N. & Glick, I. D. (2003) A meta-analysis of the efficacy of second-generation antipsychotics. *Archives of General Psychiatry*, **60**, 553–564.

Dolder, C. R., Lacro, J. P., Leckband, S., *et al* (2003) Interventions to improve antipsychotic medication adherence: review of recent literature. *Journal of Clinical Psychopharmacology*, **23**, 389–399.

Josiassen, R.C., Joseph, A., Kohegyi, E., *et al* (2005) Clozapine augmented with risperidone in the treatment of schizophrenia: a randomized, double-blind, placebo-controlled trial. *American Journal of Psychiatry*, **162**, 130–136.

Kando, J. C., Tohen, M., Castillo, J., *et al* (1994) Concurrent use of clozapine and valproate in affective and psychotic disorders. *Journal of Clinical Psychiatry*, **55**, 255–257.

Kemp, R., Kirov, G., Everitt, B., (1998) Randomised controlled trial of compliance therapy. 18-month follow-up. *British Journal of Psychiatry*, **172**, 413–419.

Munro, J., Matthiasson, P., Osborne, S., *et al* (2004) Amisulpride augmentation of clozapine: an open non-randomized study in patients with schizophrenia partially responsive to clozapine. *Acta Psychiatrica Scandinavica*, **110**, 292–298.

National Institute for Clinical Excellence (2002a) *Clinical Guideline 1. Schizophrenia: Core Interventions in the Treatment and Management of Schizophrenia in Primary and Secondary Care*. London: NICE.

National Institute for Clinical Excellence (2002b) *Schizophrenia – Atypical Antipsychotics. The Clinical Effectiveness and Cost Effectiveness of Newer Atypical Antipsychotic Drugs for Schizophrenia* (Technology Appraisal 43). London: NICE.

Nosé, M., Barbui, C., Gray, R., *et al* (2003) Clinical interventions for treatment non-adherence in psychosis: meta-analysis. *British Journal of Psychiatry*, **183**, 197–206.

O'Donnell, C., Donohoe, G., Sharkey, L., *et al* (2003) Compliance therapy: a randomised controlled trial in schizophrenia. *BMJ*, **327**, 834–836.

Shiloh, R., Zemishlany, Z., Aizenberg, D., *et al* (1997) Sulpiride augmentation in people with schizophrenia partially responsive to clozapine. A double-blind, placebo-controlled study. *British Journal of Psychiatry*, **171**, 569–573.

Small, J. G., Klapper, M. H., Malloy, F. W., *et al* (2003) Tolerability and efficacy of clozapine combined with lithium in schizophrenia and schizoaffective disorder. *Journal of Clinical Psychopharmacology*, **23**, 223–228.

Stahl, S. M. (2000) *Essential Psychopharmacology: Neuroscientific Basis and Practical Applications*. Cambridge: Cambridge University Press.

Taylor, D. (1997) Pharmacokinetic interaction involving clozapine. *British Journal of Psychiatry*, **171**, 109–112.

Taylor, D., Paton, C. & Kerwin, R. (2005) *The Maudsley 2005–2006 Prescribing Guidelines* (8th edn). London: Taylor & Francis.

Tiihonen, J., Hallikainen, T., Ryynanen, O. P., *et al* (2003) Lamotrigine in treatment-resistant schizophrenia: a randomized placebo-controlled crossover trial. *Biological Psychiatry*, **54**, 1241–1248.

Wirshing, W. C., Ames, D., Bisheff, S., *et al* (1997) Hepatic encephalopathy associated with combined clozapine and divalproex. *Journal of Clinical Psychopharmacology*, **17**, 120–121.

Yagcioglu, A. E., Akdede, B. B., Turgut, T. I., *et al* (2005) A double-blind controlled study of adjunctive treatment with risperidone in schizophrenic patients partially responsive to clozapine: efficacy and safety. *Journal of Clinical Psychiatry*, **66**, 63–72.

CHAPTER 11

Family interventions

Gráinne Fadden

The changing face of mental health provision in recent years has resulted in a greater recognition and acceptance of the key role played by family and social networks in the recovery of those who experience mental health difficulties. The development of community-based treatments and teams with specific functions such as assertive outreach and home treatment ('functionalised teams') means that contact is improved with people who are significant in the lives of individuals who access mental health services. Whereas it was easy for staff in residential psychiatric rehabilitation units to be unaware of the social supports in the lives of residents, care in the community now ensures that contact with family and friends of those using services is more likely to happen as a matter of course during home visits. The social context in which service users live is also likely to be much more visible to clinicians.

This poses issues, however, for those whose initial professional training has not prepared them for a new way of working, focusing on family and community rather than the individual. Offering services in the community involves more than changing the geography of service provision. It involves a genuine shift in thinking that recognises the importance of family, community networks, and cultural and kinship relationships. Post-qualification training has not kept pace with the fundamental changes in attitude required for this shift away from models of care in which the prime focus is the individual with the mental health difficulty. Because of this, clinicians can feel ill-equipped to work in these extended ways, and can perceive the involvement of family and friends as threatening to the long-established culture, models and processes of mental health services.

Research evidence – necessary but not sufficient for change

It is interesting that, despite the emphasis in recent years on evidence-based practice, the existence of a strong body of evidence relating to a particular topic will not in itself change practice if the change required fundamentally challenges existing models and ways of working. This is clear from the research relating to the impact on families of coping with mental health difficulties, and also the effectiveness of psychoeducational interventions.

Following the introduction of community care policies in the 1950s and the subsequent closure of large psychiatric institutions, more attention was paid to the impact on family members of supporting a relative with mental health difficulties at home. By the 1970s and '80s, there was a clear understanding of the often stressful nature of being in this situation (Creer & Wing, 1974; Fadden et al, 1987). Having a relative with a serious and long-standing mental health problem was shown to have effects on family members' work and financial situation, social relationships, household activities and children. In addition to practical effects, relatives described the emotional impact in terms of stress, a sense of loss and the general strain on family relationships. Many family members experienced mental health problems themselves because of the situation they were in. Relevant for rehabilitation services is the fact that the stress of caring increased over time. Many statutory services and voluntary agencies set up support groups for family members, but there was no fundamental change in the way mental health services were delivered to ensure that the needs of families were met.

In the 1980s, a number of research studies were published describing the outcomes of randomised controlled trials that clearly demonstrated the effectiveness of psychoeducational family interventions in terms of reductions in relapse rates and hospitalisations (Falloon et al, 1982; Leff et al, 1982; Tarrier et al, 1988). These used similar approaches emphasising factors such as the provision of information to families, encouraging effective communication among family members and helping families to develop practical ways of dealing with difficulties they faced. The efficacy of this type of approach has been confirmed by numerous studies since these early trials, and positive outcomes have been confirmed in meta-analyses of research (Mari et al, 2006). More recent reviews conclude that psycho-educational family interventions are essential to schizophrenia treatment (Pitschel-Walz et al, 2001), should be available to the majority of people who have schizophrenia (Bustillo et al, 2001) and should be offered to people with schizophrenia who are in contact with carers (Pilling et al, 2002). It was clear, however, that in spite of the evidence supporting these approaches, they were not routinely available in clinical practice (Fadden, 1997). The reasons for this will be discussed later in this chapter.

Policy – an effective driver

Over the past 10 years, the rights of family members and those in caring roles have been recognised in government policy (Department of Health, 1996, 2005). This legislation has emphasised the needs of those who provide regular and substantial care and required local authorities to

---

Box 11.1   National Service Framework – the carers' standard

'Standard six: caring about carers
All individuals who provide regular and substantial care for a person on CPA should:
- have an assessment of their caring, physical and mental health needs repeated on at least an annual basis
- have their own written care plan which is given to them and implemented in discussion with them'

(Department of Health, 1999: p. 69)

---

provide services for carers. One of the most significant factors supporting the rights of carers was the publication of the National Service Framework for Mental Health (Department of Health, 1999), which gives carers the right to have their own assessment and care plan (Box 11.1). The associated policy implementation guide (Department of Health, 2002) offers guidance on how mental health carer support services can be developed and sustained.

The National Institute for Clinical Excellence (now the National Institute for Health and Clinical Excellence, NICE) has published very clear guidelines on the provision of family interventions as a core treatment in the management of schizophrenia in primary and secondary care (Box 11.2). Services will be measured on how well these guidelines are implemented. The latest government White Paper on community services (Department of Health, 2006: pp. 123–124) highlights once again the importance of family members, and draws attention to the special needs of young carers. In addition to telephone helplines and respite support for families, the government is committed to the creation of an Expert Carers Programme that will ensure that those in caring roles have the skills they need 'to

---

Box 11.2   NICE guidelines on the treatment of schizophrenia – family interventions standard

'Family interventions to be offered to 100% of families of individuals with schizophrenia who have experienced a recent relapse, are considered to be 'at risk' of relapsing, or who have persisting symptoms, and are living with or in close contact with their family. All individuals who receive family interventions should be offered more than 10 sessions, the course of treatment lasting for more than 6 months.'

(National Institute for Clinical Excellence, 2002: p. 54)

---

take greater control over their own health, and the health of those in their care'.

Policy is now forcing a change in terms of the attention paid to the needs of families. In the past, it was possible for services to play down or ignore the research, but managers and clinicians now recognise that they must consider the needs of families and others who are important in the social networks of service users. Although this gives rise to many questions about how it can be done most effectively with the resources available, the positive side is that these issues are now being considered and confronted.

Current practice in family interventions

Many clinicians who received their training some time ago are influenced by early concepts associated with family work, such as the notion of 'expressed emotion'. There is often a lack of appreciation of how much the field of family work has moved on and developed in recent years. Literal interpretation of concepts developed for research purposes, such as the description of family members as being 'overinvolved', are not helpful in clinical settings, do not reflect a comprehensive understanding of the social context, and are often perceived as judgemental and critical by family members. For most families, the idea of not being closely involved when a close relative is experiencing difficulties would seem counter-intuitive. In our current multicultural society, Western concepts such as this do not reflect the diversity of network relationships in different cultural groups. In many cultural communities, close involvement of extended family is the norm when one individual is experiencing difficulties, and anything other than this would be considered unacceptable.

The position of families in services has changed over the years. Now, with the more widespread availability of different sources of information, particularly via the internet, families are better informed and are able to articulate their concerns. They can request the information that will allow them to make informed choices in relation to treatment. This highlights issues surrounding the sharing of information and the complexity of the whole area of confidentiality, including the rights of family members to confidentiality. Differing responsibilities to family members and to service users are therefore very pertinent. Family members need to be given time and space on their own to discuss issues.

Models of working with families is a topic of current debate: how can different approaches, such as systemic and psychoeducational, complement each other to meet the needs of families in the most comprehensive manner? The recovery paradigm influences the way in which clinicians work with service users, and the concept of recovery is important for families too. They can be traumatised by coping with odd behaviour, by their contacts with services, and worn down by years of caring. This is a developing field, and it is important for anyone involved in psychiatric rehabilitation services to keep abreast of developments.

Principles, concepts and content of family work

A number of principles are core to current family work practice and these are outlined in the following sections.

A genuinely positive attitude towards families

This includes acknowledgement of their contribution to the recovery of their relative and recognition of the impact that their loved one's experiences has on their lives. There is no place in modern mental health services for the critical, hostile, patronising or labelling approaches towards families that were commonplace in the past. These were simplistic attitudes based on limited knowledge of the family, who often were seen only at times when they were under severe stress. Now, the essence of good practice in family work is the establishment of collaborative working relationships. This requires clinicians to take account of the entire family and social situation, and of the many demands that are placed on family members, rather than seeing the situation simply from one perspective. Obviously, it is preferable for families to be involved from the earliest stages of contact with services. If positive relationships are developed with families in early intervention services, we may see far fewer people in rehabilitation services who have become alienated from their families.

Acknowledgement of the family's skill and expertise

Linked with having a positive attitude towards families is the idea of recognising that the family will have gained an extensive range of skills through their experience of dealing with mental health difficulties around the clock over a number of years. Staff from statutory and voluntary agencies bring different kinds of expertise to the situation. Together, they can establish a collaborative working relationship that capitalises on this combined knowledge and expertise.

Understanding the intention behind the action

The capacity of the family to be supportive is influenced by a range of factors – their experiences in their own family of origin, current and previous stressors and pressures, and the many demands in their life, for example having a son with psychosis and elderly parents to look after at the same time. In the absence of advice or training in how to respond to the unfamiliar behaviour common in the context of mental health problems, they may act in ways that appear unhelpful to the person who is experiencing difficulties. Mental health staff need to look beyond the actions of the family to explore their intentions and what they were trying to achieve. In most situations, families will explain that they felt their particular action would help their relative in their recovery. For example, a mother may be criticised in services for getting a bath ready for her adult son and ensuring he has clean clothes to put on afterwards. In talking to her, however, she is likely to report that she felt this might motivate him to get up and look for a job. It is likely that most families will use whatever strategies they can to assist a family member who is experiencing difficulties. If their efforts are not effective, this is usually because they have not been given advice by professionals on the best ways of responding in particular situations, and have to discover what works best through a process of trial and error.

Every family has its own culture

This principle applies to people from all cultural backgrounds. The concept of talking about broad groups, for example, 'Asian families' or 'single-parent families', belies the diversity that exists within groups. Although there may be some features common to a particular cultural group, every family within it has its own unique way of functioning. Those involved in family work need to respect how the family members manage their lives and to work with the family to bring about the changes that they feel would be beneficial. Adhering to the principle of respect for the unique way of functioning of each family means that those delivering services do not necessarily need to be from the same cultural background as the family they are working with.

Content of family work

The core content of psychoeducational family interventions is outlined in Box 11.3. The essential elements that were described when these approaches were developed remain central (Fadden, 1998). These include the emphasis on communication skills and strategies to deal with current

---

Box 11.3 Content of psychoeducational family interventions

- Establishment of a positive, respectful, collaborative working relationship between the family and the clinician
- Agreement that the service user and key family members will meet together with the clinician
- Information-sharing and an agreement about confidentiality
- Time and space for discussion of emotional issues and personal reactions to the mental health problem and its management
- Support for family members in the achievement of personal goals
- Focus on the management of practical day-to-day issues
- Enhancement of family problem-solving skills
- Agreement on relapse prevention strategies
- Development of effective communication patterns
- Agreement on the ongoing nature of the relationship between the family and mental health services

---

difficulties. As this way of working with families has developed over time, there has been a shift in relation to information-sharing. When some of these family approaches were first described, the focus was on professionals providing information to families, suggesting a one-way exchange or that professionals had more expertise than the family. There is now a greater recognition of the knowledge and skills of the service user and their family in relation to their own recovery.

There is now also greater emphasis on the need for time to process the emotional reactions different family members have to their experiences, including their feelings towards professionals in relation to the availability or absence of different treatment approaches, and the nature of the contact that service users and family members have with services. Some of these experiences can be as traumatic as the actual experience of mental health difficulties. For example, many families describe the trauma of seeing a son, daughter, husband or wife taken away in handcuffs and compulsorily admitted to hospital under a section of the Mental Health Act. Others talk of the stress of attending ward rounds and having to discuss family matters in front of a large group of professionals, many of whom have not even been introduced to them. Numerous accounts by family members can be read on the Rethink (http://www.rethink.org/get_involved/join_us/your_voice.html) and Meriden Family Programme (http://www.meridenfamilyprogramme.com) websites. The Partners in Care resource pack is also an excellent source of material (McClure, 2005).

When first provided, services to families were often disjointed, but it is now recognised that all elements of the service need to work together if the needs of the family and the service user are to be met. There is little point in agreeing a relapse prevention plan with a family if people in the services involved, including out-of-hours services, are not clear about their responsibilities should the person experience a recurrence of their difficulties.

Adapting approaches for families with varied needs

Although services for families and awareness of their needs have improved in recent years, particularly in the light of policy developments, there are still several areas in which needs are not being met in a comprehensive manner. Many children support parents who have ongoing mental health problems, but they are less likely than adults to receive support in their own right. It is often unclear who is responsible for addressing their needs. Staff in adult psychiatric rehabilitation services frequently feel ill-equipped to provide services to children, and child and adolescent services will not see these children because they are not perceived as having problems that would warrant a referral to them. The result is that children in this situation, who often take on substantial responsibilities that are not age-appropriate, such as monitoring a parent's medication, do not receive help and support.

Great sensitivity is required in adapting family approaches for young children in a caring role or where the family situation is complex. For example, it can be difficult for a child to acknowledge that they have seen early warning signs of relapse if this may result in the parent being hospitalised and the children taken into care. If parents have separated, concerns about breaches of confidentiality may stop staff from keeping one parent informed of what is happening when the other parent is admitted to hospital.

The needs of children in such situations are increasingly being recognised. Issues such as the availability of appropriate facilities for them to visit parents or other relatives on in-patient units are being addressed. *Patients as Parents* (Royal College of Psychiatrists, 2002) is helpful in prompting clinicians to reflect on their awareness of the needs of children whose parents are receiving services. The Children's Society, through its Young Carers Initiative, which is funded by the Department of Health, has created a useful database of young carers' projects in the UK (http://www.childrenssociety.org.uk/youngcarers). Innovative projects aimed at bringing together children in these situations provide hope that services to young people who find themselves in caring roles will become more widespread. Examples of such an initiative are described in *Being Seen and Heard* (Cooklyn, 2004), a training video released as part of the Royal College of Psychiatrists' Partners in Care Campaign, launched in 2004 (http://www.partnersincare.co.uk).

The close family of people receiving treatment from forensic rehabilitation services (see Davies & Abbot, Chapter 25, this volume) also have special requirements, and services are as yet underdeveloped to meet these (MacInnes, 2000). In addition to the difficulties experienced by the families of individuals in mainstream mental health services, they often have additional stresses such as living far from the forensic unit, the double stigma of the mental illness and the crime that was committed, and the fact that frequently the crime has been committed within the family. They can be exposed to violence, and often receive less support from other family members, friends and professionals. Carrying out family work in these circumstances requires effort and imagination in overcoming the many obstacles, such as restrictions on leave outside of the unit and lack of family-friendly facilities within units. This is emotionally demanding work, and staff conducting family work in these settings need to be well-trained, have appropriate supervisory structures in place and the opportunity to co-work (work in pairs).

I have already mentioned the issue of culture, and the needs of families from Black and minority ethnic groups require special attention. Stigma and the effects of racism affect family members as well as service users. Awareness of different cultural models is essential. For example, the concept of 'carer' is not meaningful in some cultures, and rehabilitation staff must appreciate the role of kinship networks and the obligations of the extended family. Translation and interpretation services are essential to work with families from diverse cultures, as are the use of a variety of media – video and audiotapes, local radio – and working through community groups.

Problems with routine implementation

Despite evidence and Department of Health policies, many services for people with long-term mental health problems struggle to ensure that the needs of families are met. This is because of a range of factors, many of which are historical. The ethos and culture of adult mental health services has for the most part been focused narrowly on meeting the needs of patients. This has been reinforced by the predominance of biological models of mental health difficulties and the emphasis on physical treatments. It is reflected in all aspects of the system, with paperwork and recording systems frequently ignoring individuals' families; for example, there will be nowhere to record family work, whether the individual has children or whether family members have been offered any services. Service settings frequently have no facilities for family work or rooms large enough for a group of people to meet comfortably. Although this is less of an issue with the development of community-based teams that provide cover 24 hours a day, 365 days a year, some services still operate a 9.00–5.00, Monday–Friday service, which makes family work difficult.

One of the big issues is in relation to the training and confidence of staff in adult mental health and rehabilitation services offering support to families. Training in the skills needed to work with families is inadequate on all professional training courses. It is striking that in an extensive multiprofessional training programme being run in the West Midlands of England, where 2200 people have been trained in family-work skills, 72% of

---

Box 11.4   Difficulties encountered by staff ($n = 208$) in implementation of family work 24 months after training

- 'Integration of family work with other demands of my case-load'
- 'Allowance of time by the service to do the intervention'
- 'Work with families using other models'
- 'Integration of family work with my own personal commitments, e.g. own family'
- 'Availability of appropriate clients and families'
- 'Engagement of clients and their families'
- 'Long-term commitment to the family that is required in this type of work'
- 'Keeping family discussions on track in meetings with them'
- 'Clash of family work with other clinical needs of the client or family'
- 'Clash of family sessions with crises with other clients on my case-load'

(Fadden *et al*, 2004)

those undertaking the training report that before entering the programme they had received no training in family work either at undergraduate or postgraduate level (Fadden & Birchwood, 2002). It is not surprising, therefore, that implementation of family work following brief training is not good. Studies of staff who have attended training courses typically indicate that about a third of those trained do not work with families at all following training, that the majority work with one or two families and that only a small proportion integrate it into their day-to-day practice (Fadden, 1997; Brooker et al, 2003). The most common implementation difficulties that staff described in the West Midlands study (Fadden et al, 2004) are listed in Box 11.4. There is now a clear recognition that the effective implementation of family work requires a systems approach, in which the issue is addressed at an organisational level with close involvement of management and those charged with operationalising services (Smith & Velleman, 2002; Fadden et al, 2004; Kelly & Newstead, 2004). In the absence of this focus on organisational issues, it is unlikely that the culture will change, or that those trained will be able to put their newly acquired skills into practice.

Integration of different family support services

A range of agencies are involved in the provision of support to families. These include key statutory health and social services agencies, and voluntary groups. Various educational programmes are in place for carers, and the UK government has recently provided funding for 700 'carer support workers' to be employed to help support the development of services for carers. A current issue is the coordination and integration of all these services to ensure that the varying needs of individual families are met. In many services, various initiatives to support families are conducted in a piecemeal fashion, with one part of the service being unaware of what is happening in other areas. Consequently, some family members have access to a range of services, whereas others have access to none – not even basic information. There is often a lack of clarity between health and social services in relation to who has responsibility for ensuring that National Service Framework Standard six assessments (Box 11.1; Department of Health, 1999: p. 69) are carried out, and completion of the assessments is emphasised rather than implementation of the associated care plan. Much work needs to be done to ensure that services to families are comprehensive and integrated, and to ensure that no one who needs support slips through the net.

Key challenges

A measure of how much services to families have yet to develop is the fact that numerous complaints to mental health services come from family members. It is also the case that carers' assessments are not taking place and that many family members have not had the opportunity to agree their own care plans. There is lack of clarity about the role of carer support workers, or indeed how many of the 700 for whom funding was agreed have been employed. It is not clear either whether the training of new types of worker is up to date with current paradigms such as the recovery model or the value of working with families. New models for service provision such as functionalised teams have not necessarily resulted in better services to families. Although the specifications indicate that they should offer services to families, many staff who lack confidence in family work and/or who have many competing work demands revert to traditional ways of working that emphasise services only for the people with mental health problems, ignoring their supportive social network and the centrality of these networks in their lives. There are still many situations where the family is seen as a resource when it is expedient, but later is excluded from services or blamed for being overprotective. The complexity of social relationships is often not taken into account.

The challenge now is to encourage clinicians to embrace family work as a fulfilling, challenging and rewarding aspect of their work. They need to move away from the idea of doing the minimum required for families (e.g. informing them about carer support groups, providing information leaflets) and from being anxious about what will happen if they explore new ways of working with families – the fear of 'opening a can of worms'. They need to grapple with the complexity of confidentiality issues and reflect on how they can respect confidentiality, yet ensure that the needs of family members are met. A change in culture is needed: staff must understand the spirit of family work, in which families are seen as genuine partners to whom they have responsibilities as they do towards individuals with mental health difficulties, and they should see working with families as a natural part of their work with these individuals.

References

Brooker, C., Saul, C., Robinson, J., *et al* (2003) Is training in psychosocial interventions worthwhile? Report of a psychosocial intervention trainee follow-up study. *International Journal of Nursing Studies*, **40**, 731–747.

Bustillo, J. R., Lauriello, J., Horan, W. P., *et al* (2001) The psychological treatment of schizophrenia: an update. *American Journal of Psychiatry*, **158**, 163–175.

Cooklyn, A. (2004) *Being Seen and Heard* (video/DVD and CD–ROM). London: Gaskell.

Creer, C. & Wing, J. K. (1974). *Schizophrenia at Home*. Surbiton: National Schizophrenia Fellowship.

Department of Health (1996) *Carers (Recognition and Services) Act 1995: Policy Guidance*. London: Department of Health.

Department of Health (1999) *National Service Framework for Mental Health: Modern Standards and Service Models*. London: Department of Health.

Department of Health (2002) *Developing Services for Carers and Families of People with Mental Illness*. London: Department of Health.

Department of Health (2005) *Carers and Disabled Children Act 2000 and Carers (Equal Opportunities) Act 2004 Combined Policy Guidance*. London: Department of Health. http://www.dh.gov.uk/assetRoot/04/11/78/66/04117866.pdf

Department of Health (2006) *Our Health, Our care, Our Say: A New Direction for Community Health Services*. London: Department of Health.

Fadden, G. (1997) Implementation of family interventions in routine clinical practice: a major cause for concern. *Journal of Mental Health*, **6**, 599–612.

Fadden, G. (1998) Family intervention. In *Serious Mental Health Problems in the Community* (eds C. Brooker & J. Repper), pp. 159–183. London: Ballière Tindall.

Fadden, G & Birchwood, M. (2002) British models for expanding family psychoeducation in routine practice. In *Family Interventions in Mental Illness: International Perspectives* (eds H. P. Lefley & D. L. Johnson), 25–41. Westport, CT: Praeger.

Fadden, G., Bebbington, P. & Kuipers, L. (1987) Caring and its burdens. A study of the spouses of depressed patients. *British Journal of Psychiatry*, **151**, 660–667.

Fadden, G., Birchwood, M., Jackson, C., *et al* (2004) Psychological therapies: implementation in early intervention services. In *Psychological Interventions in Early Psychosis: A Practical Treatment Handbook* (eds P. McGorry & J. Gleeson), pp. 261–280. Chichester: John Wiley & Sons.

Falloon, I. R. H., Boyd, J. L., McGill, C. W., *et al* (1982) Family management in the prevention of exacerbations of schizophrenia: a controlled study. *New England Journal of Medicine*, **306**, 1437–1440.

Kelly, M. & Newstead, L. (2004) Family intervention in routine practice: it is possible! *Journal of Psychiatric and Mental Health Nursing*, **11**, 64–72.

Leff, J., Kuipers, L., Berkowitz, R., *et al* (1982) A controlled trial of social intervention in the families of schizophrenic patients. *British Journal of Psychiatry*, **141**, 121–134.

MacInnes, D. (2000) Relatives and informal caregivers. In *Forensic Mental Health Nursing: Current Approaches* (eds C. Chaloner & M. Coffey), pp. 208–231. Oxford: Blackwell.

Mari, J. J., Pharoah, F. M., Rathbone, J., *et al* (2006) Family intervention for those with schizophrenia. *Cochrane Database of Systematic Reviews*, issue 1. Chichester: Wiley InterScience.

McClure, M. (2005) *Partners in Care Training Resource*. London: Gaskell.

National Institute for Clinical Excellence (2002) *Clinical Guideline 1. Schizophrenia: Core Interventions in the Treatment and Management of Schizophrenia in Primary and Secondary Care*. London: NICE.

Pilling, S., Bebbington, P., Kuipers, E., *et al* (2002) Psychological treatments in schizophrenia. I: Meta-analysis of family intervention and cognitive behaviour therapy. *Psychological Medicine*, **32**, 763–782.

Pitschel-Walz, G., Leucht, S., Bäuml, J., *et al* (2001) The effect of family interventions on relapse and rehospitalisation in schizophrenia – a meta-analysis. *Schizophrenia Bulletin*, **27**, 73–92.

Royal College of Psychiatrists (2002) *Patients as Parents: Addressing the Needs, Including the Safety, of Children Whose Parents Have Mental Illness* (Council Report CR105). London: Royal College of Psychiatrists

Smith, G. & Velleman, R. (2002) Maintaining a family work for psychosis service by recognising and addressing the barriers to implementation. *Journal of Mental Health*, **11**, 471–179.

Tarrier, M., Barrowclough, C., Vaughn, C., *et al* (1988) The community management of schizophrenia. A controlled trial of a behavioural intervention with families to reduce relapse. *British Journal of Psychiatry*, **153**, 532–542.

CHAPTER 12

Cognitive–behavioural therapy

Douglas Turkington and Renuka Arjundas

Schizophrenia is the most debilitating of psychiatric disorders. The illness course can be variable but usually manifests as periodic relapses or as chronic global deterioration. About half of people treated for schizophrenia relapse within the first 2 years (Mason *et al*, 1996). The illness can lead to long-term impairment in personal, social and occupational functioning. Although about 20% recover with treatment, a significant number are left socially isolated and unemployed, leading to poor outcome.

Antipsychotic medications remain the first-line treatment for schizophrenia, but symptom improvement is dependent on adherence to long-term medication usage. Poor adherence to medication regimens is common in people with schizophrenia. The reasons for this could include drug side-effects, impaired insight or disengagement with services because of disease-associated stigma. About 40% of patients in any treatment setting will continue to exhibit residual positive and negative symptoms. It is this group of people who could benefit from a concerted effort at rehabilitation that includes an effective psychological treatment such as cognitive–behavioural therapy (CBT).

Although originally developed for depression, CBT has been applied and studied in people with schizophrenia. The CBT approach for schizophrenia stresses the importance of understanding and coping with the symptoms of the illness. Central to this approach is the establishment of a link between the individual's thoughts, feelings and behaviours with respect to these symptoms and the re-evaluation of symptom-related thoughts and beliefs.

Over 50 years ago Beck (1952) described the successful treatment of a patient with delusions using a cognitive–behavioural approach. Since then, a number of studies, including randomised controlled clinical trials (Kuipers *et al*, 1997; Tarrier *et al*, 1998; Sensky *et al*, 2000; Turkington *et al*, 2002), have supported the efficacy of CBT in treating drug-resistant psychotic symptoms in schizophrenia. Reviews by Pilling *et al* (2002) and the National Institute for Clinical Excellence (2002) (now the National Institute for Health and Clinical Excellence, NICE) of randomised controlled trials conclude that cognitive–behavioural therapy is effective in symptom improvement in schizophrenia. The review by NICE found evidence that:

- in comparisons with 'standard care', CBT improved symptom reduction, especially for persistent psychotic symptoms
- CBT could help in improving insight and adherence to medication
- CBT for longer than 6 months and in more than 10 sessions showed greater benefit.

Consequently, NICE recommends that CBT be available as a treatment option for people with schizophrenia, particularly those with persisting psychotic symptoms. It further recommends that an adequate course of CBT that can lead to symptomatic improvement should be of more than 6 months duration and consist of more than 10 planned sessions (National Institute for Clinical Excellence, 2002).

Kingdon & Turkington (1994) and Fowler *et al* (1995) have described a process of CBT for schizophrenia that focuses on techniques to enhance engagement and collaboration, develop explanations for symptoms and an individualised formulation. This would be followed by strategies not only to manage specific psychotic symptoms more effectively and modify dysfunctional attitudes that could maintain these symptoms or impair treatment adherence, but also to prevent relapse.

In this chapter, we will describe the process and application of CBT in the treatment of persistent psychotic symptoms in schizophrenia, using two case examples.

Cognitive–behavioural therapy of schizophrenia

The process of therapy is shown in Fig. 12.1. This indicates the stages of therapy and provides a framework within which the therapist could work. However, it is important to remember that for each patient, the approach used is derived from individualised formulation of that person's problems.

Assessment

Assessment is an integral part of therapy and should continue throughout it. Initial assessment consists of a comprehensive problem list that includes both psychotic symptoms and non-psychotic conditions such as depression, anxiety and substance misuse. This enables the therapist to prioritise collaboratively with the patient which problem should be tackled first. Risk factors such as suicidality or harm to others and the level of distress should be taken into account in deciding on priority. Psychosocial factors such as social isolation, occupational status and legal problems that could affect the course of illness and treatment should be explored.

A cognitive assessment should include developing with the individual a shared understanding of their symptoms. This includes examining the antecedents and understanding the symptoms on the basis of the

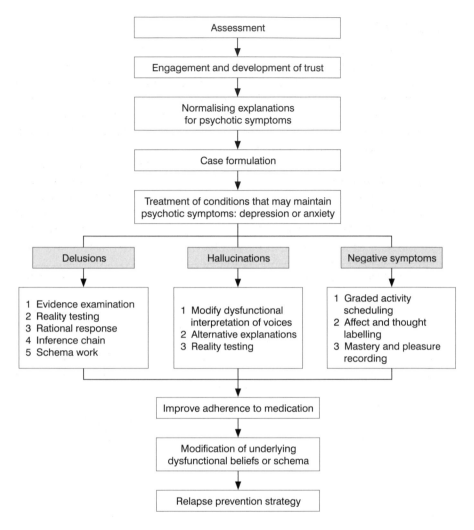

Fig. 12.1 The process of cognitive–behavioural therapy for schizophrenia (adapted from Turkington *et al*, 2004).

assumption that cognitions can influence their emotional, behavioural and physiological aspects. The patient's view of their symptoms and their coping strategies should also be explored.

Attitudes to the illness and medication should be assessed to improve the individual's insight, reduce feelings of stigmatisation and improve treatment adherence. Rating scales such as the Positive and Negative Syndrome Scale (PANSS; Kay *et al*, 1989) or the Psychotic Symptom Rating Scales (PSYRATS; Haddock *et al*, 1999) could be used to assess symptom severity. Encouraging the individual to monitor symptoms in a diary can provide further information.

Engagement

Engagement and the building of trust are important aspects of interaction between therapist and patient. The formation of a good therapeutic alliance that includes empathy, warmth and genuineness are essential in all psychotherapies, particularly so in therapy of people with psychosis. Therapists should have knowledge and experience of working with individuals with psychosis and schizophrenia, and this should come across in their interactions with the patient.

Engagement with people who have schizophrenia can be difficult. Their experience of symptoms such as delusions and hallucinations often elicits reactions of disbelief from others, making them feel discounted and not understood. It is therefore essential that therapists, in their enthusiasm to help them, do not invalidate patients' experiences by confronting their validity. Confrontation can weaken therapeutic alliance and exacerbate delusions by increasing patients' convictions in their delusional beliefs. At the same time, it is important that therapists do not collude with the beliefs.

Confrontation or collusion can be avoided by using a CBT technique called guided discovery. This aims to introduce an element of doubt in the individual's beliefs by an approach of non-judgemental guided questioning and evidence-gathering. Listening actively and empathically, summarising and reflecting what the individual has said, eliciting and responding to feedback from the person at regular intervals and appropriate use of humour all help to enhance engagement.

Engagement is a process that continues throughout therapy. Patients should feel that the therapist is genuinely interested in helping them cope with their problems.

Normalising

Kingdon & Turkington (1991) used a normalising rationale as a key component of their CBT approach in their treatment of people with schizophrenia. Normalising their psychotic symptoms increases the patient's understanding of them, thereby neutralising their catastrophic proportions (dubbed decatastrophising) and reducing the associated distress.

One method of normalising is to educate the individual about the nature of psychotic symptoms by providing information on their occurrence in non-psychotic states (Johns & Van Os, 2001). For example, providing evidence from the literature that hallucinations, illusions and paranoid ideation can occur in people who are sleep deprived could help people with psychosis, who often experience sleep disturbances at the onset of their illness, partly to explain their psychotic symptoms. Similarly, information on the occurrence of auditory hallucinations in the normal population during the transition period between sleep and wakefulness and during sensory deprivation could help patients 'decatastrophise' hallucinations.

Life events or accumulations of stressors (e.g. bullying and pressure of studies) often precede a psychotic episode. Normalising by discussing and providing information on psychological reactions normal to stressful life events can help individuals to understand their illness further. For example, hallucinations occur in normal people in the early stages of bereavement. Patients can be given literature on the common occurrence of hallucinations in Vietnam war veterans (Wilcox *et al*, 1991) and in people who have been sexually abused (Heins *et al*, 1990). Seigal's (1984) work on hallucination in hostages and the personal account of a hostage (Keenan, 1992) can be helpful. This can make patients feel less alienated and more willing to talk about their symptoms and the traumatic events they have experienced.

Exploring the link between their psychotic experiences and stressful events can lead to better understanding of the development of their symptoms. The onset of psychotic symptoms can be understood using the stress–vulnerability model (Zubin & Spring, 1977). According to this model, individuals have a personal threshold of vulnerability (genetic, psychological and social) and when they are exposed to stress that exceeds this threshold they can develop psychotic symptoms.

In addition to improving engagement and therapeutic alliance, normalising also provides a way of working with psychotic symptoms. By being given a number of possible alternative and acceptable explanations for their symptoms, patients might accept them as normal reactions to life stresses rather than signs that they are 'mad'.

The diagnostic label of schizophrenia can be very distressing for the patient. They can feel stigmatised and hold pessimistic views of their prognosis. This distress can be reduced by information on more realistic long-term outcomes of the illness and how adherence to medication and psychological treatments can improve it.

Formulation

Formulation begins during the first contact with the patient and continues throughout therapy. It is an ever-evolving process of hypothesis development, testing and refinement. It is a hypothesis that clarifies the relationship between the individual's problems and their possible origins and effects. Formulation is essential for effective planning of therapy, as it determines the goals of therapy and informs selection of appropriate intervention strategies.

Formulation also helps to predict the patient's response to interventions, understand and manage treatment failure and obstacles to response, and guide relapse prevention. It also helps the patient to gain insight into their psychotic symptoms.

Formulation is derived from cognitive models, which can be generic (Greenberger & Padesky, 1995) or specific to particular symptoms such as delusions and hallucinations (Morrison, 1998; Garety *et al*, 2001). The generic cognitive model describing the link between thoughts, feelings, behaviour and physiological symptoms can be demonstrated to patients by various methods. These include the use of case vignettes, the patient's own non-psychotic and psychotic experiences, and stories and personal disclosure from the therapist (e.g. how the therapist coped with a problem such as making a presentation to a large audience).

The initial information for formulation might include referral letters, case summaries, previous treatments and reasons for seeking treatment. A thorough assessment (see 'Assessment' above) is essential for a case formulation.

Once a formulation is arrived at, it can be offered as an alternative to the patient's explanations for their psychotic symptoms. Both the formulation and the patient's explanations could be put to the test, for example, by the use of behavioural experiments (see 'Reality testing' below).

Formulation can also help the clinician to understand the reasons behind non-adherence to medication regimens and to suggest effective strategies to overcome it.

Interventions for delusions

Delusions are traditionally defined as false, unshakeable beliefs that are not compatible with the individual's cultural and educational background. However, as with normal beliefs, the degree of conviction with which delusions are held can vary with time. Patients with delusions tend to jump to conclusions, ignoring contradictory evidence, and to hold their conclusions with greater conviction than those with normal beliefs (Huq *et al*, 1988). This would suggest that interventions used in cognitive therapy, such as collecting and evaluating the evidence supporting the individual's beliefs, considering alternative explanations and reality testing, could be effective in the management of delusions.

Collaborative empiricism, an approach central to CBT, is particularly useful in working with people with delusions. Here the therapist and patient work together as researchers testing the reality of the patient's explanations for the delusions and alternative explanations to decide on the more plausible among them.

Seven cognitive–behavioural techniques used to treat delusions are described below. These are applied and integrated within the overall framework of treatment of the schizophrenia and are informed by individualised formulation of the patient's problems.

Identification of thoughts or explanations

It is important to explore patients' explanations for the development and maintenance of their delusions in order to build trust and engagement.

Patients' explanations or thoughts can be identified using a thought diary. In this the individual records distressing feelings, the situations in which they occurred and the thoughts experienced at the time. In the early stages, this can be done during sessions, to familiarise the patient with the

175

recording of thoughts. Some people find it difficult to keep such a record, and alternative options include writing in free narrative form, from which the thoughts and feelings can subsequently be identified, or recording thoughts and feelings on audiotape.

The thought diary helps individuals to recognise that it is their interpretation of a situation (i.e. thoughts) that leads to distressing feelings rather than the situation itself.

Patients' behavioural responses to thoughts should also be identified.

Generation of alternative explanations

As people who experience delusions tend to jump to conclusions without considering all possibilities, it would be therapeutically useful to help them appreciate that for every situation that they interpret delusionally there might be a number of alternative explanations.

The therapist encourages the individual to generate as many alternative explanations as possible. Patients themselves might think some of them 'unusual', but should recognise that the therapist is willing to consider all possibilities. The patients rate their degree of belief in the explanations on a scale of 0–100%. Therapist and patient examine in detail the evidence for each of the explanations and the patient then re-rates the original thought. The process can be recorded on a grid such as that shown in the example in Fig. 12.2.

Examination of the evidence

People with delusions tend to ignore evidence contrary to their beliefs. It is therefore essential to examine closely the evidence that they offer and to explore with them all the evidence that disproves it. Sometimes they are unaware that it exists. Therapist and patient can collect contradictory evidence by looking for events or occurrences that are not compatible with the beliefs. The patient can keep a record of these as a log in a diary.

Analysis of the evidence should be sensitive and non-judgemental, to avoid alienating the individual. The therapist should encourage the patient to assess the strength of the evidence supporting their beliefs. Socratic questioning and the process of guided discovery can be used to help patients reach their own conclusions. One way might be for them to decide if the evidence supporting their beliefs is strong enough to lead to a conviction in a court of law. Alternatively, they could be asked how they would react if a friend presented the same evidence to them.

Education

Education, using both verbal and written information, about psychological processes such as cognitive distortions or thinking errors (jumping to conclusions, 'all or nothing' thinking, personalisation and generalisation) can help individuals to recognise how these might play a role in the development and maintenance of their delusional beliefs. This in turn would help them to identify these distortions and challenge their validity.

Thoughts and beliefs worksheet

Situation/trigger	Feelings	Thoughts/beliefs	Belief rate 0–100%	Evidence for belief	Evidence against belief	Re-rated belief 0–100%
I noticed my heart is beating faster	Anxious	I believe my neighbours are controlling my heart with a computer program	90%	My neighbours want to harm me because I have complained about their loud parties Whenever they are in their study, where the computer is, my heart beats faster	I don't know of any computer program that can control my heart from a distance Occasionally, I've noticed my heart beating faster when my neighbours are not around. I've never actually seen them doing it	70%
		Alternative explanations		**Evidence for alternative explanations**	**Evidence against alternative explanations**	
		Anxiety can make my heart beat faster	20%	My friend who suffers from anxiety says that his heart beats fast when he's anxious I've been in situations where I was frightened and I've felt my heart beating fast I'm constantly suspicious about my neighbours' actions, and this could make me anxious	I'm not always anxious and I've noticed a change in my heart beat even when I'm calm	40%
		Physical cause	15%	I have hypertension and it could affect my heart Maybe it's the medicine I take for my blood pressure	I've taken the medicine for many years and this didn't happen before	25%
		I'm going mad	10%	My family don't believe me, they think it is my imagination	They don't understand – after all, what I think does sound unbelievable	10%

Fig. 12.2 Cognitive–behavioural therapy for a delusion using collaborative examination of the evidence for various alternative explanations.

With education, patients could appreciate that delusions fall on the same continuum as suspiciousness, which is quite normal.

In some individuals, delusions are maintained by incomplete knowledge if not profound ignorance about the topic in question. They are therefore prone to misinterpret day-to-day occurrences in the light of their delusions. The therapist's role would be to provide factual knowledge and help correct identified knowledge gaps, with the aim of undermining the delusional belief. For example, many people with delusions involving telepathy, the US Central Intelligence Agency (CIA) or the effects of illicit drugs often have little understanding about them. Offering factual knowledge in an unemotional and practical fashion (rather than trying hard to convince patients that their beliefs are wrong) could reduce their degree of conviction.

Reality testing

Behavioural experiments such as that described in the case illustration in Box 12.1 can be used to test the validity of individuals' delusional beliefs and to provide counter-evidence. The type of experiment used would depend on the formulation of each individual's problems.

In considering a behavioural experiment the therapist should be clear about:

- its rationale: what the patient can learn from it and how it will help
- its plan
- the potential obstacles or difficulties that the patient may face: what could go wrong
- The conclusions that can be drawn from it.

The experiment should be developed as collaboratively as possible. Individuals can experience significant anxiety when carrying out behavioural experiments. Therefore, they are best attempted after patients have gone through the process of examining the evidence for their beliefs and considering alternative explanations.

Coping strategies

People can use various coping strategies to deal with their psychotic symptoms. When effective, these strategies can give them a sense of control over their symptoms, thus empowering them.

A useful coping strategy is to have rational responses to delusional beliefs. Therapists develop these collaboratively with patients after detailed examination of evidence for their delusions. Rational responses introduce doubt into a delusional belief or, if the belief cannot be shaken, 'decatastrophise' the individual's perceived consequences of it.

For example, an individual who has for the past 20 years believed that his neighbours have been conspiring to kill him could develop a rational response as follows: 'They must be pretty stupid! They haven't managed

---

Box 12.1 Testing the validity of a delusion

A 30-year-old woman believed that her face was so ugly that she looked like the Elephant Man. She further believed that her face so repulsed people that when they saw her in a restaurant they felt sick and walked out, leaving their food un-eaten. Consequently, she avoided going to restaurants.

A behavioural experiment was carried out, where the woman visited a restaurant with the therapist. The aim was to test the reality of her belief that she was so repulsive to others that they would leave the restaurant if they saw her. Evidence inconsistent with her belief was being sought.

Before the experiment was conducted the women was asked to rate her belief. She thought it 80% likely that her belief would come true. Evidence supporting her belief was evaluated. Alternative explanations for people not finishing their food and leaving the restaurant after her arrival were also considered, evaluated and rated. For example, they may have had enough to eat or had not liked the food they had ordered.

The woman and the therapist visited a reasonably popular restaurant in their city. Discreetly, both of them counted the number of people in the restaurant when they arrived and the numbers that left and those that entered. This showed that more people came into the restaurant than left it while the woman was there. Some of these people had sat on tables close to her and completed eating their food, obviously unaffected by her. All those who had left when she was in the restaurant had completed eating their food, quite oblivious to her. This provided evidence that was against her belief and served to introduce doubt into it. When asked to re-evaluate after the experiment, her conviction in her belief came down to 50%.

The experiment was repeated a number of times to reinforce the doubt in her belief and provide evidence to refute it.

---

to kill me in 20 years. What have I got to worry about?' These responses could either be written down or audiotaped to be referred (or listened) to in a crisis.

Other coping strategies involve:

- attempts at distraction from symptoms
- relaxation to deal with emotional distress caused by delusions
- the use of additional medication
- keeping busy and engaging in pleasurable activities.

Inference chaining

The aim of inference chaining is to explore the underlying meaning and significance of a delusion to the patient. Since this subconscious association is likely to be responsible for strong emotional reactions in the patient, interventions to modify it may be of benefit. This approach may be used

---

Box 12.2 An example of inference chaining

Patient   'I'm so ugly – I look like the Elephant Man.'
Therapist   'You look very distressed. You believe you are ugly; what does this belief mean to you?'
Patient   'It means that my face repulses people so much that they leave the restaurant when I enter; they feel sick looking at me.'
Therapist   'If it were true that people were repulsed by your face what would that mean to you?'
Patient   'It means that I'm not lovable. That nobody will want to know me and I'll end up being alone for the rest of my life.' (Patient starts to cry.)

Here, the meaning given to the delusional belief had a significant effect on the patient's emotions, and the therapist would next examine with the patient why being unloved held such fears for her.

---

when other techniques are either ineffective or not appropriate. It is usually employed in later stages of therapy. Box 12.2 shows an example of inference chaining using the patient introduced in Box 12.1.

Cognitive therapy for hallucinations

Auditory hallucinations are a common manifestation of psychotic illnesses, particularly schizophrenia. They account for a great level of distress and disability in people with schizophrenia.

There is now greater understanding of the development and maintenance of auditory hallucinations from the cognitive–behavioural perspective. One view is that auditory hallucinations are a result of the individual's tendency to misattribute internal events such as thoughts to an external source (Bentall, 1990). Another is that patients' interpretation of hallucinations (or the meaning given to them) could be responsible for maintaining these hallucinations and the resultant cognitive, affective and behavioural responses. Morrison (1998) has proposed that auditory hallucinations are normal phenomena and it is their misinterpretation that causes distress in the person experiencing them. Thus distressed, the person resorts to a number of safety-seeking behaviours that in turn maintain the interpretation of the hallucinations.

Cognitive–behavioural interventions based on Morrison's hypothesis tend to focus attention on the following:

- evaluation of the contents of the voices
- identification and evaluation of misinterpretations of these voices
- exploring the role of safety-seeking behaviours in the maintenance of the voices.

In the assessment of individuals with auditory hallucinations, it is first essential to determine the frequency, intensity and level of distress associated with the voices and when the individual first started hearing them. Some patients actually benefit from voices (e.g. when benevolent and supportive things are heard) and as the hallucination does not cause distress it is not a target for treatment.

The content of the voices is evaluated and interpreted in a similar manner to that of delusions. The therapist and patient collaboratively investigate the latter's explanations for the voices and generate alternative explanations. The patient's own explanations and the alternatives are evaluated by evidence examination and reality testing with behavioural experiments.

Normalising the patient's voices (as explained above) can help to reduce their belief in dysfunctional catastrophic misinterpretations of them and providing a more acceptable, less extreme rationale.

Cognitive therapy for the residual psychotic symptoms of paranoid schizophrenia is described in the case illustration in Box 12.3.

Box 12.3 Cognitive therapy for psychotic symptoms

Paul, a 30-year-old man with a diagnosis of paranoid schizophrenia, was referred for cognitive therapy for his residual psychotic symptoms. He reported hearing voices. These were predominantly negative in content and perceived as coming from both outside and within his head. The voices occurred several times a day and caused him significant distress.

The content of the voices was dependent on the situation that triggered them. For example, when he saw a child on television or outside his house, the voices would say 'You're a paedophile'; when he saw a Black person, the voices would say 'You're racist'. His appraisal of this experience was that the voices belonged to his neighbours. He did not believe that the voices could be his own thoughts, as he could not possibly think such 'bad' things. He feared that others would come to know about the content of his voices, resulting in unpleasantness. He therefore stayed home as much as possible, and when he did have to go out he would check people's facial expressions for signs of disgust or anger at him. He also attempted to suppress the voices. This resulted in his increased preoccupation with them.

A formulation of Paul's voice-hearing experiences was developed collaboratively with him. This is shown in Fig. 12.3.

An important component of Paul's treatment was informing and educating him about the nature of intrusive thoughts and their prevalence. This was done by giving him information on the normality of intrusive thoughts (Rachman & De Silva, 1978). This showed that most people experience unpleasant, unwanted thoughts and that their content is indistinguishable between people with mental disorders and the general population.

continued

Box 12.3 *continued*

The intervention assumed that Paul misattributed unwanted unpleasant thoughts to an external source to reduce the level of his distress and anxiety at thinking such things. Once Paul learned to recognise that having odd unwanted thoughts is normal in the general population and that the anxiety generated by these thoughts is caused not by the thoughts themselves but by the individual's negative appraisal of them, he could work towards reattributing his voices to his own thoughts.

The hypothesis that the voices Paul was hearing might actually be his own thoughts and not his neighbours' comments was further explored. Self-monitoring of the voices identified triggers that made them more pronounced. These included negative emotional states and behaviour such as attempting to suppress the voices. Education about common triggers for unpleasant thoughts helped Paul recognise that they were similar to his triggers for the voices he experienced. Paul was able to appreciate that the voices he 'heard' could in fact be his own thoughts. This was an important milestone in his therapy. Another milestone was his recognition that trying to suppress thoughts (voices) in fact made them more persistent. This paradoxical effect of suppression of unwanted thoughts on their persistence was demonstrated using Salkovskis & Kirk's (1997) experiment. Paul was asked to imagine a pink polar bear for 60s and then to suppress the thought of the bear for 60s. The image could not be suppressed.

For Paul, another important interpretation of the voices was that others could also hear them. This meant that other people would think he was a paedophile and racist and react to it by beating him. Understandably, Paul avoided leaving home or he checked for people's reactions by staring at their faces, which sometimes caused them to stare back, thus reinforcing his belief that they could hear his voices.

During therapy, Paul's belief that others could hear his voices was evaluated. A behavioural experiment to test this was carried out. Paul was asked to tape himself on an audiotape when he heard the voices, the hypothesis being that if his voices were audible to others they would also be recorded on the tape. Paul recorded himself several times and found that none of his voices could be heard on the tape. This reduced the intensity of his belief.

Together Paul and the therapist formulated the role of Paul's safety-seeking behaviours, such as avoidance and checking people's faces, in maintaining his interpretations of the voices. Paul was able to recognise that, since people around him could not actually hear his voices as he had previously suspected, there might be no danger of them trying to beat him up on the basis of what the voices said. In that case, he was safe and there might be no real reason to avoid contact with others or to check people's faces for angry reactions towards him. He recognised that these were safety-seeking behaviours and that his continued indulgence in them not only made him more preoccupied with his voices but also stopped him from testing the validity of his belief that others could hear them. He was gradually able to drop these behaviours, and the fact that no one reacted with disgust or violence towards him on the street reduced his belief that others could hear his voices.

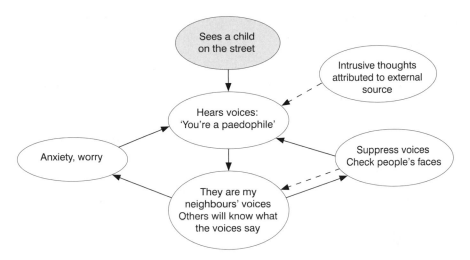

Fig. 12.3 Formulation of Paul's voices.

Negative symptoms

Negative symptoms such as poverty of speech, affective flattening, anhedonia, avolition and attentional impairment are important symptoms of schizophrenia that can adversely affect treatment response and long-term outcome. They can affect the overall functioning of the individual and make rehabilitation difficult. Therefore treating these symptoms is important.

It is essential that other conditions that can mimic negative symptoms or contribute to them be excluded. These are depression, phobias, side-effects of antipsychotic medication, extreme avoidance behaviour as a response to positive symptoms and social/environmental factors. If present, these should be managed first.

Negative symptoms can be tackled with interventions such as activity scheduling to increase activity levels and social skills training to improve social functioning. Alogia and affective blunting may gradually respond to work on affect labelling and automatic thought recognition. These are beyond the scope of this chapter but are described in Kingdon & Turkington (2004). Similarly, the coexistence of thought disorder requires specific CBT techniques (Kingdon & Turkington, 1994).

Modifying underlying beliefs or schemas

Schema-focused interventions are based on examining the validity of dysfunctional core beliefs and assumptions held by the patient. Core beliefs are strongly held beliefs about the self or the world, for example:

'I'm unlovable' and 'The world is dangerous'. Dysfunctional assumptions might include 'I must always succeed to be loved'. These beliefs are thought to have formed and been shaped by early childhood experiences. The individual is not often aware of them.

These beliefs can be identified from recurrent common themes in the person's cognitions or inference chaining (also known as downward arrowing). The chosen interventions are developed from the formulation, and they include techniques such as continuum work, examining the evidence for the beliefs, positive logging and behavioural experimentation to modify extreme beliefs (Padesky, 1994).

Schema-focused interventions are an important part of relapse prevention. Maladaptive beliefs can make a person vulnerable to relapse when exposed to stressful events.

Relapse prevention

Prevention of relapse includes identification of early warning signs, relapse signatures of the illness and potentially stressful events that could trigger symptoms. The therapist and patient together develop a detailed written plan of what the individual could do to maintain the gains achieved during therapy and to monitor early warning signs, and what they should do if they notice early signs of relapse.

The therapist might write a summary detailing all that the patient has learnt during therapy. This should include the formulation of the person's symptoms, particularly their development and maintenance, and interventions such as challenging their beliefs about symptoms, counter-evidence for beliefs and behavioural experiments. The patient can use this for self-therapy and also refer to written material noted down by the therapist during therapy sessions. Patients can also be encouraged to listen to audiotapes of sessions to remind them of and reinforce what was learnt during therapy. Keyworkers or supportive relatives can be involved in helping patients to use self-therapy to maintain their gains or to respond to stressful situations.

Patients should also be given a clear plan of whom to contact in the event of a crisis or the development of early warning signs. The service involved in the patient's care should be aware of the plans.

Conclusions

Cognitive–behavioural therapy of psychotic symptoms helps people make more meaningful sense of their psychotic experiences, enabling them to use adaptive coping strategies that empower them. It also helps in treatment adherence and can be used to complement medical treatment of psychotic symptoms. The comprehensive formulation of patients' problems that is central to CBT enables the integration of other treatments such as social skills training and family therapy as part of a formulation-driven treatment package.

The therapy can be delivered in various rehabilitation settings such as hospital, day care and the community. The therapist and the services involved in the patient's care need to work closely in the various stages of treatment planning and delivery.

Therapists who wish to deliver CBT for schizophrenia need to have basic training in the technique for non-psychotic disorders such as affective and anxiety disorders. They should also have a broad experience of working with people who have psychoses. Active supervision of the therapy and education should be available. Attendance at workshops can also help. Training in CBT should increasingly be made available to rehabilitation psychiatry staff to enhance outcome and promote recovery.

References and further reading

Beck, A. T. (1952) Successful outpatient psychotherapy of a chronic schizophrenic with a delusion based on borrowed guilt. *Psychiatry*, **15**, 305–312.

Bentall, R. P. (1990) The syndromes and symptoms of psychosis: or why you can't play twenty questions with the concept of schizophrenia and hope to win. In *Reconstructing Schizophrenia* (ed. R. P. Bentall), pp. 23–60. London: Routledge.

Fowler, D., Garety, P. & Kuipers, E. (1995) *Cognitive Behaviour Therapy for People with Psychosis: A Clinical Handbook*. Chichester: John Wiley & Sons.

Garety, P., Kuipers, E., Fowler, D., *et al* (2001) Cognitive models of the positive symptoms of psychosis. *Psychological Medicine*, **31**, 189–195.

Greenberger, D. & Padesky, C. (1995) *Mind over Mood*. New York: Guilford.

Haddock, G., McCarron, J., Tarrier, N., *et al* (1999) Scales to measure dimensions of hallucinations and delusions: the Psychotic Symptom Rating Scales (PSYRATS). *Psychological Medicine*, **29**, 879–889.

Heins, T., Gray, A. & Tennant, M. (1990) Persisting hallucinations following childhood sexual abuse. *Australian and New Zealand Journal of Psychiatry*, **24**, 561–565.

Huq, S. F., Garety, P. A. & Helmsley, D. R. (1988) Probabilistic judgements in deluded and non-deluded subjects. *Quarterly Journal of Experimental Psychology*, **40A**, 801–812.

Johns, L. C. & Van Os, J. (2001) The continuity of psychotic experiences in the general population. *Clinical Psychology Review*, **21**, 1125–1141.

Kay, S. R., Opler, L. A. & Lindenmayer, J. P. (1989) The Positive and Negative Syndrome Scale (PANSS): rationale and standardisation. *British Journal of Psychiatry*, **155** (suppl. 7), 59–65.

Keenan, B. (1992) *An Evil Cradling*. London: Arrow.

Kingdon, D. & Turkington, D. (1991) The use of cognitive behaviour therapy with a normalising rationale in schizophrenia: preliminary report. *Journal of Nervous and Mental Disease*, **179**, 207–211.

Kingdon, D. & Turkington, D. (1994) *Cognitive Behavioural Therapy of Schizophrenia*. Hillsdale, NJ: Lawrence A. Earlbaum.

*Kingdon, D. & Turkington, D. (2002) *The Case Study Guide to Cognitive Behaviour Therapy of Psychosis*. Chichester: John Wiley & Sons.

*Kingdon, D. & Turkington, D. (2004) *A Treatment Manual for Cognitive Therapy of Schizophrenia*. New York: Guilford.

Kuipers, E., Garety, P., Fowler, D., *et al* (1997) London–East Anglia randomised controlled trial of cognitive–behavioural therapy for psychosis. 1: Effects of the treatment phase. *British Journal of Psychiatry*, **171**, 319–327.

Mason, P., Harrison, G., Glazebrook, C., Medley, I., & Croudace, T. (1996) The course of schizophrenia over 13 years. A report from the International Study on Schizophrenia (ISoS) coordinated by the World Health Organization. *British Journal of Psychiatry*, **169**, 580–586.

Morrison, A. P. (1998) A cognitive analysis of auditory hallucinations: are voices to schizophrenia what bodily sensations are to panic? *Behavioural and Cognitive Psychotherapy*, **26**, 289–302.

*Morrison, A. P. (2002) *A Casebook of Cognitive Therapy of Psychosis*. Sussex: Brunner-Routledge.

National Institute for Clinical Excellence (2002) *Clinical Guideline 1: Schizophrenia. Core Interventions in the Treatment and Management of Schizophrenia in Primary and Secondary Care.* London: NICE.

Padesky, C. (1994) Schema change processes in cognitive therapy. *Clinical Psychology and Psychotherapy*, **1**, 267–278.

Pilling, S., Bebbington, P., Kuipers, E., *et al* (2002) Psychological treatments in schizophrenia: meta-analysis of family intervention and cognitive behaviour therapy. *Psychological Medicine*, **32**, 763–782.

Rachman, S. J. & De Silva, P. (1978) Abnormal and normal obsessions. *Behaviour Research and Therapy*, **16**, 233–248.

Salkovskis, P. M. & Kirk, J. (1997) Obsessive–compulsive disorder. In *The Science and Practice of Cognitive Behaviour Therapy* (eds D. M. Clark & C. G. Fairburn), pp. 179–208. Oxford: Oxford University Press.

Seigal, R. K. (1984) Hostage hallucinations. *Journal of Nervous and Mental Disease*, **172**, 264–271.

Sensky, T., Turkington, D., Kingdon, D., *et al* (2000) A randomised controlled trial of cognitive–behavioural therapy for persistent symptoms in schizophrenia resistant to medication. *Archives of General Psychiatry*, **57**, 165–172.

Tarrier, N., Yusupoff, L., Kinney, C., *et al* (1998) Randomised controlled trial of intensive cognitive behaviour therapy for patients with chronic schizophrenia. *BMJ*, **317**, 303–307.

Turkington, D., Kingdon, D., Turner, T., *et al* (2002) Effectiveness of a brief cognitive behavioural therapy intervention in the treatment of schizophrenia. *British Journal of Psychiatry*, **180**, 523–527.

Turkington, D., Dudley, R., Warman, D. M. *et al* (2004) Cognitive behavioural therapy for schizophrenia: a review. *Journal of Psychiatric Practice*, **10**, 1–12.

Wilcox, L., Briones, D. & Suess, L. (1991) Auditory hallucinations, post-traumatic stress disorder and ethnicity. *Comprehensive Psychiatry*, **32**, 320–323.

Zubin, J. & Spring, B. (1977) Vulnerability – a new view on schizophrenia. *Journal of Abnormal Psychology*, **86**, 103–126.

*Denotes suggested further reading.

CHAPTER 13

Psychodynamic considerations in rehabilitation

Sarah Davenport

Psychodynamic understanding has influenced rehabilitation practitioners for the past half century, because of the contribution such an understanding can make to longer-term management of mental illness. General mental health settings have adopted a predominantly biological model, and the use of psychodynamic principles outside of psychiatric rehabilitation services or therapeutic communities is relatively limited in the UK. This is not the case elsewhere; psychodynamic understanding has been central to the delivery of most mental healthcare in Scandinavia and within certain traditions in the USA. A review of psychodynamic treatment and the use of antipsychotic medication in Sweden (Cullberg et al, 2002) highlighted the positive impact of intensive psychosocial support on reducing the requirement for medication. The Finnish need-adapted approach (Alanen et al, 1991) requires a psychodynamic overview of the process of care that emphasises intensive individual and family psychosocial support; staff teams also have access to support and supervision. The outcome for individuals receiving care within this system revealed reduced in-patient admissions and reductions in medication usage, associated with improved service user satisfaction. Shepherd (1984) has promoted staff training and supervision to improve interactions between staff and service users in residential settings, thereby improving outcome. National guidance on the treatment of schizophrenia in the UK (National Institute for Clinical Excellence (NICE), 2002) focuses on the provision of psychological treatments such as cognitive–behavioural therapy and family work, for which there is a good evidence base. It also recommends that psychoanalytic and psychodynamic principles be considered to help professionals to understand the experience of individual service users and their interpersonal relationships.

However, not all service users engage with evidence-based approaches, and the alternatives are often psychodynamically informed therapies (Davenport et al, 2000; Van Marle & Holmes 2002).

Psychodynamically informed reflective practice is necessary for professionals working with people who have schizophrenia. Reflective practice and supervision may enable care staff to recognise and manage their own difficult feelings when working closely with people who are very disturbed or distressed over long periods. An awareness of the psychodynamic issues that affect individual patients and those closest to them, including professional carers, helps to overcome factors opposing therapeutic engagement (Davenport, 2002). A psychodynamic understanding of what has happened to each patient and those close to them during childhood and the prodrome to illness informs individual case formulation and comprehensive long-term care planning. A psychodynamic understanding can also make a helpful contribution to risk assessment and management. Helping a service user become more self-aware (or more mindful) can provide important risk information, which then forms the basis of a collaborative risk management plan. Countertransference responses may also be informative, particularly about the risk of violence (or vulnerability), and should be incorporated into risk management planning (Holloway, 2004).

The 2002 Newcastle Early Psychosis Declaration (http://www.rethink. org/newcastledeclaration) encapsulated a vision of mental health services of the future, with a strong focus on psychological understanding for service users and their families and for good psychosocial support. Psychodynamic understanding underpins many of its standards.

Murray Jackson is an Emeritus Consultant Psychiatrist at the Maudsley Hospital, London, and a psychoanalyst with long experience of the treatment and care of people with psychosis. He proposes rights of access to certain psychological approaches for people with psychosis (Box 13.1), all consistent with the Newcastle Declaration. This psychodynamic approach has implications at the level of:

- the individual service user
- the family (and carers)
- the team
- the institution where care is delivered.

It creates an agenda of change that may best be considered at the various levels at which a psychodynamic understanding can make a significant contribution.

Box 13.1 The rights of a person with psychosis

- All individuals with psychoses are entitled to the best possible psychodynamic assessment at the earliest possible opportunity
- They all have the right to be listened to and understood in terms of their past and present life, internal and external reality, and past and present conflicts
- It should be understood that the content of psychotic thinking has informative value, with important implications for the treatment and rehabilitation of people in hospital and the community

(Jackson, 2001)

The individual

Understanding thought disorder

Talking with a person who appears to have florid thought disorder is usually an upsetting experience for the person and the professional; the person may feel isolated and unable to make a meaningful connection with others, while the professional is likely to feel frustrated and unable to get through. Developing an explanatory case formulation based on the patient's history enables more effective attunement to ways of 'being with' the person, reducing arousal and increasing responsive soothing. Picking up and responding to non-verbal or vocal cues may also improve empathic understanding and attunement. Analysis of countertransference responses can lead to the identification of significant themes present in an apparently non-understandable dialogue. These themes commonly involve disempowerment, control or abuse, and neglect. Direct interpretation needs to be carefully judged, but it can be helpful to say something tentative such as 'It sounds as if you expect to be ignored', in an attempt to demonstrate a deeper understanding. Communicating that the person has been heard and is beginning to be understood can be an important step towards engaging people who feel isolated and alienated in their illness. Such psychodynamically informed attempts to engage with a thought-disordered person may also strengthen their self-worth, and reduce alienation and hopelessness.

Individual psychotherapy

The NICE schizophrenia guidelines define cognitive–behavioural therapy as the evidence-based psychological treatment of choice for all people with schizophrenia (National Institute for Clinical Excellence, 2002); however, not all service users can engage with such approaches (see Turkington & Arjundas, Chapter 12, this volume) and some will choose alternatives, where they exist.

Supportive (psychodynamically informed) psychotherapy

This type of therapy should be offered to people with chronic, severe and complex long-term difficulties, within a psychiatric rehabilitation service. It requires a long-term therapeutic relationship and supportive therapy across a variety of different settings, often over different phases and a substantial period of their life. Effective delivery requires a level of psychodynamic awareness from the practitioner to understand what is going on within the therapeutic relationship.

Many multidisciplinary staff (particularly nursing staff) have some psychodynamic understanding, and this could be better utilised. A more formal approach to training and supervision could lead to improved availability of long-term supportive psychotherapy and better practice.

Almost a quarter of a century ago Frank (1982) analysed some of the therapeutic components common to all psychotherapies. He identified some of the therapeutic aims and techniques that comprise supportive therapy; these include 'remoralisation, remediation and rehabilitation' and are just as relevant today. They are reflected in the specification of supportive therapy, which I outline here using a helpful review by Van Marle & Holmes (2002).

The therapeutic aims of supportive therapy are:

- to establish a therapeutic alliance (engage) with the patient; this often requires consideration of psychological or practical barriers to engagement
- to provide psychological holding and containing, including a safe, secure and reliable setting to serve as a structure for the work
- to understand transference and countertransference issues and their effect on the therapeutic relationship (and within the setting or treatment team).

Specific techniques used in supportive therapy include:

- certain types of communication, including empathic validation, praise and advice, affirmation and confrontation
- environmental interventions, which might include seeking help from another professional (e.g. occupational therapist, educational link worker, housing support officer, general practitioner or solicitor), encouraging voluntary work or attendance at a vocational support service
- psychoeducation to promote a better understanding of the nature of the mental disorder, its impact on the individual and its social consequences; early warning sign recognition and relapse prevention plans can be negotiated and incorporated into the therapy
- teaching the individual to recognise defences and promoting adaptive coping techniques, which can gradually improve social function and contribute to reducing social exclusion.

Supportive therapy is a complex and challenging area of work when pursued professionally and with commitment; it should not be left by default to the least experienced members of the rehabilitation team but seen as a core component of long-term care. Staff providing such therapy should be strongly encouraged to seek training, supervision and support; a psychodynamic understanding is essential to the effectiveness of these processes.

Psychodynamic interpersonal therapy: the conversational model

Psychodynamically oriented psychotherapy lacks a substantial evidence base in the treatment of psychosis. Two case studies have been published (Davenport et al, 2000) with independent outcome measures showing that a psychodynamic interpersonal therapy (Hobson, 1985) can be an effective adjunctive therapy in severe psychosis treated in long-term in-patient settings. Both patients had severe treatment-resistant schizophrenia and had not been able to engage in a cognitive–behavioural approach. Both did well enough to be able to move on to settings of lower security within 2 years.

The conversational model integrates psychodynamic, interpersonal and humanistic approaches to therapy. It exemplifies a psychodynamic interpersonal tradition and draws on the psychodynamic concepts of the unconscious or the barely conscious underpinnings of relationships.

The model assumes that people who seek psychotherapy have had to endure a disruption to their sense of personal existence, an undeniable fact for those with a severe mental illness. Recreating self-esteem, or a feeling of being comfortable with 'myself', is central to the model.

In the sense developed by Meares (2000), 'myself' grows in the context of a continuing sense of the presence of the other. The child becomes interested in physical objects in the outside world, and begins to play with them in a symbolical way. This symbolic play develops optimally if the mother is sufficiently sensitively attuned to her child to allow a space between them to grow. The space must be sufficiently wide for the child to gain a sense of his or her own boundaries, yet mother and child must remain close enough to preserve a sense of relatedness. In Hobson's terms, they are alone, but experiencing togetherness (Hobson, 1985).

Alternatively, a stable sense of self may be disrupted by traumatic attachments such as those involving sexual or physical abuse. In adult life, these traumas will live on to influence present relationships, through malignant internalisation (Meares, 2000).

The approach emphasises active exploration within a conversation. Central to the model is the notion of the therapist's task of assisting the service user towards developing a deep and whole sense of self by means of a personal 'conversation'. The word conversation is used here in its less common meaning of 'the action of living or having one's being in a place or among persons' (*Shorter Oxford English Dictionary*). This definition is particularly pertinent for people with severe mental illness, who are often socially marginalised; it demonstrates why a truly conversational approach might be particularly helpful.

In a therapeutic conversation, two individuals come together and create a relationship. Within this relationship, the patient may begin the process of personal problem-solving.

The therapeutic conversation attempts to address these traumas by the creation of a relationship within which the patient and therapist, alone and together, can discover the 'myself' who was damaged. In and between the therapeutic space, the symbolic language of play is reinvented, in order to access the inner world which has been disrupted. The key to this world lies in metaphor, 'understanding and experiencing one thing in terms of another', wherein the bridge between the inner and outer worlds is built.

191

The goal of the approach is to promote personal problem-solving. It is assumed that the service user will have been using inappropriate or maladaptive ways of avoiding pain, especially that of loss or separation. The aim is to create a situation in which the problem will be directly presented in the relationship with the therapist, rather than merely talked about. It may then be identified, explored and modified within the context of the therapeutic conversation.

This psychodynamically informed therapy has been in use for nearly a decade to treat a range of people with severe mental illness and receiving longer-term care within a secure setting. It needs to be integrated into the care plan and supported by all members of the team working with the patient, to be part of the process of recovery.

Despite its multidimensional theoretical underpinnings, the conversational model lends itself quite readily to a teaching package, which can be learned relatively quickly by trainee therapists (Margison & Moss, 1994). This could make it an ideal approach for training teams working in complex settings such as in-patient units.

The family

Family work, generally involving psychoeducation and behavioural family management, should be a central component of the recovery process for people with schizophrenia who are in regular contact with their families. It has a strong evidence base and is prioritised in the NICE schizophrenia guidelines, which stipulate that it should be available for all service users, especially those at risk of relapse or who have persisting symptoms. A psychodynamic orientation may be helpful in the provision of family work, along with the other necessary skills. Supervision of family work is enhanced by psychodynamic understanding. For a more detailed discussion of psychodynamics in family interventions see Fadden (Chapter 11, this volume).

The team

The dynamics of in-patient settings pervade treatment and those around the individual will influence that person's engagement with the team. A patient's capacity to engage in and sustain a treatment alliance is a strong determinant of outcome.

The prevalence of childhood sexual and physical abuse among psychiatric in-patients is high (Wurr & Partridge, 1996). It is particularly high in rehabilitation settings, where comorbid personality vulnerability contributes to treatment resistance and delayed recovery. Some interactions between staff and patients are therefore likely to be influenced by exposure to previous abuse. Typical dynamics of abuse (Box 13.2) include revictimisation, difficulties within power relationships, and sexualisation

---

Box 13.2 Dynamics of abuse

Difficulty with establishing trusting relationships	Manipulation of an unequal power relationship between parent and child for adult gratification leads to longer-term difficulties in negotiating trusting relationships
Difficulties with boundaries	Violation of the integrity of the child through a sexual act may lead to long-term difficulties recognising and maintaining personal boundaries
Revictimisation	Early experience creates an expectation of a repeating cycle of abuse
Low self-esteem, self-disgust and self-loathing	The experience of abuse instils the feeling that abuse is deserved
Sexualisation of therapeutic relationships	Early experience of a sexual relationship with a caregiver creates the expectation that future caregiving relationships will also be sexual
Transference and counter-transference difficulties	Working with survivors of sexual abuse may evoke powerful feelings of rage, disgust and hatred, which may be displaced by the patient or experienced as disabling, confusing and frightening by staff

---

of relationships in general and therapeutic relationships in particular (Davenport, 1997).

Most patients on an in-patient ward will be psychotic; some of their interpersonal behaviour will be driven by the psychological mechanisms underlying psychotic states. These include projection and projective identification, the suspiciousness of persecutory states and grandiose omnipotence (Box 13.3).

Both the dynamics of abuse and of psychosis have in common primitive unconscious defence mechanisms that can amplify each other, leading to an anti-therapeutic environment, characterised by scapegoating, fragmentation, omnipotent (and unhelpful) power relationships and malignant alienation. Communication is often primitive, may preclude thought and may replicate the adverse dynamics of early childhood (or current family difficulties).

Power relationships between patients living together in intimate and anxiety-provoking circumstances have the potential to become sexualised and may lead to re-enactment of the victim/perpetrator dyad. Some patients become powerless, whereas others are seen as predatory. It is most often women patients who are adversely affected.

Box 13.3   Dynamics of psychosis

Splitting	Staff and patient groups are artificially split into good *v*. bad, or victim *v*. perpetrator
Grandiose omnipotence	Patients (or staff) feel entitled to act as if they were all-powerful
Pathological projective identification	Parts of the self are experienced as intolerable and are projected onto others, who unconsciously respond in accordance with the projection. As patients often project intolerable aggression or rage, staff may be perceived as dangerous
Persecutory states	Potentially good figures are regarded with intense suspicion
Inhibition of symbolisation (failure of verbal linking)	The use of pathological projective identification may disrupt thinking and lead to disordered interpersonal behaviour

Staff find it particularly challenging to handle these difficulties with sensitivity; they may feel that they have to adopt a restrictive or prohibitive role, or become drawn themselves into sexualised and abusive re-enactments. Either scenario predicts poor outcome for staff and patient alike.

The members of the ward team therefore need to be able, on a regular basis, to reflect on how they feel about individual patients, how they themselves feel while they are at work and how they feel about their work with each other. This type of meeting needs to be facilitated, preferably by a professional who does not work on the same unit. It has to feel sufficiently safe, boundaried and protected to allow staff to express difficult countertransference feelings without fear of critical retaliation from 'management'. If these conditions can be satisfied then such a group may contain primitive aggression and hostility, by reflection on, rather than enacting of, interpersonal processes.

Case formulation

The Finnish need-adapted model developed by Alanen and colleagues (Alanen *et al*, 1991; Alanen, 1997) specifies the principles that underpin an approach to case formulation in a complex environment (Box 13.4).

Psychodynamic understanding is an important tool in creating such a formulation as the latter assumes that early relationships with a primary caregiver result in more enduring patterns of relationships as an adult. These early relationship patterns are often re-enacted within significant

> **Box 13.4** The Finnish need-adapted model
>
> - Therapeutic treatments are planned individually to meet the needs of patients and of the people nearest them
> - The psychotherapeutic attitude, with efforts to try to understand what has happened and what happens to the patient and those nearest them, characterises the treatment
> - Different therapeutic activities should support, not counteract, one another
> - The treatments are all part of a developmental and interactive process

caregiving relationships and may contribute to, or interfere with, the process of care. Understanding them is therefore central to the delivery of effective long-term care.

This method of case formulation is a particular approach for structuring the care of someone with severe mental illness within a complex setting such as an in-patient ward. It requires an understanding of the prevalent dynamics that cluster around ill people. The formulation can promote consistency in the approach that staff members take with an individual, in a setting where powerful unconscious processes make thinking difficult and the pursuit of a therapeutic intervention unclear.

In the Alanen model, 'the people nearest to the service user' are taken to mean the family and the staff team, all of whom may be in high face-to-face contact with the individual.

The formulation is developed by the team members working together with the service user, to discuss their history. The patient's view of their strengths and target problems and the manner in which they entered care is the starting point for identifying their self-view and their view of their relationships with carers. The team's views should be discussed in a multidisciplinary meeting, and can be enhanced by information from the patient's family. The views of the patient and the team are compared, to reveal explicitly how the former sees him- or herself in relationships with significant others and how those significant others are likely to respond. Countertransference reactions from staff are expected. Reflection on these should be seen as providing valuable information for the formulation. The formulation should be created in diagrammatic form, linking an aspect of the service user's self-view (expressed in their own words) with the response that this generally provokes from a carer (expressed where possible in their own words). A complex picture of a set of important interactions can then be built up, which should enable team members to adopt a consistent therapeutic response to repeating patterns of behaviour and to avoid being drawn into anti-therapeutic re-enactments. The formulation can be shared with the service user (and their family) at an appropriate time, and used like a map to negotiate the in-patient environment.

This is the key to understanding how to establish and then use a therapeutic alliance. The case formulation has many other uses. It informs the development of individual care plans. It may be used to manage the timing of a complex series of interventions to ensure that different treatments are complementary rather than competing. It can be used to focus on strengths and difficulties in clinical supervision, and in team supervision when splitting becomes a problem, as re-enactments within the staff group often replicate significant conflicts from the patient's past experience.

The formulation provides a tangible and robust method of integrating a set of psychological observations and relevant interventions for an individual service user in a setting where the complexity of the environment could otherwise obscure the therapeutic focus for the individual and their family.

The institution

Psychodynamic awareness at the level of the institution is also important, as institutional dynamics may adversely affect the care that is offered within that institution's services. The institution operates social defences to reduce the anxiety, guilt, uncertainty and doubt of those who work within it (Menzies Lyth, 1988: pp. 43–85). Psychological defence mechanisms that protect against the full experience of anxiety become incorporated into the socially structured defence system of the hospital (the way in which that particular institution works). These psychic defences are generally unconscious and primitive, and include splitting, scapegoating, ritualisation and detachment of feeling (Box 13.5). These developmentally early defences have a propensity to amplify the other dynamics prevalent within a treatment setting – the dynamics of abuse and of psychosis. Such amplification makes fragmentation and scapegoating of staff and service users more likely; and this puts vulnerable individuals (both patients and staff) at greater risk of malignant alienation. The impact felt on the ward can be dealt with through a reflective-practice group, in which ward staff consider how the ward is working. However, the overall tendency to regression (which may compromise rational thinking) can affect non-clinical groups within the institution such as service management (which may find itself re-enacting a particular difficulty that is happening on the ward, or vice versa). The capacity of staff groups for self-reflection is important to optimise their own function and therefore that of the service as a whole.

Therapeutic community approaches

Early attempts to apply psychoanalytic (or psychodynamic) understanding to social settings for the benefit of patient care originated with the famous but unsuccessful 6-week Northfield experiment (Bion & Rickman, 1943), in which Wilfred Bion and John Rickman attempted to use some therapeutic

Box 13.5 The dynamics of institutions

Ritualised task performance	Routine may lend consistency to task performance and avoid excessive decision-making, but the progression to ritual can depersonalise caregiving, replicating situations of ritualistic abuse
Avoidance of change	Familiar procedures are followed even when they are no longer relevant or appropriate, making both patients and staff feel peripheral to the process of care
Detachment and denial of feelings	The necessary professional detachment and maintenance of personal boundaries becomes extreme and characterised by therapeutic withdrawal, poor handovers, rapid rotation of staff and failure to follow through care plans
Collusive redistribution of social roles, e.g. scapegoating	Particular individuals are unconsciously chosen to fulfil a role for the ward, and then act on the role as assigned

(After Menzies Lyth, 1988)

aspects of a hospital community to treat soldiers with psychoneuroses. Bion's successor, Tom Main, realised that the first experiment failed because they had not considered the whole social system as a therapeutic agent. Main believed that a hospital in itself is the therapeutic agent. After training in psychoanalysis, he became Director of the Cassel Hospital in London, which he reorganised as a therapeutic community on psychoanalytic lines.

Maxwell Jones considered social learning to be the most important ingredient in a therapeutic community, after discovering that many of the soldiers he was treating in his cardiac syndrome unit in Mill Hill, London, began to improve after participating in group activities and group discussions.

Rehabilitation psychiatrists have long been interested in whether the principles of the therapeutic community (Box 13.6) could be adapted to improve the outcome of people in longer-term in-patient care.

Although a conventional therapeutic community approach may be too confrontational and intensive for most people in psychiatric rehabilitation, some aspects of the approach have been incorporated into longer-term treatment environments. Many have community groups to promote service user involvement and facilitate their expression of views about care and the organisation in which it is provided. Many recognise the value and effectiveness of peer support gained in ward meetings.

> **Box 13.6** The principles of the therapeutic community
>
> - Insightful learning is a curative force in overcoming personal difficulties (and it often occurs through group work)
> - The state of the organisation must be kept under continuous examination, analysis and renewal (work in a community group)
> - Communication between all community members – staff and patients – should be frank and open (unambiguous, with clear boundaries and limits)

In a helpful systematic review of therapeutic environments for psychosis, Smith (2000) observed that the most successful therapeutic environments for people with psychosis were highly supportive, with an emphasis on relationships and oriented towards the needs of individuals. There should be little expression of anger or aggression, a relaxed non-restrictive regime of care and plentiful opportunities for user involvement. She concluded that 'a therapeutic community model, modified to provide high levels of emotional support and individual care, may help such patients'. This review suggests that these components of the therapeutic community approach may be helpful for rehabilitation patients.

Conclusions

A psychodynamic understanding can make a very special contribution to the care of service users engaged in the process of longer-term recovery from severe mental illness. This approach can contribute to understanding the service users, their families and their social context; it can also support the staff who are working with them. It enables the informed practitioner to optimise crucial common therapeutic factors such as secure attachment, attunement and remoralisation and to avoid the damaging re-enactments that are likely to occur within a therapeutic setting between service users and their carers. It can be of particular benefit for individuals who find it hard to engage with other forms of psychological therapy, but it must be integrated within the overall treatment package and conducted under proper supervision. There are significant training implications in promoting a psychodynamic approach, particularly at a time when many services are struggling to train sufficient practitioners in cognitive–behavioural therapy to implement the NICE schizophrenia guidelines. However, psychodynamic awareness is also a recommendation within the same guidance. It has a valued place within psychiatric rehabilitation services and should lie at the heart of practice with service users and their families as they journey towards individual recovery.

References

Alanen, Y. O. (1997) *Schizophrenia: Its Origins and Need–Adapted Treatment*. London: Karnac.

Alanen, Y. O., Lehtinen, K., Rakkolainen V., *et al* (1991) Need–adapted treatment of new schizophrenic patients: experiences and results of the Turku Project. *Acta Psychiatrica Scandinavica*, **83**, 363–372.

Bion, W. R. & Rickman, J. (1943) Intra-group tensions in therapy. *Lancet*, **2**, 678–681.

Cullberg, J., Levander, S., Holmqvist, R., *et al* (2002) One-year outcome in first episode psychosis patients in the Swedish Parachute project. *Acta Psychiatrica Scandinavica*, **106**, 276–285.

Davenport, S. (1997) Pathological interactions between psychosis and childhood sexual abuse in in-patient settings: their dynamics, consequences and management. In *Psychotherapy of Psychosis* (eds C. Mace & F. Margison), pp. 205–219. London: Gaskell.

Davenport, S. (2002) Acute wards: problems and solutions. A rehabilitation approach to in-patient care. *Psychiatric Bulletin*, **26**, 385–388.

Davenport, S., Hobson, R. F. & Margison, F. (2000) Treatment development in psychodynamic-interpersonal psychotherapy (Hobson's conversational model) for chronic treatment resistant schizophrenia; two single case studies. *British Journal of Psychotherapy*, **16**, 287–302.

Frank, J. D. 1982) *Therapeutic Components Shared by All Psychotherapies*. Washington, DC: American Psychological Association.

Hobson, R. F. (1985) *Forms of Feeling: The Heart of Psychotherapy*. London: Tavistock.

Holloway, F. (2004) Risk: more questions than answers. Invited commentary on Psychodynamic methods in risk assessment and management. *Advances in Psychiatric Treatment*, **10**, 273–274.

Jackson, M. (2001) Psychoanalysis and the treatment of psychosis. In *The Language of Psychosis* (ed. P. Williams), chapter 2. London: Whurr Publishers.

Margison, F. & Moss, S. (1994) Teaching psychotherapy skills to inexperienced psychiatric trainees using the Conversational Model. *Psychotherapy Research*, **4**, 141–148.

Meares, R. (2000) *Intimacy and Alienation: Memory, Trauma and Personal Being*. London: Brunner Routledge.

Menzies Lyth, I. (1988) *Containing Anxiety in Institutions*. London: Free Association Books.

National Institute for Clinical Excellence (2002) *Clinical Guideline 1: Schizophrenia. Core Interventions in the Treatment and Management of Schizophrenia in Primary and Secondary Care*. London: NICE.

Shepherd, G. (1984) *Institutional Care and Rehabilitation*. London: Longman.

Smith, J. (2000) The healing elements of an environment for those with chronic psychosis. *Therapeutic Communities*, **21**, 37–46.

Van Marle, S. & Holmes, J. (2002) Supportive psychotherapy as an integrative psychotherapy. In *Integration in Psychotherapy: Models and Methods* (eds J. Holmes & A. Bateman), pp. 175–194. Oxford: Oxford University Press.

Wurr, C. & Partridge, J. M. (1996) The prevalence of a history of childhood sexual abuse in an acute adult population. *Child Abuse and Neglect*, **20**, 867–872.

CHAPTER 14

Cognitive rehabilitation

Til Wykes

Why are cognitive impairments important?

Since Kraepelin and Bleuler's early descriptions of schizophrenia it has been clear that cognitive difficulties are at the heart of the diagnosis of schizophrenia. There is still some dispute about whether these impairments are static or deteriorating, but they are present not only during and between acute episodes but also prior to the onset of schizophrenia. Recent studies of children at high risk of developing schizophrenia, conscript populations and birth cohorts have all shown that there are clear reductions in cognition that are evident prior to the onset of psychosis. In the birth cohort studies these differences seem evident at all the developmental stages that have been tested. However, although the majority of people with a diagnosis of schizophrenia do show impairments relative to what might be expected, the decrements differ in magnitude across the population and there are some people who seem little affected and a few who achieve high intellectual recognition. Dr William Chester Minor, for example, in the 19th century was a prolific contributor to an early version of the Oxford English Dictionary while a patient in the Broadmoor Asylum for the Criminally Insane.

As well as differentiating people with schizophrenia from the general population it is clear that cognitive impairments also predict functional outcomes within the population. The larger the deficits, the less likely someone is to have a job or be able to fulfil all the expected social roles. It is for this reason that over the past decade cognitive difficulties have been investigated in detail, in an attempt to understand the specific and general difficulties that are experienced.

These difficulties are also recognised by people experiencing schizophrenia. For instance, in a seminal study McGhie & Chapman (1961) asked people with the disorder to describe their experiences. One patient described the disturbance of attention as follows:

'My concentration is very poor. I jump from one thing to another. If I am talking to someone they only need to cross their legs or scratch their head and I am distracted and forget what I was saying' (p. 104).

Another young person, Michael, appeared on a UK television programme (*Inside my Head*, June 2002, UK Channel 4). He was had been studying for his examinations at age 16 and he says 'my concentration is a real problem' and reports on his memory difficulties. He shows some insight into his problem and says 'I'm just getting used to having a learning disability'.

The careful study of these cognitive difficulties carried out in the 1990s has led to the conclusion that there are general deficits in multiple functions of attention, learning and memory. Executive functions – those processes that are essential for any non-automatic activity such as planning or strategy use – have also been shown to be deficient. Although measuring differences between cognitive functions depends on the sensitivity of the tests, the general consensus is that memory difficulties are pervasive and specific. In other words they are present even when there are no obvious abnormalities in overall cognitive function.

The development of therapies for cognitive difficulties

As cognitive impairments occur before the onset of the disorder, are noticed by the patients themselves and also seem to have an impact on overall functioning it is surprising that so little attention was paid to the alleviation of these problems. This is due to two main influences, one practical and the other theoretical. The practical constraint was the effect of service configurations. When care moved from institutions, the emphasis was on teaching specific life skills to allow people to live in the community, and only later was the rate-limiting effect of cognitive difficulties on these rehabilitation programmes acknowledged.

Even when the rate limiter was exposed, the theoretical stance at the time was that cognitive difficulties were the result of a neurological problem which was similar to the effects of frontal lesions in the brain. Evidence from comparison studies of individuals with acute and chronic schizophrenia and from longitudinal follow-up studies showed that the cognitive impairments changed little over the course of the illness (evidence which is now disputed). Together with the links to brain dysfunction this produced a model of cognitive difficulties which were immutable and which were present even when symptoms had waned. Therapeutic pessimism reigned and the main rehabilitative efforts focused on discovering what sorts of support were necessary to allow people to achieve their highest level of independence.

Eventually the theoretical model of immutability gave an unexpected boost to the development of therapy for cognitive problems. It occurred because Terry Goldberg in the USA carried out a study in which he showed that it was impossible to teach in-patients with chronic schizophrenia how to carry out the Wisconsin Card Sorting Test – a neuropsychological task measuring flexibility of thought (Goldberg *et al*, 1987). In Fig. 14.1

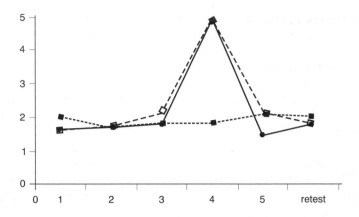

Fig. 14.1 Card Sort performance with and without training. ■-----■ No training; ●———● explicit instructions and feedback order 1; ▫--▫ explicit instructions and feedback order 2 (data from Goldberg *et al*, 1987).

it is clear that both of the two training conditions were not successful in improving performance until the groups were provided with specific card-by-card instructions. However, as soon as this learning support was removed performance returned to baseline and was no different from that of the group who had merely carried out the test repeatedly. The reason this study produced a boost to therapy development was that many researchers investigated this particular task and tried to show that some form of instruction could change task performance. Although many found similar results, no change in cognitive performance, a few showed that it was possible under some conditions to get not only improved performance following training but that these improvements were durable over several weeks. These results produced a chink of therapeutic optimism and cognitive remediation therapy was born.

What should be a target for cognitive rehabilitation?

Clearly we need to intervene in cognitive difficulties that will have the most impact on a person's life, but these may differ for different real-life functions. In a comprehensive review Green and colleagues (2000) set out the evidence on the associations between different cognitive functions and social outcomes and, more recently, McGurk & Mueser (2004) have reviewed similar literature for work outcomes. Both reviews commented on the difficulty of making general conclusions, as few studies carried out a comprehensive assessment of all cognitive functions and few carried out similar tasks to measure the same function. However, both concluded that memory and executive functions are important in predicting overall functioning and that some basic functions such as sustained attention also show some relationship, although this may be as a result of poor executive control.

But it is not just that cognition is related to overall outcome: we need to know whether particular cognitive domains interfere with the rehabilitation of social or occupational functions. The learning of social skills has been found to be impaired by memory difficulties. Supported employment programmes seem to be able to fully compensate for impairments in basic cognitive functions, including attention and psychomotor speed, but are only partially effective at compensating for the effects of the higher-order cognitive processes of learning, memory and executive functions. In these work schemes, overall work outcome is affected mainly by memory and executive functioning. Specific cognitive problems also seem to affect people at different times during a rehabilitation programme. For instance, Bryson & Bell (2003) found that during the first half of a supported work programme run on the 'place and train' principle, 28% of the variance was accounted for by cognitive variables, but in the second half only 19%. Initially, sustained attention, response inhibition and idiosyncratic thinking were important, but this switched to attention, verbal memory and psychomotor speed in the latter parts of the programme. At the beginning of the programme there is a need to concentrate on instructions, but later in the programme practice and speed of response are important as the person begins to become an expert in the relevant tasks.

It is therefore important when designing cognitive rehabilitation to understand the nature of the rehabilitation task and the way that cognition might impede progress. However, it must be remembered that all the associations that have been reported so far are only correlations and that it has until recently been a leap of faith to assume that improvements in these cognitive functions will actually lead to improvements in real-life functioning or remove the rate limiter on rehabilitation. There are several issues which can be resolved only through empirical investigation, a few of which are listed below:

- Is it an improvement in all or some cognitive domains that is vital to produce change in functioning?
- Does cognition have to improve just a little to produce a direct effect in function or does it have to improve above a threshold?
- Will the same cognitive functions that are associated with functioning statically be associated with dynamic improvements?

The method for investigating the effects of cognition also affects the results. For instance, when testing several putative predictors in an exploratory regression analysis, what is produced is the effects of single independent predictors. However, it may be that some factors, for example symptoms, affect whether cognitive factors have an impact. These interactive effects would be hidden in the data in the current literature. In fact, data from my own laboratory suggest that there are synergistic effects of symptoms and cognitive problems that result in increased difficulties with community functions that cannot be accounted for by the two factors alone.

Not all of these questions have received conclusive answers but that does not mean that cognitive rehabilitation has failed. Rather, we need to do further investigations to be able to develop therapies that are even more effective.

The development of the technology of cognitive rehabilitation

The initial studies on cognitive rehabilitation were designed to test whether it was possible to find some techniques that would change performance on single cognitive tests. I will call these 'laboratory studies', and they are important because they tell us about not only the techniques that worked but also those that did not work. This is unusual in the development of a therapy because usually only positive data is in the public domain. This situation results from the original scientific reasons for carrying out the studies – the assumption that changing cognition in people with schizophrenia was impossible. The studies that reported negative results – i.e. agreed with the current scientific zeitgeist – found favour with the editors of journals and so we can benefit from what would otherwise be 'bottom-drawer' studies that never get published.

Most of the laboratory studies concentrated on the Wisconsin Card Sorting Test, but some also investigated memory and attention tasks. One meta-analysis concluded that there are large positive effects of cognitive remediation but that some functions, such as attention, are more difficult to train (Kurtz *et al*, 2001). This set of studies also provided data on the types of training that seem to have the most beneficial effects. Errorless learning (reducing the error rate when teaching the task), scaffolding (providing tasks where effort is required but the solution still lies within the person's competence) and verbal monitoring (overtly rehearsing the task rules and strategies for solution) were all found to be successful. However, just rehearsing the task and just receiving instruction did not produce benefits, and neither did receiving payment when it was provided without the other beneficial elements of training.

The second generation of studies moved on from attempts to influence performance on a single test to the rehabilitation of a variety of cognitive functions that might have an effect on real-life functioning. Again positive results were found for the improvement of cognition, although the effect sizes were considerably reduced. Figure 14.2 shows the range of effect sizes in three meta-analyses. The meta-analysis by Krabbendam & Aleman (2003) also tried to distinguish the effects of different types of training. They found that the effect of rehearsal-based training was less than when strategic processing was targeted. In fact, the confidence interval for the

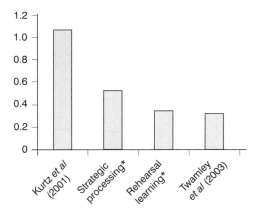

Fig 14.2 Average effect sizes from meta-analyses for cognitive outcomes following cognitive remediation therapy (*data from Krabbendam & Aleman, 2003).

effect of rehearsal learning crossed zero, suggesting that this is not even a robust effect.

There have now been more than 15 randomised control trials of cognitive training to improve cognition and these show moderate effect sizes (0.45) identical to that of cognitive–behavioural treatments (effect size is here defined as the mean difference between treatment and control conditions divided by the standard deviation of the measure employed). But the other assumption for the effect of cognitive remediation is that these cognitive improvements will lead to improvements in real-life functioning. There is some evidence that there are modest effects on positive and negative symptoms (an effect size for overall symptom severity of 0.26; Twamley *et al*, 2003) and more robust effects for social functioning (0.51). There are also emerging data that cognitive remediation affects the number of hours worked.

So there is evidence of positive effects on functioning outcomes. Model 1 in Fig. 14.3 shows what is currently being tested. This assumes that the remediation acts on cognition, leading to an improvement that then changes real-life functioning. However, the empirical data are now pointing to a different model, one in which improvements in cognition have to be moderated by cognitive rehabilitation. The reason for this is that there are few overall group effects on functioning outcome following remediation. Cognition does have to improve before functioning improves, and people who do not respond to cognitive remediation do not improve their functioning. But cognition sometimes improves as a result of non-specific methods – medication changes or the effects of a control therapy – and these non-specific improvements do not have an effect on outcome. The effect is solely when the cognitive improvements have been produced

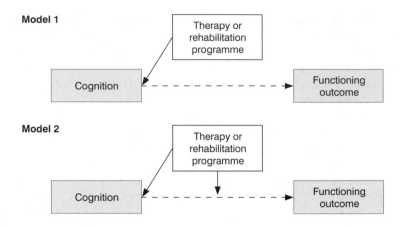

Fig. 14.3 The relationship between cognitive remediation and functioning.

by rehabilitation therapy. This type of effect is shown in the second model in Fig. 14.3. Clearly whatever is learnt within these cognitive programmes is the key to success, and the next obvious question is to ask what it is that we are teaching that is effective.

What is cognitive remediation therapy?

This question has come rather late in this chapter because it is the most difficult to answer. Cognitive rehabilitation has so far been led by pragmatic studies to show that it is possible to achieve cognitive improvement. The processes adopted have had some face validity, but there have been many different approaches. The factors that differentiate programmes include:

- individual or group treatment
- computer-driven presentation or paper-and-pencil tasks
- therapist present or automated presentation (or both)
- frequency of therapy (weekly or intensive daily sessions)
- type of training (rehearsal or strategic processing).

All these factors have been used in every combination, making it almost impossible to separate the successful from the unsuccessful characteristics. The therapies may also have specific effects and so cannot be compared across cognitive functions. A therapy that is useful for memory may not be useful for flexibility of thinking. The list of unanswerable questions is endless. However, some general points can be made. Both laboratory and clinical studies have shown that concentration solely on rehearsal learning is unlikely to produce large cognitive improvements. Therapy needs to be tailored to an individual's needs and goals, and this is difficult when providing group therapy. There is little current evidence on the efficacy of computer- *v.* therapist-driven therapy, but it seems highly likely that some supervision from a clinical specialist will be needed to aid engagement in the task and to help specify the strategic information processing necessary, at least until we can produce a computer that will sensitively respond to information overload or realise when a cup of tea and a break are needed.

The interaction between therapy and participant also needs to be further investigated in order to reduce the failure rate. However, because most studies have been pragmatic all these subsequent analyses are exploratory at best and at worst are fishing exercises by clinical scientists trying to pull a significant result out of a hat. What cognitive remediation needs now is a theory on which to base therapy. Clare Reeder and I have developed such a theory, which we think has relevance not only to cognitive remediation but to all therapies that try to improve real-life functions. This theory, and the clinical model that we derived from it, are outlined below and described in more detail with case studies in Wykes & Reeder (2005).

A model for therapy

Our starting point was to look at the relationship between cognition and functioning. Adopting the extremely simple model shown in Fig. 14.4, most of the effort in the past decade has been to unpack the cognition box to find out which cognitive processes are important. But it now seems obvious that the arrow in the diagram is also important. For remediation to be effective it is not enough for cognitive improvement to occur, this improvement has to be mediated by therapy. Changes in real-life functioning do not occur when the cognitive improvements are produced in a non-specific way. What we need is a model that will explain how cognitive processes actually affect real-life functions such as shopping. The one we have produced considers what sorts of behavioural response are required. We have defined them as either routine or non-routine. Routine actions are those that are specified as soon as the intention or goal is specified because there is a cognitive schema that is activated that defines the behaviours that need to be carried out. So, for instance, if you are watching TV and a film appears that you want to watch then the behaviours necessary for watching the film are specified by your intention to watch the film. You direct your eyes to the screen and sustain your attention. Attention is sustained by some additional cognitive

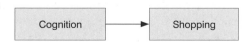

Fig. 14.4 The relationship between cognition and functioning.

control mechanisms, probably similar to executive functions, but the main behaviours follow relatively automatically from your intention.

Most actions, however, are not routine. If I intend to make a meal, I need to decide what kind of meal I would like to make, look in a recipe book, consider what ingredients are available and so on. I must reflect on my intention, my goals, my past experience and the way in which these interact with the current circumstances in order to select a certain set of appropriate actions which will allow me to achieve my goal. This ability to reflect on and regulate one's own thinking is referred to as meta-cognition. Metacognition is the key to carrying out these non-routine actions successfully. Improvements in cognitive processes will have a direct effect on routine actions as they will improve the efficiency of the cognitive schema. However, they may not have an effect on non-routine actions because metacognitive skills are also needed. So to ensure improvement in non-routine actions metacognition must be a target.

We need to add one more factor because, although we can improve cognition in one setting, for example for a neuropsychological test, these same skills might not be used in everyday life. This was a problem encountered in social skills training, where skills learnt in group therapy were not generalised or transferred. Transfer is not a new concept to psychology: it was mentioned in the very earliest textbooks and has been more recently defined as the ability to use knowledge, experience, motivations and skills in a new situation. Figure 14.5 shows this final model, where the broken lines distinguish the course for routine actions and the unbroken lines that for non-routine actions. The role of cognitive remediation therapy is to train for this essential transfer if functioning is to improve.

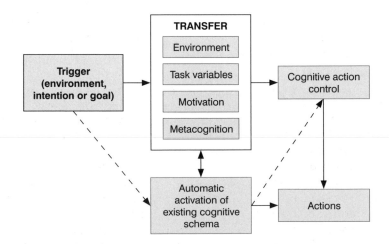

Fig. 14.5 A model for cognitive remediation therapy (after Wykes & Reeder, 2005).

A clinical model of cognitive remediation therapy

Training for transfer has been the focus of studies in two entirely different fields of psychology, management training and teaching mathematics and scientific concepts to children. There is now a growing evidence base that certain types of training enable transfer to take place, particularly the type of transfer denoted as 'far transfer', in which the learning situation differs from the situation in which the skills need to be used. This is vital because if we were to attempt to train the cognitive schemas that specify each possible situation in which the person will find themselves it would be tedious for the learner as well as the trainer.

Our theoretical model relies on the engagement of metacognitive processes in order for far transfer to be achieved. So for strategy instruction to contribute to transfer, the learner must be (a) shown the value of effortful processing, (b) be encouraged to modify and personalise the general heuristic and (c) given opportunities and incentives for such activity.

Training methods should explicitly promote the development of the personal resources needed for successful transfer. Participants may be encouraged to articulate their cognitive and motivational processes during learning and problem-solving to promote metacognitive processing and knowledge. The development of broad, generic schemas may be facilitated by the use of multimedia learning environments and helping people to connect verbal explanations to visual representations.

In our current therapeutic manual (Wykes & Reeder, 2005) we carry out a series of pencil-and-paper tasks that encompass different types of strategic processing. There are three main modules: cognitive flexibility, memory and planning, and the 1 h one-to-one sessions occur daily over a period of 12–16 weeks in a total of 40 sessions. This model is intensive and requires much therapist time. We employ graduate psychologists as cognitive remediation therapists; they are trained over a period of weeks and are supervised by a qualified clinical psychologist. This clinical implementation means that special expertise is developed which is separate from generic skills usually required within the participant's care team and makes therapy feasible in terms of time and cost.

Cognitive remediation therapy aims to provide the participant with a comprehensive cognitive structure to reduce stimulus overload and facilitate efficient cognitive processing. Initially, the responsibility for providing this structure lies with the therapist, but it is gradually surrendered to the participant as his or her skills improve.

We teach people to adapt flexibly and efficiently to novel situations. First, we provide different sorts of tasks that use similar sets of strategic skills. The skills learnt are therefore not context-bound, thus allowing the development of a new style of thinking which can be used in all aspects of the participant's life. Then we emphasise throughout the therapy how the skills might be used in the real world, with prompts and discussions about their use. These transfer skills need to be further reinforced by integrating them into different rehabilitation or life skills programmes. The general principles for successful generalisation need to be followed in a comprehensive rehabilitation service if we are to enable our clients to achieve their full potential. What is clear from the current programmes is that we can be much more optimistic about realising this potential given the development of these new cognitive rehabilitation technologies.

References

Bryson, G. & Bell, M. D. (2003) Initial and final work performance in schizophrenia. Cognitive and symptom predictors. *Journal of Nervous and Mental Disease*, **191**, 87–92.

Goldberg, T. E., Weinberger, D. R., Berman, K. F., *et al* (1987) Further evidence for dementia of the prefrontal type in schizophrenia? A controlled study of teaching the Wisconsin Card Sorting Test. *Archives of General Psychiatry*, **44**, 1008–1014.

Green, M. F., Kern, R. S., Braff, D. L., *et al* (2000) Neurocognitive deficits and functional outcome in schizophrenia: are we measuring the 'right stuff'? *Schizophrenia Bulletin*, **26**, 119–136.

Krabbendam, L. & Aleman, A. (2003) Cognitive rehabilitation in schizophrenia: a quantitative analysis of controlled studies. *Psychopharmacology*, **169**, 376–382.

Kurtz, M. M., Moberg, P. J., Gur, R. C., *et al* (2001) Approaches to cognitive remediation of neuropsychological deficits in schizophrenia. A review and meta-analysis. *Neuropsychology Review*, **11**, 197–210.

McGhie, A. & Chapman, J. (1961) Disorders of attention and perception in early schizophrenia. *British Journal of Medical Psychology*, **34**, 103–113.

McGurk, S. & Mueser, K. (2004) Cognitive functioning, symptoms, and work in supported employment: a review and heuristic model. *Schizophrenia Research*, **70**, 147–173.

Twamley, E. W., Jeste, D. V. & Bellack, A. S. (2003) A review of cognitive training in schizophrenia. *Schizophrenia Bulletin*, **29**, 359–382.

Wykes, T. & Reeder, C. (2005) *Cognitive Remediation Therapy for Schizophrenia: Theory and Practice*. London: Routledge.

CHAPTER 15

Managing challenging behaviour

Dominic Beer

There have been various attempts to define challenging behaviour. Emerson (1995), for example, describes it as intense, frequent or prolonged culturally abnormal behaviour that is a serious risk to the safety of the individual or others, or greatly limits the individual's use of or access to ordinary community services and facilities. This definition came from learning disability services, where a great deal of expertise in the management of challenging behaviours has been developed, particularly in terms of behavioural approaches to its analysis and management (Xenitidis *et al*, 2001). General mental health services have expanded on Emerson's description, leading our own local services (Oxleas National Health Service Trust) to the following definition:

'Behaviour of such frequency, duration or intensity that the physical safety of the person or others is likely to be placed in serious jeopardy and where all the following apply:

- the behaviour has occurred over a period more than six months, appears chronic and not easily remedied
- the behaviour is likely to recur because the causes have not yet been identified and/or cannot yet be remedied
- the behaviour is requiring detention under secure conditions and/or is requiring very close supervision and/or frequent restraint (by staff or protective devices)
- the behaviour has led to convictions in court (or could have done so were it not for the person's learning disabilities and/or mental health needs) but is not so serious that the person would be currently accepted by the forensic services (for self-injury, people do not have to meet this fourth criterion)'

Challenging behaviours in mental health services

Challenging behaviour commonly found in mental health services can be divided into behaviours that pose a risk of harm to others (Box 15.1) and those that pose a risk of harm to the self (Box 15.2). It may be helpful to subdivide these behaviours further into 'mild', 'moderate' and 'severe'. The

---

Box 15.1   Behaviours that pose a risk of harm to others

Severe
- Sexual assault
- Physical assault
- Fire-setting (deliberate)

Moderate
- Property damage
- Inappropriate sexual behaviour
- Intimidation (minor) or bullying
- Fire-setting (accidental)

Mild
- Verbal abuse
- Overactive or aroused state
- Impulsivity
- Making constant demands of staff

---

grading of severity is to some extent arbitrary, but is based on the degree of professional intervention required to manage the behaviour. It is also cumulative, in that individuals posing multiple mild or moderate risks will 'challenge' the service more intensely. Challenging behaviour may be compounded by other problems, such as substance misuse and acquisitive offending (which itself is often instrumental, as the person needs to find funds to maintain a substance misuse habit). Some forms of challenging behaviour are markedly less common in contemporary mental health services – notably, the most extreme forms of self-neglect and socially unacceptable behaviour – than they once were in the era of the large mental hospital.

Box 15.2   Behaviours that pose a risk of harm to self or to health

Severe
- Self-harm
- Absconding

Moderate
- Self-harm
- Non-adherence to treatment regimen
- Self-neglect

Mild
- Non-engagement with professionals/rehabilitation plan
- Threats of self-harm

Services that manage individuals with challenging behaviour

The service that a patient is placed in will depend on the risks that the individual poses, measured along two dimensions: the severity of the risk and its probability and immediacy. The more severe the risk (particularly to others), the higher the level of perimeter security required. The more probable and immediate the risk (either to self or others), the higher the degree of supervision (Procter, 2001). At each level of security and supervision there are various types of service for different lengths of treatment, for example acute day hospitals, supervised accommodation, acute wards, hospital hostel wards and high secure hospital care (Fig. 15.1).

Most people exhibiting the more severe or chronic forms of challenging behaviour in mental health services are placed in hospital hostels, rehabilitation wards or low secure units. However, such patients are also found on acute wards and in psychiatric intensive care units (PICUs). Those exhibiting severe challenging behaviour tend to be placed in low secure units and those with mild/moderate challenging behaviour are usually housed in an open rehabilitation setting. However, some individuals who exhibit multiple challenging behaviours of a moderate nature may need to be managed in low secure units, unless the open facilities are especially well staffed and can supervise them adequately.

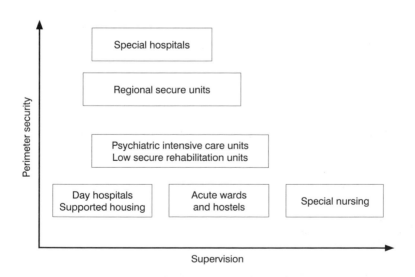

Fig. 15.1 Relationship between components of risk and characteristics of units in which a person can be appropriately supported (after Procter, 2001).

Shepherd (1999) estimated between 10 and 30 individuals per 100 000 total population are 'difficult to place' patients who challenge services. He identified three broad types: young men with schizophrenia; middle-aged women with affective psychoses; and a heterogeneous group, most of whom have organic brain syndromes (acquired brain damage, borderline learning disability, alcohol-related brain damage). To these three groups can be added a fourth: young women with borderline personality disorder.

Approaches to understanding challenging behaviour

Links between history, diagnosis and challenging behaviour

Challenging behaviour occurs in the context of the individual's mental disorder. Understanding the mental disorder requires a detailed assessment of the person's developmental, family, occupational, psychosexual, forensic, medical and psychiatric history as well as their personality structure. Table 15.1 describes the links between aspects of the history and underlying psychiatric and neuropsychiatric disorders.

Some of the challenging behaviour that is encountered in mental health services is clearly and directly linked to a primary diagnosis. Thus, verbal abuse may be linked to the hallucinatory symptoms of a chronic paranoid schizophrenic illness. Inappropriate sexual behaviour or assault is associated with a chronic difficult-to-treat hypomanic or mixed affective disorder. Physical assault is associated with the persecutory delusions and command hallucinations of schizophrenia. The risk of this behaviour is exacerbated in people with antisocial personality disorder and substance misuse. However, when a behaviour has become entrenched it is likely that it has come to serve a purpose for the individual. The approach to understanding such 'functional' behaviour has its origins in learning theory.

Functional behaviour and reinforcement

Consequences of behaviour that shape or maintain it are called reinforcers. Positive reinforcers lead to an increase in the behaviour when a reinforcing stimulus is present. Negative reinforcers lead to an increase in the behaviour as a result of the withdrawal (or prevention of occurrence) of a reinforcing stimulus. It is important to divide functions and consequences into what the patient perceives them to be and what they actually are.

Case history 15.1

Ms A is 25 years old and has a history of schizoaffective disorder, substance misuse, some dependent personality traits and self-harm. Her concentration is impaired because of her mental illness and she finds it hard to participate in ward activities. She is feeling anxious and this is exacerbated when she sees other patients participating in activities and receiving attention from nurses. She starts to shout and threaten self-harm, causing the nurses to come over to her to calm her.

Table 15.1 Assessment areas, key questions and potential underlying psychiatric and neuropsychiatric disorders

Area	What to ask	Possible diagnoses
Developmental history	Antenatal or perinatal insult/injury	Brain damage
	Postnatal depression in mother or separations in childhood	Adverse effects on personality development and vulnerability to depression
	Childhood emotional disorders, e.g. bedwetting, school refusal	Possible personality disorder, anxious/dependent types
	Childhood behavioural disorders, e.g. truancy, conduct disorder	Possible anti-social personality disorder
	Childhood sexual, physical or emotional abuse	Borderline personality disorder
	Childhood difficulties in socialising, communication	Autistic-spectrum disorder
	Medical history	Epilepsy, acquired brain injury
	Education:	
	Special schooling for:	
	(a) behavioural problems	(a) Possible anti-social personality disorder
	(b) learning difficulties	(b) Learning disability
	If level of attainment tails off	Major mental illness possible
	If CSE/GCSE attained rules out learning disability	
Family history	Psychiatric illness, especially first-degree relatives, e.g. schizophrenia, bipolar affective disorder, depression	Psychiatric illness more likely
	Alcohol problems	Alcohol disorder
	Personality disorders	Personality disorder
	Medical conditions, e.g. thyroid	Medical condition
	Learning disability	Learning disability
Medical history	Epilepsy, head injury, thyroid	Psychiatric disorder, including cognitive damage related to medical condition

continued overleaf

Table 15.1 *Continued*

Area	What to ask	Possible diagnoses
Psychosexual history	Childhood sexual abuse	Borderline personality disorder, eating disorders, paedophilia
	Poor social skills leading to inappropriate sexual behaviour	Learning disabilities or chronic schizophrenia of adolescent onset
	Side-effects of psychotropic medication	Sexual frustration
	Frequent unsatisfactory relationships	Possible personality disorder
Occupational history	What level attained and stability: if frequent arguments, dismissals	Anti-social personality disorder
Psychiatric history	Schizophrenia	See disorder from the history
	Bipolar affective disorder	
	Depression	
	Personality disorders	
	Learning disabilities	
	Substance misuse	
	Post-traumatic stress disorder	
	Anxiety disorders	
	Organic disorders	
Forensic history	If frequent offences against another person	Anti-social personality disorder
	Sexual offences	Anti-social personality disorder
Personality	Development interrupted before adulthood	Learning disability, schizophrenia
	Conduct disorder, criminality, childhood sexual abuse	Anti-social personality disorder Borderline personality disorder
	Frequent changes in job, relationships	Anti-social personality disorder

Ms A's challenging behaviour thus served the function of attracting the nurses' attention, and she received positive reinforcement for it. However, their planned intervention might have been that she was to be ignored or told briefly that she would be seen for a one-to-one session in half an hour, when staff had finished the planned ward activity.

Another patient may have threatened self-harming behaviour to avoid the planned activity and, had the nurses removed the person from the group, the behaviour would have served as a negative reinforcer.

According to operant conditioning theory reinforcement will lead to a worsening of undesirable behaviours. These behaviours can be weakened by two processes, 'extinction' and 'punishment'. In extinction, a particular behaviour is weakened by the consequence of not experiencing a positive condition or stopping a negative condition (i.e. the reinforcement is removed). In punishment, a particular behaviour is weakened by the consequence of experiencing a negative condition, either something directly aversive (such as a verbal reprimand) or by the deprivation of something positive (as in time out in one's own room).

Behavioural assessment

A behavioural assessment can further the understanding of a particular challenging behaviour. It involves addressing a number of questions: What is the behaviour? Where does it take place? What is its frequency, duration and intensity? What factors in the person may be important? Is there a relationship with psychiatric or medical conditions, sleep cycles, eating routines, tiredness, medication, caffeine, drugs, alcohol? What environmental factors are important? Is the behaviour related to a time of day, setting, activity, presence of carer, staffing patterns, other patients, staff attitudes? What are the consequences of the behaviour for the patient and others?

To develop a treatment plan a further set of questions need to be addressed. What is the supposed function of the behaviour for the patient? What methods have been employed in an attempt to manage it? For how long? In what ways were they successful, if at all? What baseline measurements are needed? How will these be made? A chart such as that shown in Fig. 15.2, recording antecedents, behaviours and consequences (an ABC chart) provides a tool for a detailed analysis of a problematical behaviour (for further details see Emerson, 1995: chapter 6).

In the case of Ms A, it was found that her shouting and threats of self-harm occurred most frequently before scheduled ward activities that she disliked. Thus, her challenging behaviour was maintained by negative reinforcement involving avoidance of, and escape from, demands. Her biological state was a feeling of anxiety and the environmental state was seeing other patients receiving help from nurses. These two factors combined to produce in her a desire for reassurance and attention through interaction with nurses (her motivational state). She exhibited the challenging behaviour (screaming)

Name _____

Date _____

	Behaviour	Antecedents			Function			Actual consequence	
	Threat to self-harm	Request made	Difficult task	Alone (no attention)	Obtains attention	Avoids activity	Ignored by staff	Time out
Time of day								
No. of occasions behaviour occurs								

Fig. 15.2 An ABC behavioural chart.

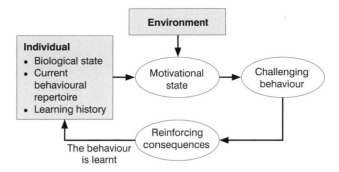

Fig. 15.3 Interactions between the individual and the environment in the development and maintenance of challenging behaviour (after Emerson, 1995: p. 41).

and received attention (reinforcing consequences). She has learnt this behaviour and incorporated it into her 'learning history'. Figure 15.3 describes the interrelationships that can occur between the individual, their environment and challenging behaviours.

Cognitive theory

It is not only from behavioural therapy that we need to bring in concepts – cognitive therapy is also helpful. Faulty cognitive styles using cognitive schemas or patterns of thought may lead to challenging behaviour.

Case history 15.2

Mr B is a 25-year-old man who has had schizophrenia since he was 15 and who also has antisocial personality disorder. He has no criminal record because the police declined to charge him, in view of his concurrent psychosis whenever he was aggressive. Mr B was referred because he was repeatedly getting into fights in social situations. He has a history of ridicule and rejection from his father and being bullied and teased at school. Ultimately, he had fought back and developed a reputation for violence. Now when he walks into a social situation he feels tense and aroused with the expectation of confrontation. A glance from another man he interprets as a challenge and a threat. He broods on it, believing that he cannot let the challenge pass as it would mean he was 'less than a man; in fact, worthless'. This thought would cause him to feel bad about himself and eventually he would react angrily and challenge his perceived rival. If a fight ensued all negative thoughts and feelings would disappear.

According to Beck & Freeman (1990), people with personality disorder try to use a schema to manage both interpersonal events (external) and feelings (internal). When the schema – which is maladaptive – fails, anxiety results. The patient then tries to control the anxiety by further disturbances of affect, behaviour and cognition. Beck & Freeman see this as a problem of

219

internal control. This is similar to the concept proposed by Linehan (1993) in her study of self-harm by people with borderline personality disorder, where the core problem is affect intolerance. Patients cannot tolerate feeling and they substitute behaviours such as self-harm for the affect.

Case history 15.3

Ms C is a 28-year-old woman with an affective disorder and borderline personality disorder. She has made a number of serious attempts on her life and carried out severe acts of self-injury. She said she did this to get rid of persecuting memories of serious sexual, physical and emotional abuse that she had suffered as a child. These thoughts brought on 'black feelings', especially self-hatred and low self-esteem, which made her feel terrible. Harming herself brought relief.

This woman appears to substitute physical pain, of which she was in control, for psychic pain.

In Mrs D (below), we can see an entrenched schema that appears to organise her mode of thought and provoke behaviour whenever she feels rejected. She cannot tolerate rejection and can deal with it only through an explosion of anger and the taking of revenge.

Case history 15.4

Mrs D is a 33-year-old woman with a history of bipolar affective disorder and borderline and dependent personality traits. She would often glance over at the nursing station and try to catch the eye of a nurse busy at work. The nurse would look away and return to her paperwork. This would arouse feelings in Mrs D of rejection and exclusion. She would then knock on the door of the nursing station, sometimes angrily, and demand something that she knew the nurse had the authority to arrange, for example an escorted trip to the patients' bank. The nurse, often under pressure, would say that nothing could be done at that time. An angry altercation would follow and Mrs D would storm off to her room; she would brood about the injustice of the matter. Later in the day, she would react violently to a seemingly trivial incident with unwonted ferocity.

Commenting on this case, McKenzie (2001: p.113) suggested that Mrs D's unexpectedly violent outbursts can best be understood (and treated) as the result of emotional dysregulation, problems of internal control and affect substitution.

Analytic theories

Theories derived from analytical work can also shed light on challenging behaviour (for a fuller discussion see Davenport, Chapter 13, this volume). McKenzie (2001) states that about 4% of infants show a pattern of attachment defined as insecure or disorganised. Disturbed bonds between child and caregiver may be carried on as a model for interpersonal functioning in adult life. This may be evidenced in an extreme form by repeated absconding from hospital, treatment for which will need to address issues of trust. Alternatively, overdependency may be the main issue, and this can very easily become hostile. The individual experiences overwhelming dependency needs which are not met by carers and which are relieved by attacking them. This leaves the individual more isolated, anxious, vulnerable and dependent.

Synthesis

No single perspective has adequate power to explain the diversity of challenging behaviour encountered among users of mental health services. The task for the clinician working within a service setting seeking to address such behaviour is to be able to develop a formulation of the patient's problems that draws on the full range of theoretical approaches available. The pragmatic aim is to identify approaches that will modify the behaviour and therefore improve the quality of life of the individual. This is identical to the aim of risk assessment (a task that is central to the operation of a service purporting to address challenging behaviour), where the aim must go beyond quantification of the risk to a case formulation that identifies approaches to addressing risk factors.

Approaches to treating challenging behaviour

The role of medication

When challenging behaviour occurs in the context of treatment-resistant schizophrenia, clozapine is without doubt the drug of choice. However, patients often do not want to take it, despite education about its risks and benefits. Concerns often focus on the need for regular haematological monitoring, as required by the product licence. I have found the following procedure useful for individuals who have refused clozapine therapy (Pereira *et al*, 1999).

Review the individual's history and response to medication, previous mental states and the accounts of carers. Review the current mental state. Exclude overmedication, organic causes such as epilepsy or affective disorder, substance misuse and personality disorder, and treat accordingly. Confirm that appropriate trials of typical and atypical antipsychotics (using *British National Formulary* maximum doses (British Medical Association & Royal Pharmaceutical Society of Great Britain, 2006)) have been undertaken for an adequate time (perhaps 3 months) and that adjunctive strategies have been tried (e.g. lithium or electroconvulsive therapy). If psychological treatments have not been used, consider whether they would be appropriate.

Once these approaches have been exhausted, consider compulsory treatment under the relevant Mental Health Act 1983. It may be necessary to review the treatment setting and transfer the patient to a locked unit to prevent absconding. Further educate the patient and carers about benefits of clozapine and offer incentives for accepting treatment: these might include leave and special activities as part of the therapeutic programme, when safety permits. If the individual continues to refuse clozapine, their needs should be further discussed thoroughly within the multidisciplinary team and with relatives and carers. It may be helpful to set out formally the risks and benefits to the patient associated with a trial of clozapine and to consult with your peers, experts and specialist units.

Under the Mental Health Act 1983, which applies to England and Wales, the next step is to consult a 'second opinion approved doctor' (SOAD), who will make an independent assessment of the case. There is no doubt that, with the agreement of a SOAD, compulsory treatment with clozapine of a dissenting patient (including compulsory blood testing and the use of restraint if necessary) is lawful. Some clinicians find it helpful to consult their trust's solicitors and their medical defence organisation before taking what appears to be a dramatically coercive step.

It is important to be aware of the need for antidepressants and mood stabilisers in patients with schizophrenia. Often there are no readily discernible biological symptoms of depression because of the effects of antipsychotic medication; for example, appetite enhancement and sedative effects can mask appetite and sleep disturbance. The negative symptoms of schizophrenia may be hard to distinguish from the cognitive symptoms of depression, for example lack of drive, anergia and anhedonia. Often, the best clues come from the content of delusions and hallucinations. These can be very unpleasant, catastrophic, frightening. In these situations an antidepressant is often indicated.

Not every patient with treatment-resistant schizophrenia responds adequately to clozapine. The medication of schizophrenia and schizo-affective disorders, including non-response to clozapine, is discussed in detail by Sweeting (Chapter 10, this volume).

Although schizophrenia is the most common diagnosis in people with challenging behaviour in psychiatric settings, refractory depression, mania and rapid-cycling bipolar affective disorder can also be the cause. The Maudsley Prescribing Guidelines provide regularly updated evidence-based advice for these situations (Taylor et al, 2005). Despite its regular prescription, medication plays a relatively limited role in the management of challenging behaviour that occurs in the context of acquired brain injury, autistic-spectrum disorder and dementia, although it is clearly indicated for the treatment of comorbid psychiatric disorder and epilepsy. There is some evidence for the use of the atypical antipsychotic risperidone in autism and autistic-spectrum disorders (Barnard et al, 2002), although its use in dementia is discouraged because of an increased risk of stroke. Selective serotonin reuptake inhibitors may have a role to play in ameliorating the repetitive and aggressive behaviours seen in autistic-spectrum disorders (Taylor et al, 2005: p. 219.)

Pharmacological approaches to managing violent and disturbed behaviour are described in the Maudsley Prescribing Guidelines (Taylor et al, 2005:

pp. 313–318). However, the response to impending violence should always first involve an attempt to understand what is happening from the individual's perspective, de-escalation and other forms of psychological and social manipulation, such as time out or transfer to a more secure facility.

Psychological approaches

One important aspect of managing challenging behaviour is to change the context in which it occurs by manipulating its antecedents (Emerson, 1995: chapter 7). This includes such general measures as increasing the level of stimulation in the setting, providing opportunities for physical exercise and expression and offering increased opportunities for making choices. If a particular behaviour has been thoroughly assessed, a functionally based approach can be adopted. This involves initially avoiding antecedents that set the occasion for the behaviour and basing activities on the individual's preferences. The antecedents are then gradually re-introduced (stimulus fading). Task varieties can be increased and antecedents that precipitate the behaviour can be embedded in a reinforcing context. It is also possible to precede antecedents with requests that normally elicit cooperation. Clearly, such an approach is possible only within a unit that is both highly structured and has access to sophisticated analysis of behaviour.

In planning behavioural treatments it is valuable to ask a number of questions. What interventions are you planning to make? How and when will these be measured? How will you know the success of any intervention? What resources – human and material – are available? What do the staff think about the behaviour? What are staff's reactions to the behaviour? What alternative strategies are used by the patient?

Pure behavioural approaches, which are based on the principles of operant conditioning, are unfashionable in adult psychiatry, although they are central to the workings of services supporting people with challenging behaviour that has resulted from brain injury. Cognitive–behavioural therapy, however, is fashionable and has been shown to be effective for a very wide range of disorders (for a detailed description of its use in the treatment of schizophrenia see Turkington & Arjundas, Chapter 12, this volume). In the context of a challenging behaviour, the cognitive approach would be to identify problematic schemas or automatic thoughts underlying the behaviour (e.g. 'If staff don't pay attention to me, they don't like me', 'I cannot bear not to be liked', 'If I'm not liked I'm worthless'). Problematic beliefs can then be challenged in therapy. In motivational interviewing, a technique developed within substance misuse services, the patient is encouraged to consider the advantages and disadvantages of change. The therapist adopts a non-directive, non-confrontational approach, showing warmth and empathy. Compliance therapy (Kemp *et al*, 1998) applies motivational interviewing techniques to adherence to medication regimens.

Mental health services are treating increasing numbers of people with borderline personality disorder. Linehan (1993) has developed a sophisticated set of therapeutic interventions targeted at the (self-) destructive behaviours that are a feature of the disorder under the rubric of dialectical behaviour therapy. These interventions include:

- mindfulness skills: teaching the patient to take a non-judgemental stance;
- distress-tolerance skills: teaching how to tolerate and accept distress and how not to 'catastrophise' or be overjudgemental (this can lower impulsive and reactive destructive behaviour);
- emotional regulation skills: emotions are initially validated, then identified and labelled, from the patient's perspective; then the patient is taught to understand the connection between the emotion and destructive behaviour;
- interpersonal skills, as taught in assertiveness training or interpersonal problem-solving groups;
- self-management skills: behavioural targets with realistic goals are set.

Linehan (1993) sees the dialectic as balancing the reasons for the behaviour with the goals for less destructive behaviour. The therapist accepts the patient's position, yet teaches him or her to change.

Psychodynamic understanding may be particularly helpful in approaching the problem of non-engagement with the therapeutic process. Campling & Lodge (1999) use attachment theory. They suggest that time be taken in the assessment phase to examine the patient's fears about therapy. It is useful to explain that progress may be slow and things may get worse at times. A therapeutic contract should be drawn up which clarifies the staff's responsibilities, the patient's responsibilities and joint staff–patient responsibilities. Therapeutic forbearance is important. The patient is in proximity to an attachment figure (the therapist), and feels safe and able to engage in exploratory behaviour. The therapist can help the patient to progress from insecure to secure attachment to the treating team.

Applying theories to clinical practice

The following case examples show how these ideas may be put into practice.

Case history 15.5

Mr E has a long history of schizophrenia with extreme self-neglect and staying in his room. The degree of self-neglect currently makes placement out of hospital impossible.

In this case psychiatric treatment will be geared towards optimal antipsychotic, mood-stabilising and antidepressant medication. The primary nurse/keyworker and nursing care team will seek to engage Mr E. In individual therapy, cognitive schemas need to be identified and trust needs to be engendered, both of which take time. A crucial breakthrough may come from the involvement of occupational therapy staff to identify a hobby or interest that Mr E has, with staff interviewing the family to ascertain any hobbies from the past. Behavioural strategies can be employed. Positive reinforcers such as being taken out to a fast-food restaurant may be offered if hygiene and self-care improve. The social worker can show pictures of accommodation Mr E might be able to move to if he makes progress, and a visit could be arranged to a possible placement.

Case history 15.6

Mr F is 45 years old and has schizoaffective disorder. He has been repeatedly admitted to hospital and has a long-standing history of absconding and angry outbursts in which verbal abuse and damage to property occur. Many behavioural programmes have been put in place without much success. Mr F's keyworker tried to keep rapport going but with little success, as Mr F would rarely participate in a conversation for long. He could be talkative at times, although this behaviour could end unpredictably. He seemed an impulsive law unto himself.

When the keyworker suggested and presented a behavioural contract, Mr F stormed out of the room in anger. However, he returned an hour later and agreed to sign it. The contract set clear goals but tolerated a level of failure. It also required regular update and brief feedback sessions that emphasised positive reinforcement. Much to the surprise of the team, Mr F began to use this contract to relate to all staff members. It appeared that he had found a useful and safe way to relate. He became far less verbally abusive.

Case history 15.7

Mr G is a 35-year-old with chronic paranoid schizophrenia and a long history of intimidation and property damage. His aggressive behaviour occurs frequently on the ward.

The team decide on a plan to impose strict boundaries with respect to his verbal and physical aggression, supported by a programme of positive reinforcement. Mr G was known to enjoy socialising at a hospital social centre. The nursing shift was divided into short time periods. For every period he completed without showing aggression he would be rewarded with time to visit the social club. This was the primary reinforcer. During regular keyworker sessions he would be helped to use previously learnt strategies to deal with his verbal and physical aggression.

When the team presented the plan to Mr G his reply was 'I know what you're up to. You can fuck off. There is no way I'm going to work for my ground leave. You and your behavioural programme can get stuffed'. However, after some weeks of explanation and encouragement, he eventually agreed to try the plan. There were many problems but after some months his behaviour had improved.

225

Case history 15.8

Mr H has a history of schizophrenia, substance misuse and aggressive behaviour. Whenever he goes out on leave from the ward he returns intoxicated and aggressive. If he is not allowed leave he is threatening towards staff and then absconds.

In this case a low secure ward is required so that firm boundaries can be maintained. Principles of management similar to those used in cases 15.6 and 15.7 would be useful, but in addition motivational interviewing will be needed to address the substance misuse. Here the therapist can help Mr H explore the benefits of remaining abstinent while acknowledging the difficulties in so doing.

Whole-ward approaches

Any service that tries to support people who are exhibiting challenging behaviour will itself face multiple challenges. The staff involved have to provide a therapeutic environment that combines sophisticated understanding of each patient's problems and perspective, which requires above all flexibility of conceptual approach, with a highly consistent response to any particular behaviour.

RAID

The RAID programme for challenging behaviour (Davies, 1993) is a method for maintaining a positive style by all treating staff in the face of difficult behaviour. The acronym is derived from the approach that it recommends: 'reinforce appropriate (behaviour), ignore difficult or disruptive (behaviour)'. The focus is on the positive aspects of the individual's behaviour, and less emphasis is placed on the disruptive elements. This creates an environment in which more positive interaction occurs and helps staff to think positively of patients despite the difficult behaviours that they exhibit. Reinforcing positive behaviour makes future positive action more probable and builds on the patients' sense of competence. Ultimately, therefore, success on the ward should strengthen the relationship between staff and patients.

The following attitudes underpin RAID. First, staff should not focus on disruptive behaviour and its consequences. Second, they should be ready to reinforce the next appearance of appropriate behaviour, even if it comes very soon after disruptive behaviour. Even the most difficult-to-manage or disruptive in-patients will be behaving appropriately for about 85% of the time. The temptation for staff, of course, is to focus on the remaining 15%, during which the patients cause trouble, thereby unconsciously reinforcing this mode of personal interaction. The task of the staff is to positively reinforce each instance of appropriate behaviour, which they can do by identifying and targeting such behaviour – situations such as talking to others, watching television, smiling, cooking, playing, doing repairs, eating appropriately, using the bathroom appropriately and sleeping.

Staff–patient groups

Ward meetings should represent the entire ward, with all its subgroups. Patients should be free to raise subjects of their own. Group leaders must often provide structural help. As far as possible, the ward should run on collaboration and agreement, so that staff and patients become partners. In practice, there should be agreed minute-takers, chairpersons and a formal process for referring decisions to the appropriate hospital manager or clinician if the matter cannot be dealt with at the ward meeting.

Conclusions

The causes of challenging behaviour are numerous and not always obvious. Eliciting causes and manifestations can take time, and the management of such behaviour requires skilled intervention from a united multidisciplinary team. Professionals charged with this role need the support of each other and of their local managerial colleagues to effectively address and treat this hard-to-engage group of patients.

Progress can be slow, setbacks are inevitable and failures will occur, but the rewards are seen when very ill and difficult individuals begin to respond to a team that displays therapeutic optimism, delineates clear boundaries and behaves with compassion.

Acknowledgement

Some of the case histories included in this chapter are based on examples given in McKenzie (2001) and are used with permission.

References

Barnard, L., Young, A. H., Pearson, J., *et al* (2002) A systematic review of the use of atypical antipsychotics in autism. *Journal of Psychopharmacology*, **16**, 93–101.

Beck, A. T. & Freeman, A. (1990) *Cognitive Therapy of Personality Disorders*. New York: Guilford Press.

British Medical Association & Royal Pharmaceutical Society of Great Britain (2006) *British National Formulary*. London & Wallingford: BMJ Books & Royal Pharmaceutical Society of Great Britain.

Campling, P. & Lodge, F. D. (1999) Chaotic personalities: maintaining the therapeutic alliance. In *Therapeutic Communities: Past, Present and Future* (eds P. Campling & R. Haigh), pp. 127–139. London: Jessica Kingsley.

Davies, W. (1993) *The RAID Programme for Challenging Behaviour*. Leicester: Association for Psychological Therapies.

Emerson, E. (1995) *Challenging Behaviour. Analysis and Intervention in People with Learning Difficulties*. Cambridge: Cambridge University Press.

Kemp, R., Kirov, G., Everitt, B., *et al* (1998) Randomised controlled trial of compliance therapy. 18-month follow-up. *British Journal of Psychiatry*, **172**, 413–419.

Linehan, M. (1993) *Cognitive–Behavioral Treatment of Borderline Personality Disorder*. New York: Guilford Press.

McKenzie, B. M. (2001) Psychological approaches to longer-term patients presenting with challenging behaviours. In *Psychiatric Intensive Care* (eds M. D. Beer, S. M. Pereira, & C. Paton), pp. 107–132. London: Greenwich Medical Media.

Pereira, S. M., Beer, M. D. & Paton, C. (1999) When all else fails. A locally devised structured decision process for enforcing clozapine therapy. *Psychiatric Bulletin*, **23**, 654–656.

Procter, A. W. (2001) Setting up a new PICU: principles and practice. In *Psychiatric Intensive Care* (eds M. D. Beer, S. M. Pereira, & C. Paton), pp. 263–276. London: Greenwich Medical Media.

Shepherd, G. (1999) Social functioning and challenging behaviour. In *Handbook of Social Functioning in Schizophrenia* (eds K. T. Mueser & N. Tarrier), pp. 407–423. Boston, MA: Allyn and Bacon.

Taylor, D., Paton, C. & Kerwin, R. (2005) *The Maudsley 2005–2006 Prescribing Guidelines* (8th edn). London: Taylor & Francis.

Xenitidis, K., Russell, A. & Murphy, D. (2001) Management of people with challenging behaviour. *Advances in Psychiatric Treatment*, **7**, 109–116.

Part 3

Services and organisational perspectives

CHAPTER 16

Pulling it all together: the care programme approach at its best

Frank Holloway

The origins of the care programme approach

The care programme approach (CPA) was introduced as a direct result of the Inquiry into the Care and Aftercare of Sharon Campbell, a woman with a psychotic illness who killed her former social worker (Spokes, 1988). This documented failures in after-care very similar to those later identified in the better-known Clunis Inquiry (Ritchie, 1994). Healthcare is a devolved function in the UK and the CPA is a specifically English initiative, although similar policies are in place in Scotland and Wales, but not Northern Ireland. The Spokes Inquiry recommended clarification of the responsibilities of health and local authorities to provide after-care for discharged psychiatric in-patients and the publication by the Royal College of Psychiatrists of a document setting out good practice for discharge and after-care. In the event, perhaps wisely, the Department of Health opted for regulation binding on service commissioners and providers rather than exhortation by one of the many professional bodies concerned with the care of people with mental illnesses.

The CPA was one element of a range of reforms to health and social care published in 1989 and 1990 (Thornicroft, 1994). Many other aspects of these reforms are now only of historical interest, having been overtaken by further shifts in policy: who regrets or even recalls the demise of general practice fundholding, the mental illness specific grant or care management? That the CPA survives, albeit after modification and elaboration, is due to the simplicity of the underlying idea: that people in contact with mental health services have their needs assessed, treatment and care is provided and their needs are regularly reviewed.

Reactions to the CPA

When the initial guidance outlining the CPA was issued (Department of Health, 1990) it was greeted with a mixture of indifference and frustration by specialist rehabilitation services, which uniformly believed they were already assessing, treating and reviewing their patients/clients. These tasks are an elementary part of good rehabilitation practice (Shepherd, 1983). In fact there was good evidence from epidemiologically based studies as well as the formal inquiries into rare tragedies that arrangements for the treatment and support of people with severe mental illness were haphazard at best, even after discharge following prolonged hospital stays. The views of staff working in hard-pressed acute psychiatric services about the introduction of the CPA were never adequately documented: there was certainly profound resistance to its introduction from many psychiatrists, who perceived it as a bureaucratic infringement on their clinical practice. Few practitioners would have been reassured by the statement in the original circular that health authorities were 'expected to meet any … costs arising from the introduction of more systematic procedures from existing resources' (Department of Health, 1990). Most would not have agreed that introducing the CPA 'places no new requirement to provide services'.

The evolution of the CPA

The CPA, as initially defined, involved:

- assessment of health and social care needs
- a keyworker to coordinate care
- a written care plan
- regular review of the plan
- interprofessional collaboration
- consultation with service users and carers (Kingdon, 1994).

The central aim was to stop people falling through the net of care (or control). Services were required to develop registers of people cared for under the CPA. Tiers of CPA were subsequently elaborated. At the lowest level were those in contact with specialist services who required assessment and management from one professional ('standard CPA'). At a higher level were patients who required multidisciplinary care, including the now-defunct 'care management' from social services, and in receipt of after-care under section 117 of the Mental Health Act 1983 ('enhanced CPA'). At the top were people who were deemed particularly problematical or vulnerable and enrolled on the Supervision Register, which was introduced in 1994 as part of the response to the Clunis Inquiry (Ritchie, 1994). Policy required services to develop computerised information systems to identify and track those 'known to be at significant risk or potentially at significant risk of committing serious violence, or suicide or of serious self-neglect as the result of severe and enduring mental illness' (Department of Health, 1994a). Detailed guidance was published on the discharge of patients from hospital and their after-care, including a mandatory risk assessment. The guidance provided considerable detail on the content and process of the risk assessment (Department of Health, 1994b).

Although the Supervision Register itself, with its sinister and negative overtones, was dropped, much was retained when the CPA was most recently relaunched (Department of Health, 1999). The focus on risk assessment as a central task of specialist mental health services was further emphasised. The commitment to an electronic patient record deepened. Language changed subtly – 'keyworker' became 'care coordinator'. Service users and, with their agreement, carers were to receive copies of the care plans agreed at CPA reviews. Two tiers of CPA were defined: 'minimal' and 'complex'. In reality the older terminology of 'standard' and 'enhanced' CPA has prevailed. Everyone in contact with rehabilitation services should, by definition, be on enhanced CPA, including those placed in residential and nursing homes and in hospitals as 'out-of-area treatments' in order to ensure that the needs of those who are living in the 'virtual mental hospital' that has replaced the traditional asylum are receiving appropriate and cost-effective care. One very important change was to unravel in a formal way the deeply pernicious divide between health and social care for people with mental illnesses that was introduced in 1989 by subsuming care management into the CPA. Integrated mental health services, where health and social services staff work under joint management, have now become the norm.

The CPA and rehabilitation practice

In many ways the CPA has been an astonishingly successful policy. In little more than a decade it has moved from being a clumsy neologism invented by an anonymous committee for an essentially bureaucratic process to its current pivotal role in the life of all specialist mental health services in England. The contemporary model for secondary mental health care is that, following the CPA principles, after an assessment all patients receive a care plan that aims to meet their identified needs. The care plan is delivered either by a single professional or a multidisciplinary team, often in partnership with other agencies, and is always regularly reviewed.

Many would argue that this approach is just a restatement of good rehabilitation practice, extending this practice to all specialist mental health services. The CPA can, in this context, be seen as providing a helpful framework to pull together the multiple strands of care identified in this book. In this chapter I seek both to define how the CPA can be used as a tool for improving patient care and to warn of the dangers of the CPA becoming a routinised, sterile and bureaucratic exercise.

Elements of the CPA

Core principles

The core principles of enhanced CPA have changed little since its inception: identification of a keyworker, assessment of need and the elaboration of a care plan and its regular review. How these principles are put into practice varies markedly between mental health services, individual teams within each service and, indeed, the practitioners who come together within the team. All mental health services in England have developed and refined a CPA policy, procedure and documentation in conjunction with their local social services authorities. These are rarely shared between services: Burns (2004: pp. 64–67) provides an example of the documents and procedures to be followed in one large National Health Service (NHS) trust, where a decision was made to capture key CPA information on a single sheet of A4 paper. Despite the differences between services there are some core commonalities, which largely stem from evolving mental health policy. These include an expectation that, for people on enhanced CPA, there are review meetings that bring together key actors involved in the care programme. These meetings can be routine (for example 6-monthly or yearly reviews) or convened because of a crisis or at a significant change-point, for example transfer of care between services or before planned discharge. (Formal CPA meetings are also required on all detained patients who are about to have appeals heard by a mental health review tribunal or the hospital managers to discuss what support plans would be put in place should the patient be discharged from their detained status.) There is an expectation that routine outcome measures such as the Health of the Nation Outcome Scales (HoNOS) will be measured and recorded at the time of a CPA.

The CPA and the electronic care record

It is becoming increasingly common for CPA documentation to be captured on an electronic care record that is readily available throughout the service, wherever and whenever the patient presents. (The long-term vision is for this information to be available across service boundaries within the National Programme for Information Technology, with appropriate safeguards for patient confidentiality: see http://www.connectingforhealth.nhs.uk/) Electronic records provide the opportunity, and the temptation, to elaborate the information collected within the CPA documentation. This documentation will routinely be shared with the patient, their carer(s) and other agencies, although all information-sharing is governed by the patient's right to confidentiality, which can only be overridden in uncommon and particular circumstances that largely relate to risk issues.

The CPA summary documentation for the South London and Maudsley NHS Trust provides an illustration of the areas that need to be addressed within the process. It records simple but vital basic information about the patient, key professional staff (who are defined as being clinically responsible), other involved professionals and carers. Mental and physical health needs are identified, as are a range of social needs. These are broken down into domains: (a) relationships, (b) occupation and education, (c) accommodation, (d) activities of daily living, (e) ethnicity/culture/spirituality, (f) child need and risk, and (g) finance (domains that are very similar to those identified in tools assessing need or quality of life). Risk issues are recorded, with reference to more elaborate risk assessment tools used within the trust. There follows the care programme, a set of actions or interventions that aim to address the key needs. The care programme seeks to specify who will be doing what and how often. The summary also includes details of current medication, diagnoses and, very importantly, a contingency plan and a crisis plan. The contingency plan sets out actions that need to be taken to avoid crises, for example by maintaining regular contact with the patient and carers and identifying how services can be contacted early should concerns be emerging. The crisis plan sets out early-warning signs and relapse indicators specific to the individual and the nature of the service response to be offered in a crisis both during and out of working hours. Within the South London and Maudsley Trust this information is available in the electronic patient record for all individuals on enhanced CPA (which can also include all correspondence generated about the patient). The record is accessible at all trust sites and within the local accident and emergency department, so that basic information is available to any staff required to respond to a request for treatment or support.

Risk

The rise of risk

We live in a society that is obsessed with risk, its avoidance and the identification of someone to blame should things go wrong. The CPA grew out of the recommendations of a homicide inquiry, and risk lies at the heart of contemporary psychiatric practice. Although professionals understandably perceive the focus on risk as a worrying burden, risk issues raise many important and interesting questions about the nature of mental healthcare (Box 16.1). Mental health trusts are required to develop and implement frameworks for the assessment and management of risk, and, as part of Twelve Points to a Safer Service (Appleby et al, 2001: p. 162), to ensure that their staff receive regular training in risk assessment.

Risk assessment methodologies

The risk assessment tools that are employed in general adult psychiatric practice tend to be locally developed and be based on checklists of features that are known to be predictive of risky behaviour (such as past behaviour and demographic and clinical factors robustly associated with self-harm and violence). There are isolated examples of risk assessment methodologies that have been developed in a systematic fashion (e.g. Watts et al, 2004). The most useful aspect of these tools is to encourage staff (and service users and carers) to think about risk issues, to review past risky behaviours and to identify plans that might decrease the likelihood of adverse outcomes in the future.

Box 16.1   Why risk is not just a burden: some issues raised by questions of risk

The social policy of mental health
- How are policy decisions made?
- How does professional opinion influence decision-making?
- How are decisions implemented?

Epistemology
- On what basis can we predict the future?
- How can we draw valid causal inferences?

Epidemiology
- What are the risks?
- What are the predictors/correlates of risk?

Evidence-based mental health
- What is the evidence for risk statements that are made?
- How do risk assessment tools work in practice?
- Does risk management reduce bad outcomes and if so how?
- What are the effective strategies for reducing bad outcomes in psychiatry?

Risk communication
- How do we inform ourselves and others of risk?
- Ethics
- How do we conceptualise personal responsibility for bad actions that are committed?
- What master do mental health professionals serve in making risk decisions?
- Is defensive practice ethical?

Medicolegal issues
- What comprises negligence?
- How do we avoid criticism when things go wrong?

Clinical practice
- The phenomenology of violent and self-harming behaviour
- Risk management: good practice in care planning
- Patients as parents
- Risk-sharing
- The value of taking risks

(From Holloway, 2004*a*)

Even where a tool has admirable sensitivity and specificity it may not be useful in predicting at an individual level serious adverse outcomes in environments where the base rate of the target event is low, as are serious violence, suicide and homicide within routine clinical practice (Szmukler, 2003). The situation is rather different in forensic practice, where validated tools such as the 20-item Historical/Clinical/Risk Management scale HCR–20 may usefully be employed to identify individuals who are likely to reoffend (Dowsett, 2005) (whether this knowledge helps community forensic services alter the pattern of reoffending is moot).

Box 16.2   Risk issues for mental health services

Risks due to the patient's behaviour
Self-harm; self-neglect; suicide; violence to others; homicide

Risks that the patient poses to carers and dependants
Harm to children; harm to elderly carers; harm to partners

Risks of abuse/exploitation of the patient by carers or services
Financial exploitation; sexual, physical and emotional abuse

Risks to the patient from treatments
Obesity; diabetes; cardiac disease; tardive dyskinesia

Risks from the care environment
Violence; abuse; loss of dignity; loss of skills

Risks that the patient poses to the public
Violence against strangers; socially unacceptable and antisocial behaviour

Risks faced by mental healthcare staff
Violence or abuse during home visits; violence from patients and carers; staff stress

Risks to the service/organisation
Complaints; serious untoward incidents; breach of confidentiality; litigation; failing to reach government targets

---

The practice of risk assessment and risk management

Whatever intellectual doubts professionals might hold about the rise of the risk industry, a systematic approach to the assessment, recording and management of risk is now mandatory. The risks that services are expected to address are ever-widening (Box 16.2). Most recently, in an era of community care where people with severe mental illness are commonly undertaking the role of parent, the issue of child welfare has come to the fore. It must also be acknowledged that patients experience significant risk of harms stemming from the treatments and services they receive, perhaps the most pervasive but least recognised risk being that of deteriorating social functioning within impoverished and understimulating care environments.

There are a number of practical points to be made about risk assessment and management within a rehabilitation service. The first, and most important, is not to lose sight of the positive value of informed risk-taking. We all learn and change by exercising choice and embracing the unknown. There is an ethical imperative for mental health professionals to promote the autonomy of those with whom they are working. This imperative must, of course, be balanced against the potential for harms that might occur should someone make bad decisions by, for example, running away from hospital, killing themselves, spending to excess or engaging in violent behaviour. Rehabilitation practitioners constantly walk a tightrope between being too restrictive, thus limiting autonomy, and allowing people to harm themselves and others. The hospital closure programme proved that in the past services had erred on the side of restrictiveness.

The next point is the importance of detail in risk assessment and risk management. Risky behaviours tend to fall into a pattern typical for an individual, so a detailed history is important. Risk associated with psychosis may stem from the individual's psychopathology, hence the need for a detailed and contemporaneous understanding of the contents of a person's mental state. Risky behaviours tend to be contextual: staff need to be fully aware of the person's social environment. Most of the excess in risk of violence associated with a severe mental illness occurs in individuals with comorbid substance misuse (and much of the suicide risk too). Risk management therefore requires a detailed understanding of a person's use of alcohol and other psychoactive substances, both prescribed and non-prescribed. (The biggest risk psychiatric patients face is that of an early death due to life-style issues such as smoking.) The increasingly close relationships between rehabilitation and forensic practice allow a cross-fertilisation between the two areas, with rehabilitation practitioners learning much about the value of detail. The importance of detail extends, of course, into the daily fabric of a rehabilitation service. The service must assess the ability of an individual to live safely and well in a particular environment, ranging from independent accommodation to high security, and must develop strategies to allow the individual to live in the least restrictive setting.

It is also important to emphasise the value of the therapeutic relationship in managing risks. This is akin to the concept of relational security emphasised by forensic practitioners. At its simplest level, people who are engaged in a therapeutic relationship with a practitioner are less likely to harm themselves than those who feel alienated from services. They are also more likely to report changes in circumstances and symptomatic deterioration that will increase risk and to adhere to recommendations for treatment if they know and trust the treatment team. Similarly, families and carers will be better able to report their concerns and have them effectively addressed if they are engaged with the service.

A few brief statements about risk management are also appropriate:

- if in doubt, share the risk: difficult decisions are best undertaken after full discussion within the multidisciplinary team, drawing in others as appropriate
- if concerned, communicate the risk (within the boundaries of confidentiality): the homicide inquiry literature is replete with reports that document and criticise the quality of communication between interested parties

- always document the risk and risk decisions: medico-legally it is difficult to defend decisions that were not properly recorded
- always pay attention to the duty of care that services and individual professionals hold towards their patients.

In practice, professionals are much more likely to receive censure for sins of omission, such as not detaining a suicidal patient who subsequently takes their own life, than sins of commission, such as detaining a patient who is later released by a mental health review tribunal. This comment should not be seen as encouraging inappropriately defensive practice.

Using the CPA effectively

It is perhaps inevitable, but unfortunate nevertheless, that the CPA is perceived less an approach to care than in terms of the regular reviews it mandates. The CPA review has come to dominate practice, rather than act as a tool for meeting the overall objective of developing, delivering and coordinating effective services to patients and their carers. Care programme approach documentation such as that used within the South London and Maudsley Trust serves as a helpful shorthand reminder of the areas of need that services should be addressing.

The CPA review

Teams vary widely in how they conduct CPA reviews (Burns, 2004: pp. 88–90), which may be incorporated into multidisciplinary team meetings or, surely preferable for the patient/client and their carers, involve only the key actors in the review. There are, however, some pointers to good practice in undertaking a CPA review. The first is that adequate preparation is vital. This requires a considerable amount of groundwork by the care coordinator, not only in inviting relevant people to the review but also in drafting documentation and identifying issues for discussion at the review with the participants. It is very helpful if the care coordinator has gone through the documentation with the patent/client before the meeting: this is particularly important where the individual experiences a degree of cognitive impairment or is distressed.

The second aspect of good practice is that the review should be structured. This ensures that all areas are addressed and long-held assumptions are questioned. Appropriate documentation helps provide this structure, although if it is too long or used too rigidly it can reduce a review to a bureaucratic exercise within which the patient/client, carers and others present can feel railroaded by a process that appears to take no genuine account of their views. It is vital that all participants feel involved in the review and have a chance to express their views. Here both good chairing of the review and adequate intelligence about the potential concerns of participants is required. The care coordinator role is a complex and demanding one and it is usually appropriate for another person (such as a team leader or consultant) to chair large-scale reviews involving multiple agencies and many participants.

Attention to the conduct of the CPA review is clearly important. Clear ground rules, good agenda-setting, a comfortable location, sensible time-keeping and effective minuting of agreed actions are all important. Disagreements also need to be acknowledged, as do certain potentially uncomfortable givens such as the role of the Mental Health Act. The precise conduct of the review is likely to vary between settings. Large and formal meetings tend to be the norm in in-patient settings, particularly as discharge is planned. Small, informal meetings are more appropriate when the review is being held in a community setting such as the individual's home. On occasion it will be appropriate for the care team to hold a review in the absence of patients or carers, particularly in emergencies or when the individual has made a decision to withdraw from services. If this does occur, common courtesy and common sense suggest that the patient/client and other key actors should be informed of the outcome of the review.

Misuses of the CPA

The corollary of good practice in using the CPA is bad practice, which is surprisingly easy to slip into. Aspects of bad practice include meetings where preparation is poor, an agenda is pushed through without adequate reflection, communication with users and carers is inadequate, a superficial approach to complex issues is adopted and there is a lack of attention to detail. Surveys of users and carers suggest that they generally do not feel involved in the process and, indeed, many service users report that they do not know the name of their care coordinator and were not involved in developing their care plan.

Some ethical issues

Rehabilitation practice is an ethical minefield. There is a daily ethical dilemma facing staff who are committed to promoting their client's autonomy but in doing so may have to engage in potentially coercive practices. When does prompting to engage in basic self-care become bullying? When does allowing an individual to engage in risky behaviour become neglect? When is it appropriate to take control over a person's financial affairs? How does one respond when someone's recovery goals defy common sense or appear unattainable?

Concerns over criticism if things should go wrong may cause staff to be excessively restrictive of patient freedom and choice. A particularly difficult dilemma is produced by the substance-misusing in-patient who is involved in drug dealing within a rehabilitation unit: how does one balance the duty of care that is held to this patient against the duty of care towards vulnerable fellow residents? (The pragmatic answer is generally the exclusion of the dealer unless they can be educated to change their ways.) There is a major unmet need for services that can address the needs of individuals with comorbid substance misuse and severe mental illness (for a useful discussion of the issues see Burns & Firn, 2002: pp. 192–203).

A further ethical difficulty that has already been identified is how to respect the rights of the individual to confidentiality. A very vexed issue is that of communication between services and informal carers when the patient states they do not want the carer involved. Although professional regulators such as the General Medical Council have not changed their traditional views towards confidentiality, there is no doubt that public policy is currently undermining our traditional rights to confidentiality, particularly if we have a mental illness (Holloway, 2004b). In addition to the CPA policy, which expects good information-sharing between agencies and with carers, there are demands to engage in arrangements and develop protocols with the criminal justice system that will ensure public protection.

By their nature ethical questions generally defy clear-cut dogmatic answers. Practitioners should be aware of the problems that their work raises and be prepared to discuss them with colleagues. The presence within a multidisciplinary team of individuals with a variety of professional and personal backgrounds should enrich an ethical debate within a rehabilitation service. If necessary, colleagues from outside the service should be consulted (for example the Caldicott guardian). Useful texts are available that provide general methodologies for addressing particular problematical issues (e.g. Bloch *et al*, 1999; Dickenson & Fulford, 2000) and professionals have recourse to codes of conduct, although these may well be out of date.

Conclusions

The CPA is, in many ways, an astonishingly bold statement about how mental health services should work. There is nothing like it in any other country in the world. In essence it sets out a requirement on mental health services that applies to everyone accepted for specialist care to adopt a holistic approach to need, to follow people up and to be concerned about their long-term welfare. These aims are totally consistent with the long-held principles of psychiatric rehabilitation. People on the case-loads of rehabilitation services invariably have complex needs and usually have lengthy histories of engagement with mental health services. The relatively slow throughput of rehabilitation services means that there is no excuse for anything other than the adoption of best practice in undertaking the requirements of the CPA.

References

Appleby, J., Shaw, J., Sherratt, J., *et al* (2001) *Safety First: Five Year Report of the National Confidential Inquiry into Homicides and Suicides by People with a Mental Illness.* London: Department of Health.

Bloch, S., Chodoff, P. & Green, S. A. (1999) *Psychiatric Ethics.* Oxford: Oxford University Press.

Burns, T. (2004) *Community Mental Health Teams. A Guide to Current Practices.* Oxford: Oxford University Press.

Burns, T. & Firn, M. (2002) *Assertive Outreach in Mental Health. A Manual for Practitioners.* Oxford: Oxford University Press.

Department of Health (1990) *The Care Programme Approach for People with a Mental Illness Referred to Specialist Psychiatric Services* (HC(90)23). London: Department of Health.

Department of Health (1994a) *Introduction of Supervision Registers for Mentally Ill People* (HSG(94)5). London: Department of Health.

Department of Health (1994b) *Guidance on the Discharge of Mentally Disordered People and their Continuing Care in the Community* (HSG(94)27/LASSL(94)4). London: Department of Health.

Department of Health (1999) *Effective Care Coordination in Mental Health.* London: Department of Health.

Dickenson, D. & Fulford, K. W. M. (2000) *In Two Minds. A Casebook of Psychiatric Ethics.* Oxford: Oxford University Press.

Dowsett, J. (2005) Measurement of risk by a community forensic mental health team. *Psychiatric Bulletin*, **29**, 9–12.

Holloway, F. (2004a) Risk: more questions than answers. Invited Commentary on... Psychodynamic methods in risk assessment and management. *Advances in Psychiatric Treatment*, **10**, 273–274.

Holloway, F. (2004b) Confidentiality in mental health. *Psychiatry*, **3**(3), 11–14.

Kingdon, D. (1994) Care Programme Approach. Recent government policy and legislation. *Psychiatric Bulletin*, **18**, 68–70.

Ritchie, J. H. (1994) *The Report of the Inquiry into the Care and Treatment of Christopher Clunis.* London: TSO (The Stationery Office).

Shepherd, G. (1983) Planning rehabilitation for the individual. In *Theory and Practice of Psychiatric Rehabilitation* (eds F. N. Watts & D. H. Bennett), pp. 329–348. Chichester: John Wiley & Sons.

Spokes, J. (1988) *Report of the Committee of Inquiry into the Care and After-care of Miss Sharon Campbell.* London: TSO (The Stationery Office).

Szmukler, G. (2003) Risk assessment: 'numbers' and 'values'. *Psychiatric Bulletin*, **27**, 205–207.

Thornicroft, G. (1994) The NHS and Community Care Act 1990. *Psychiatric Bulletin*, **18**, 13–17.

Watts, D., Bindman, J., Slade, M., *et al* (2004) Clinical Assessment of Risk Decision Support (CARDS). The development and evaluation of a feasible violence risk assessment for routine psychiatric practice. *Journal of Mental Health*, **13**, 569–581.

CHAPTER 17

No place like home: accommodation for people with severe mental illness

Paul Wolfson

Aside from its use to describe institutions for groups such as elderly people and orphans, the word 'home' has almost entirely positive associations. Playing at home is a recognised and distinct advantage for a football team. As the saying goes, 'home is where the heart is'. It is at the core of our emotional life, and 'Make yourself at home' is an invitation to be relaxed and unrestrained. A home offers not just protection from the elements but cosiness, privacy and autonomy. It is a place where the decor is customised and there is a door to keep out unwanted people. Home is where we can be 'both most and least ourselves', but it is more than just a place: it is an idea. 'Our homes are yoked to identities, both personal and political, as much as to experience' (Wilson, 2004).

When the Wizard of Oz orders Dorothy to repeat 'There's no place like home', her journey to Oz is revealed as a delirium secondary to a head injury. Home is where she will recover. The healing qualities of the living environment have long been recognised in the treatment of mental illness. The asylums were constructed with the humanitarian aim of reversing the community neglect of people with mental illness and to provide healthy, light and airy accommodation in leafy rural settings. In the ongoing debate about what type of accommodation is best for mentally ill people in the 21st century there is a tension between a home as an entitlement and home as a treatment environment. A review of the literature on housing and mental health concludes that, although 'the quality of life benefits of improving housing satisfaction can be justified on humanitarian grounds, public investments ... will remain difficult to justify unless it can be demonstrated that satisfaction is cost effectively related to improved mental health outcomes' (Newman, 2001). Such evidence has proved difficult to obtain.

This chapter traces the transition of home from a single bed with a bedside cupboard, enclosed by a plastic curtain, in a mental hospital ward to independent accommodation for some and a placement in a family, in a shared house or in a variety of institutions for others.

The heyday of the British mental hospital – and its decline

Jones describes how, after the Second World War, mental hospitals in the UK evolved into a unique blend of English public school, Royal Air Force base and holiday camp. The typical hospital contained 2000–3000 beds. The medical superintendent had supreme authority over the lives of patients and the workforce. Hospitals had elite first teams in football and cricket that mixed staff and patients, and highlights of fixtures between rival hospitals would be recalled years afterwards. Each institution had its own traditional way of celebrating Christmas and 'sports day'. Discharged patients were encouraged to come back and visit staff and fellow patients like ex-pupils returning to school (Jones, 1993: pp. 145–147).

There was a darker side to mental hospital life, apparent even in as bland a source as the minutes of Bexley Hospital Medical Staffing Committee. The hospital prided itself on public demonstrations of unmodified electro-convulsive treatment using 'mental defectives' from a nearby institution. The minutes record numerous requests from eminent physicians for the hospital to 'provide' patients with diverse medical conditions for unspecified purposes. There are no references to today's preoccupations with aggression or suicide, but much alarm and despondency about devastating outbreaks of dysentery and the spread of tuberculosis. The strongest impression is of a lack of accountability to the world outside: 'A preliminary meeting was held (in 1960) to discuss the implications of the 1959 Mental Health Act. It was decided to defer any action until these became clear' (Wolfson *et al*, 2002).

Things were moving faster at Westminster. Only 2 years after the 1959 Act, the Health Minister Enoch Powell announced a startling new policy initiative in his 'Water Tower' speech. It was presented as a ground-breaking humanitarian leap of the imagination, but the aim was rather more mundane – to cut the cost of the NHS to the taxpayer. The mental hospitals would be stripped of at least 75 000 beds over the next 15 years, from a total of over 130 000. Further policy developments occurred over the next couple of years. The plan was that all acute care would be provided in district general hospitals, and all 'chronic patients' would be treated in community settings (Jones, 1993: pp. 145–147).

Sociology and the mental hospital: the Three Hospitals Study

When Erving Goffman published his collection of essays on mental asylums (Goffman, 1961) he created a new concept – 'the total institution', dehumanising and Kafkaesque. His great strength was 'in pinpointing and naming institutional practices. Like a botanist in a forest of strange plants, he identified, classified and listed' (Jones, 1993: pp. 145–147). Goffman was a leading member of a new school of sociology emerging in the USA that was interested not specifically in mental illness but in all types of perceived social deviance.

Polsky, whom Goffman supervised at university, has described the methodology of the developing social science (Polsky, 1971). It had much in common with modern investigative journalism. Detailed personal observations were collected from field studies, the validity of existing literature was scrupulously checked and the approach to research was 'value free', i.e. not biased by any official line or policy. This new approach was combined with traditional medical research methods in the landmark Three Hospitals Study in England.

Although before the Three Hospitals Study there had been descriptions of the impact of an institutional environment on long-stay hospital patients, no one had 'addressed the important problem of cause and effect' (Wing & Brown, 1970). The authors, psychiatrist John Wing and sociologist George Brown, wished to examine 'the interaction between social and clinical events'. The views of Goffman, who, they wrote, 'tends to explain patients' behaviour purely in terms of their reaction to the social environment' were contrasted with 'biological' interpretations of the negative symptoms of schizophrenia, and both approaches were found wanting. Wing & Brown adopted a stress/vulnerability model, the key hypothesis being that many people with schizophrenia are 'biologically vulnerable to under-stimulating environments'. They are 'liable to respond to them by a marked increase in social withdrawal', which along with blunting of affect and poverty of thought, the authors named 'the clinical poverty syndrome'.

The study had many innovative features. It occurred over an impressively long time scale and used data from three hospitals: Mapperley in Nottingham, Netherne in Surrey and Severalls in Essex. These hospitals were selected because they were thought likely to be the most contrasting on measures of social environment. The principal finding of the study was a strong association between measures of poverty of the social environment and the severity of the clinical poverty syndrome. Box 17.1 shows a summary of the findings.

Almost 30 years later, using the same instruments, Curson et al (1992) re-examined the association at a fourth English hospital, Horton in Surrey. They found it to be much weaker than in the Three Hospitals Study. Differences in the population and statistical problems make interpretation of the results complex, but the main findings were challenging to our belief in progress. Ward restrictiveness was much lower at Horton and more patients – 80% – spent over 5 h a day doing nothing than did in the most restrictive environment of the Three Hospital study 30 years previously. This occurred despite much improved staff/patient ratios. Medication doses in chlorpromazine equivalents were up to five times higher at Horton than in the three hospitals three decades earlier.

Box 17.1   Summary of conclusions of the Three Hospitals Study

- Environmental poverty was strongly correlated with clinical poverty syndrome
- The hospital with the richest social environment (Netherne) housed the patients with the fewest negative symptoms
- Patients with the fewest personal possessions were least likely to be in touch with relatives or friends outside and more likely to spend most of the time doing nothing
- Improvements in negative symptoms occurred following improvements in the social environment at Netherne and Mapperley, but reversed as social conditions deteriorated
- New developments in drug treatment did not account for the findings
- The longer patients had been in hospital, the greater the likelihood that they had a negative attitude to discharge
- The single most important factor associated with improvement of negative symptoms was a reduction in time spent doing nothing
- Ward restrictiveness seemed to play an independent role in promoting or maintaining negative symptoms

(Wing & Brown, 1970)

People and services in transition (1970s–1990s)

Inspired by Goffman and the Three Hospitals Study, progressive mental health workers formed an uneasy alliance with politicians to close hospital beds. A series of scandals involving ill treatment captured the public imagination and accelerated the process. Early results were far from encouraging. A follow-up study of 120 people discharged from a mental hospital in the early 1970s (Johnstone *et al*, 1984) found that nearly half were living with relatives, who felt that psychiatric services were ill equipped to help people with chronic disabilities. A quarter were out of contact with all services. Half had 'definite psychotic symptoms' and 'severe emotional, social and financial difficulties were commonplace'. Despite this no former in-patients wished to return to hospital, and few relatives wanted this either.

While hospital managers had to draw up plans for closure that many thought would never be implemented, small local schemes began to attract finance. The psychiatrist Jim Birley recalled how in the early 1970s, with the backing of a local philanthropist, who had donated the cash deposit, and the borough, which provided 100% mortgages,

'we started the housing association … and it's been running ever since. … We always bought houses that had multiple occupancy and instead of a resident warden we had a manageress who lived locally. That way we were not changing the use of the house and didn't have a public inquiry and all the ensuing palaver. … It was quite novel, in those days to set up a house like this without any resident staff' (Birley & Wilkinson, 1995).

Resettlement teams were set up in some hospitals to assess need and work with staff and residents. Three sometimes conflicting philosophies or ideologies were predominant influences on both the planning of new services and clinical practice on hospital wards preparing residents for hospital closure – deinstitutionalisation, rehabilitation and social role valorisation (Box 17.2).

Clifford described some of the conflicts involved when preparing a small group of residents of a large mental hospital for transfer to a community home in the 1980s:

'T2 ward became designated a rehabilitation ward ... it slowly assumed its own identity and became more independent of its base institution. Not surprisingly it met with resistance from the hospital – as exemplified by battles over uniform and nursing hours. The issue of dependence was played out in terms of the catering arrangements. T2 wanted to do its own catering. The hospital objected. It was decided to postpone implementing the new arrangements ... [until] the move into the community' (Clifford, 1988: p. 261).

Service users were not involved in the planning and design of the new facilities, although their views were beginning to be sought in the form of 'satisfaction' surveys. A survey was undertaken in 1995 in the hospital described by Clifford, now with a much depleted population, and about to close. Extracts contrast some of the opinions of those remaining on the long-stay wards with those of a small group of residents living in a 'shadow unit', Sycamore House, in the hospital grounds prior to the move to a staffed community home (Butler & Salter-Ling, 1995):

Box 17.2 Philosophies and conceptual frameworks influencing reprovision and resettlement in the 1980s

Deinstitutionalisation Used in North America to describe the replacement of isolated large institutions for the care of mentally ill people with smaller settings that have close ties to the community. This approach was modified by British researchers, who diverted the focus away from changing the locus of care to improving its quality by developing 'resident-oriented' management practices.

Rehabilitation The acquisition of new skills and the maintenance of existing skills following a multidisciplinary assessment and care plan. This should not be confused with the 'ladder model' of resettlement – a stepwise progression to increasingly independent accommodation that can be very disruptive. When progress is made, the support should move rather than the person.

Social role valorisation Principles associated with Wolfensberger, who developed them in the context of learning disability services. They can be applied to services for all care groups at risk of social devaluation, and imply that people with mental disorders should live in dispersed, accessible, ordinary housing rather than clustered special schemes.

(After Garety, 1988)

On the ward:

'I wait for things to come along. I don't do much. I sit here wondering if I'm going to get my next meal.'

'I do smoking and reading.'

'Got only one dress, wore it last week as well.'

'Sometimes I don't feel safe when men are asking me for sex. … Mike, if I don't give him cigarettes he goes like he's going to hit me. Feel threatened all the time.'

'Can't be by myself. Not in here.'

'Live like a normal human being, if I was in a group home, I'd be happy as the day is long.'

In Sycamore House:

'Bit scared of being here … like at night, all dark and spooky. Wake up at night and you're by yourself.'

'I go gardening now, all day, nearly every day, up at 9.00, go gardening at 1.00, get back 3.00 or 4.00.'

'Got to take my own [medication] now. Little better. I sort my own.'

'If you want to be by yourself go to your room. I spend a lot of time alone. Like it sometimes.'

'They talk about the community. I'll find out where that is later.'

The TAPS hospital closure study

The Team for the Assessment of Psychiatric Services (TAPS) was established in 1985 with the aim of evaluating the closure of Friern and Claybury Hospitals in north London. During the course of the study, the regional health authority decided it could no longer afford to close both hospitals, so the Claybury closure was halted. Meanwhile, the admission wards at Friern stayed open and continued to accumulate patients until the hospital closed in 1993, by which time one-third of the patients in the acute ward had lengths of stay of over 1 year.

Hospital residents were discharged to a wide range of community provision. Wherever possible the group settings were in ordinary-looking accommodation, not recognisably connected with mental illness, and preserved existing relationships, mixing men and women of different ages and social abilities. 'Difficult-to-place' residents tended to be discharged much later in the closure process.

The conclusions were mainly reassuring, although the savings that the closure policy was expected to produce did not occur. There was a marginal but significant increase in cost of community care compared with hospital care. The increased cost was most marked for those who left the hospital in the final year (Beecham et al, 1997). There were few adverse events, modest clinical improvements and significant gains in the social sphere. The key findings for residents without dementia are summarised in Box 17.3.

Box 17.3 Summary of findings of the TAPS study of former in-patients without dementia

- The death rate over 5 years was nearly twice as high as in the general population, a common finding in this population and unlikely to be due to hospital closures. The suicide rate was low. Contacts with the police were more likely to be as victims of crime than as perpetrators of aggressive behaviour. Only 7 out of 737 were lost to follow-up after 1 year, and may have become homeless.
- There was a small but significant improvement in negative symptoms in the early cohorts of discharged patients, almost all in the first year, lending some support to the findings of the Three Hospitals Study, but overall they were unchanged. Active delusions and hallucinations were found in nearly half throughout the follow-up period. Attitudes to medication improved significantly in the first year and persisted over 5 years.
- Community skills improved at 1 year and were maintained. Gains in domestic skills at 1 year had declined by 5 years but were still above baseline.
- Social networks remained the same size but improved in quality. The increase in the number of friends at 1 year was sustained and the number of confidants increased steadily over the next 4 years. Contact with relatives reduced over the period of the study.
- The social environment was dramatically less restrictive than hospital: 84% wanted to stay in their community homes; of the 21 individuals who wanted to leave their community homes, only three wished to return to hospital.
- 15% of patients discharged from hospital were readmitted within the first year, but the majority returned to their original community home. Stability of tenure at 5 years was reported for the majority (61%) of those resettled.
- 40% of a group of difficult-to-place patients could be discharged into community settings 5 years after baseline.

(Leff, 1997; Leff & Trieman, 2000; Trieman & Leff, 2002)

Other closure studies were undertaken in the UK, but none so comprehensive as TAPS. There were similar generally positive findings (e.g Donnelly *et al* ,1996), but some negative consequences. High mortality rates were associated with relocation of elderly residents, especially those who were the most dependent (Holloway, 1991). Warnings about fragmentation and inadequacy of community services, particularly day care, were born out by experience. The Hampstead Schizophrenia Survey reported that the percentage of people with no daytime activity rose from 50% to 61% between 1986 and 1991, in one of the areas affected by the closure of Friern Hospital (Jeffreys *et al*, 1997).

The relatively smooth progress of the hospital closure policy in the UK may have been assisted by its slow pace compared with that in the USA. When President Reagan suddenly cut federal funding to the mental health programmes that were to replace the rapidly disappearing mental hospitals, visible and distressing consequences were immediately apparent:

'When I was at college in Boston in the early eighties, mental patients started to gather most days at Boston Common near the Park Street subway station. They would dance round and round the fountain. I remember one woman with a very long pink feather sticking out of her hair would always be there. She followed me down into the subway and wanted to go home with me. Other students had similar experiences' (L. Windemuth, radio journalist, personal communication, 2004).

The virtual asylum

As early as 1985, attention was drawn to a group of patients who presented difficulties for hospital closure programmes (Levene et al, 1985). Mann & Cree (1976) identified a group of 'new long-stay' patients in British hospitals a decade later, defined as people under 65 with hospital stays of 1–5 years. After a series of failed community placements, these individuals gradually accumulated on acute wards, where they remained hard to manage. A planning blight was identified (Hirsch, 1992). A 1991 survey of five hospitals scheduled for run down or closure found that a third of the population of these hospitals was now 'new long-stay', and identified three main subgroups: younger men with schizophrenia, women over 65 with affective disorders and people with cognitive impairments secondary to learning difficulties or organic illness (Clifford et al, 1991).

'Wards in a house' or 'hospital hostels' on the perimeters of hospital grounds were developed in specialist centres to meet the needs of these individuals. They combined a highly structured behavioural rehabilitative approach with more autonomy and responsibilities for residents than is possible in traditional hospital settings. The outcomes were generally favourable (e.g. Creighton et al, 1991), but despite Department of Health support they remained in short supply.

The TAPS study demonstrated what could be achieved locally when appropriate facilities were available for hospital residents who were 'difficult to place' (Trieman & Leff, 2002). Although there was no change in the first year, problem behaviours gradually improved over the next 4 years, and physical aggression practically disappeared. As a result, 40% of a group of 72 long-stay in-patients, previously assessed as unsuitable for community placement, were able to move to more independent care homes.

Meanwhile, at a national level, the effects of the 'planning blight' were becoming increasingly evident. 'The lack of NHS facilities for patients whose behaviours are intractably difficult to manage or require specialist placements has been exploited as a market opportunity' thundered an editorial in the British Medical Journal (Poole et al, 2002). The authors claimed that patients are isolated, far from family and friends, in the care of poorly trained staff, and are only offered rehabilitation which is focused on acculturation to institutional life. They described a network of private facilities – 'a virtual asylum, dispersed, invisible, and inadequately regulated'.

The chief executive of a private health care company responded: 'They are not invisible: they are shiny, clean, proud, quasi public institutions that devote huge efforts to visibility to attract in-patient and out-patient customers' (Hughes, 2002), and the dispute spread to the business section of *The Sunday Times*, an indicator of its importance to the health economy. The fact remains that spot-purchased out-of-area treatments, generally within the independent hospital sector, are a significant drain on local mental health finances, are difficult to monitor and may require new posts specifically for this purpose (Ryan *et al*, 2004). The experience of isolation from families and community is a source of distress, especially for people from minority ethnic or religious groups, and will continue until there is effective regional planning for specialist services, perhaps in partnership with the private sector.

A spectrum of care settings for a mental health service

To meet the diversity of local need, every mental health service requires access to a range of accommodation, including rehabilitation facilities in hospital as well as in the community, and a network of staffed homes and supported housing for the longer term. For a guide to the terminology, see Box 17.4. This can only be a guide, as the meaning of these terms varies according to local custom and over time. Alternative typologies have been developed (e.g. Macpherson *et al*, 2004).

Falling bed availability and the aversive environment on acute psychiatric wards (e.g. Mind, 2000) have led to important developments in alternatives to hospital admission. New community services such as home treatment teams need to be supplemented by residential crisis facilities for situations where relapse can be managed safely outside hospital. Flexible access criteria are crucial as local resources tend to be limited. Priorities may be conflicting: what appears to be the ideal residential home for someone on clinical grounds can be too distant from a close relative or too near them, or has a long waiting list. In residential settings, the potential impact of a new arrival on the welfare of existing residents can pose ethical dilemmas. Even when a staffed home would offer greater supervision and monitoring, ordinary housing with external support may be the only community option available to someone with a psychosis who deals in street drugs or poses a risk to vulnerable women.

An ideal size for a residential setting has yet to be identified. There is some evidence that there are better mental health outcomes in settings where there are fewer occupants (Newman, 2001). Larger settings attract economies of scale, but may be more difficult to manage. Problems with staff retention and training are useful indicators of dysfunction. Placement costs are only partially dependent on resident characteristics; geography and market forces play a significant role, and NHS facilities are generally

---

Box 17.4 A typology of residential and housing facilities for people with severe mental illness

Rehabilitation ward Hospital-based setting for people whose needs cannot be met on the acute ward and who require a longer in-patient stay with specialised multidisciplinary team interventions before they can acquire the skills necessary to leave hospital

Ward in a house/hospital hostel Units on a domestic scale for people with behavioural problems that are hard to contain in ordinary community settings

Core and cluster housing Staff are based in a core setting that houses residents with greatest need for support; satellite (cluster) housing accommodates other residents, grouped by need for support

Hostel Non-specific term for a staffed community setting which is usually rehabilitative rather than providing a permanent home

Family placement From an idea originating in Belgium, residents become part of a family. This may particularly suit people with educational underachievement or cognitive difficulties

Adult placement A private landlord provides support to tenants renting rooms in a house. May be a temporary arrangement before moving to more independent accommodation

Group home Generally for older people, providing mutual support for those who value it, staffed or unstaffed. Residents hold their own tenancies

Supported housing Ordinary housing with support from an outreach team, or a specialist housing scheme with a warden

Dispersed intensive supported housing A specialised form of supported housing providing an alternative to residential care. Staff/patient ratios similar to those found in hospital and therefore able to provide support several times a day (Howat *et al*, 1988)

Crisis or respite beds Short-term provision, usually within a hostel or staffed house, for unplanned emergencies such as relapse or respite (e.g. if the carer is taken ill)

---

more costly than private or voluntary sector provision (Chisholm *et al*, 1997).

To help ensure equity of access and the best use of resources, placement panels have been established in many services. They may mix housing providers from the public and voluntary sectors with clinicians, managers and, ideally, a commissioner. If the panel is unable to make financial decisions, it can cause frustrating and costly delays in decision-making. A panel should regularly review out-of-area placements and ensure that they are agreed only when local solutions have been fully explored. The clinical team who know the client well are best placed to make the recommendations to a panel. For guidelines on good practice for submitting to a placement panel see Box 17.5.

> **Box 17.5** Guidelines for presenting housing recommendations to a placement panel
>
> - Following discussion with the client, relative and consultant at CPA review, the care coordinator compiles a housing care plan
> - The care coordinator submits a report to the panel, including psychiatric history, risk assessment and the agreed housing recommendation
> - The report also provides the multidisciplinary team's view of the likely consequences if the recommendation is not accepted by the panel
> - It is important that the care coordinator presents the report to the panel in person
> - A decision is made and a review date is agreed

Supported housing

An early study of people with schizophrenia and a history of multiple hospital admissions discharged from hospital in New York City opens with the statement that 'housing is a primary element in the community care of the mentally disabled' (Goldstein & Caton, 1983). The study failed to demonstrate that the type of accommodation had any effect on readmission rate or mental state. It was the psychosocial environment they returned to, the available social support and interpersonal stress, that best predicted readmission and was a more important factor even than the availability of out-patient treatment. The authors drew on the findings of 'expressed emotion' research in families to explain the findings. Since then high expressed emotion has been identified in the staff of residential homes, where it has been associated with patient characteristics such as attention-seeking behaviour, aggression and reduced social interaction (Moore *et al*, 1992).

In recent years there has been a reluctance to place people in institutional environments just because there is a history of 'revolving-door' admissions. Supported housing (Box 17.4) has become a less restrictive alternative. It is popular with a new generation of people diagnosed with schizophrenia, who may not feel they derive any benefit from group living, especially when the composition of the group is determined by a diagnosis which is disputed.

Surveys of people with schizophrenia living in Nithsdale, a rural area of south-west Scotland, are a useful barometer of trends in community care. A comparison of living arrangements in 1981 and 1996 showed that supported accommodation grew from nothing to provide support to 20% of non-in-patients. Many of these were severely ill and many of the staff employed by a voluntary agency had only basic training in mental health care (Kelly *et al*, 1998).

A growing problem, particularly in London, is accessing suitable housing for mentally ill refugees – an important socially excluded group. On arrival in the UK they may be detained in prison or special holding centres, often because of mental illness. Their treatment and care can be interrupted by sudden and arbitrary dispersal to other parts of the country, where they are isolated from their communities. Suitable housing and mental health delivery can thwarted by difficulties in accessing interpreters, primary care services, housing and other benefits, as well as coping with the humiliations of the support system, which is subject to frequent and arbitrary change (Murphy *et al*, 2002).

Supported housing in the UK takes two major forms: self-contained flats in a dedicated housing scheme on one site with professional support or dispersed ordinary housing with outreach team support. Residents of schemes who no longer require intensive support usually remain where they are, as there is little incentive to move. The practical advantages of outreach support are that it offers more focus. Support follows the person when and where they need it. A Cochrane review has concluded that research evidence for the superiority of either arrangement is weak because no studies met the inclusion criteria of a properly conducted randomised controlled trial (Chilvers *et al*, 2002). The choice should therefore be based on 'personal preference, professional judgment and available resources'. The reviewers point out that 'the safe haven of stability and support' offered by housing schemes must be balanced against 'the risks of dependency on professionals and prolonging social exclusion'.

Research into the relationship between mental health and housing has suffered from difficulties in randomisation due to the large number of variables, a lack of a shared conceptual framework between researchers and a tendency to use local measurement tools designed by the authors, with the result that the findings cannot be easily generalised (Newman, 2001).

Conclusions

Currently, people who experience disabilities as a result of their mental illness in the UK live in four broad kinds of setting. They may live entirely independently or with their family, with or without support from mental health services; they may live in some form of supported housing; they may be cared for in a residential care home or nursing home; or they may be an in-patient in a hospital, within either the NHS or the independent sector. Funding streams and regulatory arrangements for these settings are radically different. Independent living is largely unregulated and commonly paid for through state-funded housing benefit. Supported housing, for all client groups, is currently funded and regulated through Supporting People, an initiative that is centrally funded but locally managed through the housing departments of local councils. Residential and nursing home care is funded through local social services departments and monitored by the

Commission for Social Care Inspection (CSCI), which publishes detailed reports on facilities (see http://www.csci.org.uk/). Hospital care is funded by the Department of Health and monitored, at the time of writing not very effectively, by the Healthcare Commission. The CSCI and the Healthcare Commission are due to merge by 2008.

Chaplin & Peters' (2003) survey of mental hospitals built before Powell's 'Water Tower' speech in 1961 in two large areas of England found that 25% remain open and operational. The past is still with us. Where hospitals have been sold, preserved buildings have commonly been converted to luxury housing. Wealthy home-buyers who value segregation from the community can now purchase property on old asylum sites in gated communities protected by private security firms and closed-circuit television (Chaplin & Peters, 2003). Meanwhile, all over the UK, former institutions such as convents, old people's homes and primary schools are being acquired at bargain prices and given a new role. Ever-increasing demand for 'challenging behaviour beds' and the higher standards for space per resident now required by inspectors of residential homes make developing facilities for people with complex needs attractive to the private sector.

Many people with less challenging or complex needs, who a generation ago would have spent their lives in a mental hospital, now live in supported housing. Despite concerns about the quality and intensity of support, independent accommodation is highly valued and associated with better quality of life (Newman, 2001). A tenancy agreement for supported housing outlines the rights and responsibilities of both provider and tenant. Although the agreement may not be fully honoured by either party, there is at least 'a legal right to a home' and a right to 'live peacefully and quietly in your home' (Housing Corporation, 1998). There are strong political, financial and ethical drivers towards increasing the supported housing sector, which is where the most exciting innovations in housing for people with a severe mental illness are occurring.

References

Beecham, J., Hallam, A., Knapp, M. *et al* (1997) Costing care in hospital and in the community. In *Care in the Community: Illusion or Reality* (ed. J. Leff), pp. 37–47. John Wiley & Sons.

Birley, J., & Wilkinson, G. (1995) Jim Birley in conversation with Greg Wilkinson. *Psychiatric Bulletin*, **19**, 33–39.

Butler, D. & Salter-Ling, N. (1995) *Reprovision within the Bexley Hospital Site: The Clients' Views*. Dartford: Oxleas NHS Trust.

Chaplin, R. & Peters, S. (2003) Executives have taken over the asylum: the fate of 71 psychiatric hospitals. *Psychiatric Bulletin*, **27**, 227–229.

Chilvers, R., MacDonald, G. M. & Hayes, A. A. (2002) Supported housing for people with severe mental disorders. *Cochrane Database of Systematic Reviews*, issue 3. Oxford: Oxford Update Software.

Chisholm, D., Knapp, M. R., Astin, J., *et al* (1997) The mental health residential care study: predicting costs from resident characteristics. *British Journal of Psychiatry*, **170**, 37–42.

Clifford, P. (1988) Out of the cuckoos nest: the move of T2 ward from Bexley Hospital to 215, Sydenham Road. In *Community Care in Practice: Services for the Continuing Care Client* (eds A. Lavender & F. Holloway), pp. 257–274. Chichester: John Wiley & Sons.

Clifford, P., Charman, A., Webb, Y., *et al* (1991) Planning for community care. Long-stay populations of hospitals scheduled for rundown or closure. *British Journal of Psychiatry*, **158**, 190–196.

Creighton, F. J., Hyde, C. E. & Farragher, B. (1991) Douglas House. Seven years' experience of a community hostel ward. *British Journal of Psychiatry*, **159**, 500–504.

Curson, D. A., Pantelis, C. & Ward, J., *et al* (1992) Institutionalism and schizophrenia 30 years on. Clinical poverty and the social environment in three British mental hospitals in 1960 compared with a fourth in 1990. *British Journal of Psychiatry*, **160**, 230–241.

Donnelly, D., McGilloway, S., Mays, N., *et al* (1996) Leaving hospital: one and two year outcomes of long-stay psychiatric patients discharged to the community. *Journal of Mental Health*, **5**, 245–255.

Garety, P. (1988) Housing. In *Community Care in Practice: Services for the Continuing Care Client* (eds A. Lavender and F. Holloway), pp. 143–160. Chichester: John Wiley & Sons.

Goffman, E. (1961) *Asylums. Essays on the Social Situation of Mental Patients and Other Inmates*. New York: Anchor Books.

Goldstein, J. M. & Caton, C. L. (1983) The effects of the community environment on chronic psychiatric patients. *Psychological Medicine*, **13**, 193–199.

Hirsch, S. R. (1992) Services for the severe mentally ill – a planning blight. *Psychiatric Bulletin*, **16**, 673–675.

Holloway, F. (1991) 'Elderly graduates' and a hospital closure programme: the experience of the Camberwell Resettlement Team. *Psychiatric Bulletin*, **15**, 321–323.

Housing Corporation (1998) *The Shorthold Tenants Charter*. London: Housing Corporation.

Howat, J., Bates, P., Pidgeon, J., *et al* (1988) The development of residential accommodation in the community. In *Community Care in Practice: Services for the Continuing Care Client* (eds A. Lavender and F. Holloway), pp. 275–293. Chichester: John Wiley & Sons.

Hughes, J. (2002) Misconceptions are naïve. *BMJ*, **325**, 1300.

Jeffreys, S. E., Harvey, C. A., McNaught, A. S., *et al* (1997) The Hampstead Schizophrenia Survey 1991. 1: Prevalence and service use comparisons in an inner London health authority, 1986–1991. *British Journal of Psychiatry*, **170**, 301–306.

Johnstone, E. C., Owens, D. G., Gold, A., *et al* (1984) Schizophrenic patients discharged from hospital – a follow-up study. *British Journal of Psychiatry*, **145**, 586–590.

Jones, K. (1993) *Asylums and After. A Revised History of the Mental Health Services: From the Early 18th Century to the 1990s*. Atlantic Highlands, NJ: Athlone Press.

Kelly, C., McCreadie, R. G., MacEwan, T., *et al* (1998) Nithsdale schizophrenia surveys. 17. Fifteen year review. *British Journal of Psychiatry*, **172**, 513–517.

Leff, J. (1997) *Care in the Community: Illusion or Reality?* Chichester: John Wiley & Sons.

Leff, J. & Trieman, N. (2000) Long-stay patients discharged from psychiatric hospitals. Social and clinical outcomes after five years in the community. The TAPS Project 46. *British Journal of Psychiatry*, **176**, 217–223.

Levene, L. S., Donaldson, L. J. & Brandon, S. (1985) How likely is it that a district health authority can close its large mental hospitals? *American Journal of Psychiatry*, **147**, 150–155.

Macpherson, R., Shepherd, G. & Edwards, T. (2004) Supported accommodation for people with severe mental illness: a review. *Advances in Psychiatric Treatment*, **10**, 180–188.

Mann, S. & Cree, W. (1976) 'New long-stay' psychiatric patients: a national sample survey of fifteen mental hospitals in England and Wales. *Psychological Medicine*, **6**, 603–616.

Mind (2000) *Environmentally Friendly? Patients views on Conditions on Psychiatric Wards*. London: Mind.

Moore, E., Ball, R. A. & Kuipers, L. (1992) Expressed emotion in staff working with the long-term adult mentally ill. *British Journal of Psychiatry*, **161**, 802–808.

Murphy, D., Ndegwa, D., Kanani, A., *et al* (2002) Mental health of refugees in inner-London. *Psychiatric Bulletin*, **26**, 222–224.

Newman, S. J. (2001) Housing attributes and serious mental illness: implications for research and practice. *Psychiatric Services*, **52**, 1309–1317.

Polsky, N. (1971) *Hustlers, Beats and Others*. Harmondsworth: Penguin Books.

Poole, R., Ryan, T. & Pearsall, A. (2002) The NHS, the private sector and the virtual asylum. *BMJ*, **325**, 349–350.

Ryan, T., Pearsall, A., Hatfield, B., *et al* (2004) Long term care for serious mental illness outside the NHS. A study of out of area placements. *Journal of Mental Health*, **13**, 425–429.

Trieman, N. & Leff, J. (2002) Long-term outcome of long-stay psychiatric in-patients considered unsuitable to live in the community: TAPS Project 44. *British Journal of Psychiatry*, **181**, 428–432.

Wilson, F. (2004) Review of 'Home: the story of everyone who ever lived in our house', *The Guardian Review*, 15 May.

Wing, J. K. & Brown, G. W. (1970) *Institutionalisation and Schizoprehenia: A Comparative Study of Three Mental Hospitals 1960–1968*. London: Cambridge University Press.

Wolfson, P., Paton, C. & Jarrett, P. (2002) Clinical governance in the asylum. *Psychiatric Bulletin*, **26**, 430–432.

CHAPTER 18

Gender-sensitive services

Sarah Davenport

British psychiatry has been influenced historically by the biomedical model, an emphasis that has neglected the social determinants of mental ill health. These social factors differ markedly between men and women, and an understanding of these differences might therefore be regarded as central to gender-sensitive service development. Until recently, mental health services have largely reflected the biomedical emphasis, with a focus on the delivery of evidence-based biological interventions, at the expense of psychosocial or gender-sensitive approaches. However, rehabilitation services have always paid attention to sociocultural perspectives; the earliest research into social determinants of outcome from schizophrenia were studied in women patients in the famous Three Hospitals Study (Brown & Wing, 1962). This was the first systematic attempt to understand how the social environment (of the hospital) affects people who have severe mental illness; but it has taken nearly half a century since then for the gender differences in social determinants of mental ill health to become accepted and incorporated into mental health service planning.

In this chapter I will examine some of the gender differences in the prevalence, presentation and prognosis of mental disorders, comment on some of the different social determinants of mental ill health for men and women, and then make recommendations on the development of gender-sensitive rehabilitation services, where the service user might need to expect lifelong, high-quality contact.

Gender differences in the prevalence of psychiatric disorders

There are significant gender differences in the prevalence of some mental health problems (Box 18.1), with some disorders being exclusive to one gender; post-partum psychosis is an obvious example; alcohol dependence has a much higher prevalence in men, whereas women represent 90% of people with anorexia nervosa (Meltzer *et al*, 1995).

> **Box 18.1** Gender differences in presentation of mental disorder
>
> • Depression twice as common in women
> • Women represent 90% of people with anorexia
> • Severe mental illness usually has later onset in women
> • Oestrogen may play a part in aetiology

The mental health of women also differs from that of men in terms of the greater incidence of specific illnesses such as depression; the latter is twice as common in women than in men. The chronologies of some psychiatric disorders differ between genders; serious mental illness tends to have a later onset in women, and there are overall differences in prognosis. Men with schizophrenia appear to have a more severe form of the illness, characterised by early age at onset, poor premorbid adjustment, more positive and negative symptoms and poor outcome, whereas women have a more marked affective component (Castle & Murray, 1991). These differences may be related to aetiology, with men being more likely to have a neurodevelopmental form of the disorder, whereas in women there appears to be a stronger genetic component.

Women with bipolar affective disorder appear to have a later onset; they tend to have more features that predict poor prognosis (rapid cycling and depression). They respond to mood stabilisers at lower dosage and tend to have a deteriorating course after the menopause. There has been interest in the role of oestrogen as central to this differing psychopathological profile of men and women across the life span. Specifically, oestrogen may have a protective effect on neuronal systems. It can potentiate the neuroleptic effects of antipsychotics (Gold, 1998). It may also affect the function of the hypophyseal–pituitary axis (HPA) or the 'stress axis'. Oestrogen appears to make the HPA axis hypersensitive to catecholamines and some other neurotransmitters in some circumstances (such as early childhood trauma). These observations may turn out to be important clues in the puzzle to explain the gender-specific biological determinants of psychiatric disorder.

Gender differences in the social risk factors for mental ill health

The social context in which mental ill health arises is different for men and women. Women face an increased prevalence of the social risk factors for mental ill health (Box 18.2). These include the high prevalence of violence against women as children: 50% of children on at-risk registers experience domestic violence. Women as adolescents also experience an increased risk of domestic violence, particularly if they become pregnant (the risk

Box 18.2 Gender differences in social risk factors

- Women experience more childhood sexual abuse
- Women experience more domestic violence
- Women experience more poverty and unemployment
- The social disadvantages of women's role include powerlessness, discrimination and stigma
- Women's mental health seems to be more strongly correlated with social environmental factors than men's

(1992 Health and Lifestyles Survey: Cooper *et al*, 1999)

of interpersonal violence to pregnant adolescents is double that to their non-pregnant peers) Between 18% and 30% of adult women experience domestic violence during their lifetime (Dobash, 1992). Domestic violence is a powerful risk factor for mental ill health, but enquiry about domestic violence is rarely part of a screening interview during presentation to mental health services; much therefore goes undetected.

There is a high prevalence of childhood sexual abuse among children, but the prevalence for female children is much higher than for male children. Childhood sexual abuse is a powerful predictor of adult mental ill health (Mullen *et al*, 1994) right across the range of minor and major mental illness and personality disorder, particularly where it is part of a complex matrix of social disadvantage.

The impact of earlier (usually childhood) trauma on the pathogenesis of mental disorders is often overlooked by mental health professionals in both men and women; like domestic violence, sensitive enquiry is infrequently made into childhood adversity and abuse. Consequently, therapeutic opportunities are lost.

There are disproportionately higher levels of poverty and unemployment among women, both of which contribute to the risk for mental ill health. The social disadvantages of women's role in society still include powerlessness, discrimination and stigma, all of which are risk factors for mental ill health (Cooper *et al*, 1999).

Being a female child in care increases the chance of becoming a lone single young mother, so perpetuating the cycle of social and economic disadvantage (1 in 7 girls leaving local authority care are either pregnant or already mothers. Being a young single mother carries three times the risk of a mental health problem compared with young single fathers) (West, 1995).

More women than men are primary (or lone) carers for older or disabled family members; this role too carries an increased risk of psychological morbidity (Great Britain, Office of Population Censuses and Surveys, 1992).

Lesbian and bisexual women have higher rates of mental ill health than gay men (Gilman *et al*, 2001). The persisting discrimination and stigma attached to homosexuality may be experienced as more damaging by women, or society's prejudice towards lesbians may be more marked.

The 1992 Health and Lifestyles Survey found that community involvement and social support varied with socioeconomic status, and that women's health appeared more strongly correlated with the social environment than men's (Cooper *et al*, 1999). This must have major implications for the social inclusion agenda.

Gender differences in interactions with services

Men and women tend to express their mental health problems in different ways, and will therefore interact with and access services differently. An understanding of how some of these gender differences are expressed may be important in planning services that are gender sensitive.

Women present to their general practitioner with both psychological and physical complaints more frequently than men (Abel *et al*, 1996). However, men seem to arouse more anxiety and fear when they do present; more men than women are referred to secondary psychiatric services, and they are more likely to be regarded as in need of physical containment. There are differences in the use of the Mental Health Act 1983, with men comprising 53% of the detained population in 1998–1999 (Department of Health, 2000). The overall number of detained patients is rising, but the number of women being detained is rising at a slower rate than the number of men.

In a study of psychiatric rehabilitation service users by Perkins & Rowland (1991) older women received less intensive input than men, and a higher proportion of women than men were receiving day care in services designed for people functioning at a lower level, suggesting that stigma is still operating to discriminate against some groups of mentally ill women.

Planning services to respond sensitively to the gender differences in mental health must therefore embrace biological, social and psychological perspectives, if the needs of men and women are to be met appropriately. One might argue that this is particularly important for rehabilitation service users, as their experience of mental health care is essentially long term and should be transforming for recovery.

Gender issues in severe mental illness

Schizophrenia is an illness of young adults; its onset usually occurs at a crucial stage of social development when the impact is likely to be highly disruptive to the attainment of normal adult adjustment (Box 18.3). Separating from family as an independent autonomous adult is a key developmental task potentially at odds with an illness that can create dependency in many areas, including the interpersonal, financial and social.

Making and sustaining supportive adult peer relationships may become very challenging during an illness in which interpersonal hypersensitivity

---

Box 18.3   Gender issues in severe mental illness

- Age at onset of schizophrenia is maximally disruptive to the attainment of adult adjustment (therefore more damaging for men with earlier onset)
- Sexual roles and relationships may be compromised
- High prevalence of childhood abuse has longer-term implications for engagement and re-enactments
- Side-effects of medication affect social and sexual role performance
- Severe and persisting impairments contribute to social exclusion

---

and suspiciousness interfere with normal social intercourse. Men may be more compromised than women, as their average age at onset of schizophrenia and other major mental illnesses is earlier.

The development of sexual roles and relationships is another key developmental task likely to be interrupted or disrupted by the onset of illness, leaving the individual struggling at a time when most young adults would expect to be sexually very active.

There is a high prevalence of childhood sexual abuse among people with serious mental illness. This form of early childhood adversity affects both genders, although the prevalence is higher for women. Women are predominantly victims, whereas men are predominantly perpetrators (although there must be sensitivity to the small group in which this relationship is reversed). The early experience of sexual abuse predicts difficulty within intimate and power relationships, so services need to be sensitive to the risk of abusive re-enactments between patients, and between staff and patients.

Abuse, either physical or sexual, is likely to have a longer-term impact on personality development (Mullen *et al*, 1994). Service users with a history of abuse usually generate powerful interpersonal dynamics that influence the way in which a professional team functions; this is particularly marked in in-patient settings, where the dynamics of psychosis and the dynamics of the institution have the potential to interact with the dynamics of abuse. There is often amplification of primitive projection, splitting and scapegoating, which has the potential to make the therapeutic environment toxic for both staff and patients (Davenport, 1997). Services should have systems for self-reflection and clinical supervision to ensure that the ward milieu remains therapeutic.

Side-effects of medication have an impact on sexual and social role performance, and may affect fertility and therefore limit the opportunity to become a parent. (Some psychotropic medication cannot be prescribed during pregnancy and breast-feeding).

Some impairments associated with illness (especially schizophrenia) compound social dysfunction, for example frontal dysexecutive syndrome can lead to sexual and social disinhibition, which may make new learning and social skills training more difficult. Mood-related disinhibited behaviour may have a similar impact, and increase the vulnerability of the individual to exploitation or abuse.

Single-gender provision

Hospital admission creates an unnatural social environment where people are expected to live together in non-family groupings, and often with little respect for the safety of vulnerable patients or the requirements imposed by different cultural or religious backgrounds.

In many areas there is a relative absence of respect for cultural and religious differences in relation to gender. There are particular constraints expected within a domestic environment, for example for Muslim and Jewish women; these are often not provided for in in-patient settings, but should be considered as central to the planning and modernisation of any in-patient service.

Historically, there has been poor attention paid to physical and psychological safety. Women (and much less often, men) may experience sexual harassment and bullying, lack of privacy and infringement of their personal boundaries (a loss of personal dignity) within in-patient settings.

Bedrooms may not be lockable, and there may not be separate day, dining or smoking areas, offering no choice to those who are vulnerable and who find coping with unequal power relationships difficult. Forced socialisation may then create the opportunity for sexual harassment and coercion.

Some units have difficulty scrutinising visitors or public access, making the continuation of domestic violence or opportunistic exploitation a real threat while in hospital.

Lack of privacy and appropriate facilities (crèches and family visiting rooms) to maintain relationships with children are frequently problems that hinder recovery and promote social isolation.

There is often little choice regarding the gender of the doctor advising on mental or physical health issues, or the gender of the care coordinator,

---

Box 18.4 Single-gender provision

- Safety, dignity and privacy are paramount
- Choice of gender of keyworker, therapist and psychiatrist
- Same-sex chaperoning and for all 'hands on' procedures
- Robust policies to reduce sexual coercion and investigate complaints
- Gender-sensitive team training and reflective practice
- Gender-sensitive prescribing and good reproductive healthcare
- Gender-sensitive advocacy service

primary nurse or therapist. This contributes to the prevailing experience that service users report: they feel that their views are not taken into account by planners.

Some of the central difficulties experienced by women during periods of in-patient care were highlighted in *Safety, Privacy and Dignity* (National Health Service Executive, 2000) and confirmed by user surveys and listening panels across the country. These difficulties included feeling unsafe, and actually being unsafe, for example because of sexual harassment and coercion, lack of privacy, lack of female staff for chaperoning purposes, and lack of choice in the gender of the professional with whom they were expected to work closely. The launch of the women's mental health strategy 'Into the Mainstream' (Department of Health, 2002) has provided a policy framework for the development of gender-sensitive mental health services for women. It has also provided a framework for debate about the needs of men for gender-sensitive services.

Essential components of gender-sensitive care environment

The choice of gender of the named nurse, doctor and therapist or other multidisciplinary team members is very important to some service users. The high prevalence of abuse predicts difficulties with engagement, and the gender of particular care staff is likely to be an issue for service users with an history of abuse.

Dependent patients with psychosis should have access to same-sex carers if they wish it, particularly for the execution of intimate self-care or medication administration. This should also apply to the implementation of any 'hands-on' technique such as the use of restraint.

Prescribing should be gender sensitive (see next section).

The gender composition of the workforce should reflect the gender of the patient group (e.g. in the healthcare region in which I work, the standards for in-patient care for women stipulate staffing with 70% female nurses and care staff to 30% male nurses and care staff. These proportions are usually difficult to achieve, but do provide aspirational guidance). Staffing should be sufficient always to provide a same-sex chaperone as required.

The physical environment should optimise safety, privacy and dignity by providing good observation and separate sleeping, bathing, toilet and living facilities for men and women. Sufficient therapeutic living space and access to fresh air are essential, as are child and family visiting facilities.

The provision of gender-specific psychological therapies (e.g. women's and men's groups, and work on the longer-term impact of childhood trauma) are important components of a gender-sensitive service. Good-quality physical and reproductive healthcare is a central component of any gender-sensitive service, which also needs to be responsive to diversity.

Team reflective practice and clinical supervision should be available to all staff. Staff should have the opportunity for gender sensitivity training, to recognise the impact of trauma on the genesis of mental disorder and to recognise how social inequalities and institutional powerlessness affect the delivery of care. There should also be access to a gender-sensitive advocacy service.

Gender-sensitive prescribing

Some antipsychotic medications, particularly those with a high D_2-receptor occupancy (e.g. flupentixol, haloperidol, sulpiride and amisulpride) interfere with the normal feedback mechanisms controlling prolactin secretion in the anterior pituitary. This results in high levels of circulating prolactin, which can produce sexual/reproductive side-effects and loss of bone density. These issues are discussed later in the section on sexual dysfunction.

Some psychotropic medications interfere with the effectiveness of oral contraceptives, some are contraindicated in pregnancy or are excreted in breast milk. Conventional antipsychotic medication is associated with an increased risk of tardive dyskinesia in older women. The prevalence of tardive dyskinesia in men is lower than in women (21.6% v. 26.6%; Yassa & Jeste, 1992), although subsequent work suggests that young men with chronic psychotic illnesses are at greater risk of tardive dyskinesia than young women (van Os et al, 1999).

Oestrogen is thought to influence the pharmacokinetics of many psychotropic medications; in particular, it appears to enhance the neuroleptic activity of antipsychotics. Women are likely therefore to require lower doses than men and to be less tolerant to their side-effects. Plasma clozapine levels in women are about 30% higher than in men on equivalent doses (Lane et al, 1999). An increase in age of 1 year appeared to be related to a 1% increase in the plasma levels for both genders. Smoking reduces the plasma concentration of clozapine in both genders, but the effect is greater in men than in women (Haring et al, 1989). These results should assist in optimising dosing strategies for antipsychotic medication.

Men and women with chronic depression show different responsiveness to and tolerability of selective serotonin reuptake inhibitors (SSRIs) and tricyclic antidepressants. The differing response rates occur primarily in premenopausal women. Some studies have suggested that female sex hormones may enhance response to SSRIs but inhibit response to tricyclics (Kornstein et al, 2001).

Some studies report a difference between men and women in the pharmacokinetics of antidepressants; women taking antidepressants exhibit a different adverse event profile and generally require lower doses than men. Dosage should therefore be carefully adjusted to take account of gender in order to ensure a favourable drug response, optimised adherence and minimised risk of side-effects and adverse events (Frackiewicz et al, 2000).

The literature does not support a differential response to lithium between women and men in the treatment of bipolar affective disorder. Women with the disorder tend to be diagnosed later than men, which results in a

---

Box 18.5 Gender-sensitive prescribing

- Prescribe prolactin-sparing antipsychotic medication as far as possible (because of sexual dysfunction and bone-density loss)
- Women need lower doses of antipsychotics generally than men
- The risk of tardive dyskinesia is greater in older women on conventional antipsychotics
- Women tend to be more sensitive to SSRIs and tricyclics and therefore need lower doses

---

corresponding delay in initiating lithium maintenance therapy, but their response appears equally as good (despite lower serum concentrations) (Viguera *et al*, 2001).

It is clearly important to be aware of these gender differences in response to psychotropic medication so as to optimise prescribing and reduce the associated side-effects and adverse event profile in both genders.

Men's and women's groups

The provision of gender-specific groups for men and for women can make a significant contribution to the development and consolidation of social roles. These groups may be run along psychoeducational lines, with participants choosing their own agenda and inviting professionals to contribute within their field of expertise. Such groups usually run on 'slow-open' lines with two facilitators. Individual service users join an existing group, where members then expect to leave at their own pace.

Some groups are more psychotherapeutically focused, and may deal with the gender-specific implications of childhood sexual abuse, the management of anger and violence or alcohol misuse. Some gender-specific groups are run on analytic principles, with either one or two facilitators, and address difficulties in interpersonal relationships in general.

Sex offenders

Most sex offenders do not have a major mental illness (Gordon & Grubin, 2004). However, people with schizophrenia or related psychoses may commit sex offences or show abnormal sexual behaviour; these may be related to the psychosis itself, either directly or indirectly through, for example, the secondary effects of frontal lobe disinhibition. The behaviour may be related to deviant sexual fantasies. Affective disorder is not usually associated with serious sexual offending, although in hypomanic episodes individuals may behave in a sexually disinhibited manner, leading to indecent exposure or assault.

A history of childhood sexual abuse, long-standing social isolation with comorbid personality disorder, and alcohol misuse all increase the risk of sexual offending in severe mental illness. It is likely that rehabilitation services will have a small proportion of service users with sexual offending behaviour. Rehabilitation psychiatrists therefore should expect to be able to make a basic assessment of abnormal sexual behaviours and refer as appropriate to a multi-agency multidisciplinary team that can make use of the full range of clinical, psychotherapeutic, psychometric and psycho-physiological methods available. These teams are usually allied to forensic psychiatry services.

Sexual dysfunction

Sexual dysfunction is unfortunately very common in people with severe mental illness. The aetiology is likely to be multifactorial, but the prescrip-tion of antipsychotic and antidepressant medications is probably the one of the most important factors. The social difficulties and social exclusion experienced by people with severe mental illness are likely to contribute to sexual dysfunction; the longer-term impact of childhood sexual abuse, which has a high prevalence in in-patient populations, will contribute to sexual dysfunction in other, more complex ways.

The Nithsdale Schizophrenia Survey (Macdonald *et al*, 2003) measured rates of sexual dysfunction in people with schizophrenia and a community control sample, using a self-rated gender-specific questionnaire. At least one sexual dysfunction was reported by 82% of men and 96% of women with schizophrenia. Male patients reported less desire for sex, were less likely to achieve and maintain an erection, were more likely to ejaculate too quickly and were less satisfied with the intensity of their orgasms. Female patients reported less enjoyment than the control group; in women, sexual dysfunction appeared to be associated with negative symptoms and high levels of psychopathology in general.

Many antipsychotic drugs induce hyperprolactinaemia (Wieck & Haddad, 2002), which can cause breast enlargement and milk secretion and also loss of libido in both genders. Loss of fertility and hypo-oestrogenism are particular problems in women. Low oestrogen levels cause atrophic changes in the urethra and vagina and can lead to dyspareunia. (Low oestrogen levels also predispose to bone-density loss and increase the risk of osteoporosis.)

These side-effects clearly relate to sexual dysfunction for both genders and can be powerful determinants of adherence to treatment. Many young people with schizophrenia say that the treatment makes them feel rather worse than the illness; prolactin-sparing novel antipsychotics such as quetiapine and aripiprazole should be considered for this group.

Antidepressants also have an adverse effect on sexual function; tricyclics have an antimuscarinic effect and can produce constipation, urinary retention and difficulties with erection and ejaculation. Some SSRIs

> **Box 18.6**   Sexual dysfunction
>
> - Very high levels of sexual dysfunction are reported by both genders being treated for serious mental illness
> - Antidepressants interfere with erectile and ejaculatory function in men
> - Hyperprolactinaemia provoked by antipsychotics with high D_2-receptor occupancy is problematic for both genders
> - Antimuscarinics can also cause sexual dysfunction

are associated with impotence, ejaculatory failure or delayed orgasm; fluvoxamine appears to be associated with the lowest prevalence of sexual dysfunction and paroxetine with the highest.

Antimuscarinics are also linked to sexual dysfunction, and should be avoided wherever possible.

Taking a sensitive history of sexual dysfunction and providing information about medication should guide a collaborative approach with the service user. The most appropriate antipsychotic and antidepressant prescribing should then be jointly agreed, after taking into account the particular circumstances and the alternatives.

Sexual needs and freedom

People with serious mental illness have sexual needs just like the rest of us, but these are rarely specifically considered as part of a holistic needs assessment. They are more likely to be considered during a risk management plan for more vulnerable service users, but the basic human rights to privacy and a family life are often neglected. This is a particular issue for longer-term in-patients, particularly if they are detained and living in single-gender settings. Services rarely consider how conjugal rights can be respected, even for married service users. There is a general paucity of guidance in relation to consenting sexual activity conducted between in-patients; generally the guidance comes from secure services and is restrictive, with an embargo on same-sex and heterosexual contact.

In legal terms, women who are detained for treatment are regarded as if they do not have capacity to give consent to sexual intercourse; this is, of course, nonsense as detained women may well have demonstrable capacity in relation to their sexual activity.

Good practice suggests that the sexual needs of all rehabilitation service users should be considered as part of a routine needs assessment; a sensitive history of relationships, use of contraceptives, reproductive health and the capacity to give informed consent to sexual intercourse should be discussed at an appropriate time, and with a professional of the service user's choice; the gender of the professional may be important here.

It should be assumed that sexual activity between in-patients will occur, despite the existence of restrictions. Service users may therefore need advice about practising safe sex and education about sexually transmitted disease and the use of contraceptives. The opportunity to discuss contraceptive options, and their provision, should be freely available. This should include the provision of condoms, prescription of the morning-after pill, insertion of intra-uterine contraceptive devices and depot medroxyprogesterone.

Some service users wish for a child; both men and women are entitled to information about the heritability of their disorder to help them make up their mind. The potential involvement of child protection services may also need discussion. They will need information about the medication they are taking, the potential for teratogenic effects on a foetus, and the risk of relapse associated with their disorder during pregnancy and after delivery, particularly if they cease medication.

In-patient rehabilitation services should consider how to provide safe and private facilities for the pursuit of mutually consenting sexual activity between regular partners.

Services should also have in place protocols to guide the investigation of any complaints or allegation of sexual misconduct, between patients or between staff and patients. Complaints procedures should be easy to access, culturally sensitive and operate within a short timescale, to provide a clear outcome to the complainant.

Conclusions

The important social considerations surrounding gender differences in mental ill health have been neglected and have only recently been accepted into the mainstream of service development. These considerations are key to the provision of service systems which are sensitive to the gender-dependent needs of longer-term service users, their families and their carers. Rehabilitation services attuned to gender can make a real contribution to recovery, social inclusion and the reduction of stigma.

References

Abel, K., Buscewicz, M. & Davison, S. (1996) *Planning Community Mental Health Services for Women. A Multiprofessional Handbook*. London: Routledge.

Brown, G. W. & Wing, J. K. (1962) A comparative clinical and social survey of three mental hospitals. In *Sociology and Medicine: Studies within the Framework of the British National Health Service* (ed. P. Halmos). Keele: University of Keele.

Castle, D. J. & Murray, R. M. (1991) The neurodevelopmental basis of sex differences in schizophrenia. *Psychological Medicine*, **21**, 565–575.

Cooper, H., Arber, S. & Fee, I. (1999) *The Influence of Social Support and Social Capital on Health*. London: Health Education Council.

Davenport, S. (1997) Pathological interactions between psychosis and childhood sexual abuse in in-patient settings: their dynamics, consequences and management. In *Psychotherapy of Psychosis* (eds C. Mace & F. Margison), pp. 205–219. London: Gaskell.

Department of Health (2000) *Patients Formally Detained in Hospitals under the Mental Health Act 1983 and Other Legislation, England: 1988–89 to 1998–99*. London: Department of Health.

Department of Health (2002) *Women's Mental Health: Into the Mainstream*. London: Department of Health.

Dobash, R. (1992) *Women, Violence and Social Change*. London: Routledge

Frackiewicz, E. J., Sramek, J. J. & Cutler, N. R. (2002) Gender differences in depression and antidepressant pharmacokinetics and adverse events. *Annals of Pharmacotherapy*, **34**, 80–88.

Gilman, S., Cochran, S., Mays, V., *et al* (2001) Risk of psychiatric disorders among individuals reporting same sex partners in the National Co-morbidity Survey. *American Journal for Public Health*, **91**, 933–939.

Gold, J. H. (1998) Gender differences in psychiatric illness and treatments. *Journal of Nervous and Mental Disease*, **186**, 769–775.

Gordon, H. & Grubin, D. (2004) Psychiatric aspects of the assessment and treatment of sex offenders. *Advances in Psychiatric Treatment*, **10**, 73–80.

Great Britain, Office of Population Censuses and Surveys (1992) *General Household Survey: Carers in 1990* (OPCS Monitor, no SS92/2). London: OPCS.

Haring, C., Meise, U., Humpel, C., *et al* (1989) Dose-related plasma levels of clozapine: influence of smoking behaviour, sex and age. *Psychopharmacology*, **99** (suppl.), S38–S40.

Kornstein, S. G., Schatzberg, A. F., Thase, M. E., *et al* (2001) Gender differences in treatment response to sertraline v imipramine in chronic depression. *American Journal of Psychiatry*, **158**, 1531–1533.

Lane, H. Y., Chang, Y. C., Lin, S. K., *et al* (1999) Effects of gender and age on plasma levels of clozapine and its metabolites analysed by critical statistics. *Journal of Clinical Psychiatry*, **60**, 36–40.

Macdonald, S., Halliday, J., MacEwan, T., *et al* (2003) Nithsdale Schizophrenia Surveys 24: sexual dysfunction. Case–control study. *British Journal of Psychiatry*, **182**, 50–56.

Meltzer, H., Gill, B., Petticrew, M., *et al* (1995) *OPCS Surveys of Psychiatric Morbidity in Great Britain. Report 1. The Prevalence of Psychiatric Morbidity among Adults Living in Private Households*. London: TSO (The Stationery Office).

Mullen, P. E., Martin, J. L., Anderson, J. C., *et al* (1994) The effect of child sexual abuse on social, interpersonal and sexual functioning in adult life. *British Journal of Psychiatry*, **165**, 35–47.

National Health Service Executive (2000) *Safety, Privacy and Dignity in Mental Health Units. Guidance on Mixed Sex Accommodation for Mental Health Units*. Leeds: NHS Executive.

Perkins, R. E. & Rowland, L. A. (1991) Sex differences in service usage in long-term psychiatric care. Are women adequately served? *British Journal of Psychiatry*, **158** (suppl. 10), S75–S79.

van Os, J., Walsh, E., Van Horn, E., *et al* (1999) Tardive dyskinesia in psychosis: are women really more at risk? *Acta Psychiatrica Scandinavica*, **99**, 288–293.

Viguera, A. C., Baldessarini, R. J. & Tondo, L. (2001) Response to lithium maintenance treatment in bipolar disorders: comparison of women and men. *Bipolar Disorders*, **3**, 245–252.

West, A. (1995) *You're on Your Own: Young People's Research on Leaving Care*. London: Save the Children Fund.

Wieck, A. & Haddad, P. (2002) Hyperprolactinaemia caused by antipsychotic drugs. *BMJ*, **324**, 250–252.

Yassa, R. & Jeste, D. V. (1992) Gender differences in tardive dyskinesia: a critical review of the literature. *Schizophrenia Bulletin*, **18**, 701–715.

CHAPTER 19

Working to recovery: meaningful occupation and vocational rehabilitation[†]

Jed Boardman and Brian Robinson

Psychiatric rehabilitation emphasises the improvement of supports, opportunities, skills and community integration for people with long-term mental illness. People with mental illness have long been excluded from mainstream participation in society, and recent policy initiatives have stressed the importance of measures to promote social inclusion (Office of the Deputy Prime Minister, 2004). Occupation and work have been given a central place in these initiatives and this reflects a long-standing recognition of their therapeutic role and their importance in linking people to civil society.

This chapter examines the background and importance of occupation, work and employment for people with severe and enduring mental illness, and vocational rehabilitation approaches.

When reflecting on the role of occupation and employment in rehabilitation, consider:

- the role and importance of work in social inclusion
- the fact that the overwhelming majority of people with mental illness want to be occupied and work, and the need to recognise service users as central to choosing their own goals, approaches and settings
- that good evidence for the effectiveness of vocational schemes exists and that service development should utilise this existing evidence base.

Background

Occupation, work, employment and leisure

The traditional definitions of work emphasise that it is an activity that involves the exercise of skills and judgement, taking place within set

---

[†]This chapter is a modified version of Boardman, J. (2003) Work, employment and psychiatric disability. *Advances in Psychiatric Treatment*, **9**, 327–334. Reproduced with permission.

limits prescribed by others (Bennett, 1970). Work is therefore essentially something you 'do' for other people. By contrast, in most leisure activities you can 'please yourself'.

'Employment' is work you get paid for. Most childcare, housework, looking after elderly or sick relatives is clearly 'work', in the sense that the tasks and outcomes are defined by others, but they do not, at present, usually attract formal payments. This distinction between 'work' and 'employment' is very important in the context of mental health because the overwhelming majority of people with mental health problems want to 'work', that is to be engaged in some kind of meaningful activity which uses their skills and meets the expectations of others. However, not all wish to be 'employed', with all the additional stresses and responsibilities that entails. Occupation may be considered as a general term that refers to engagement in activities, tasks and roles for the purpose of meeting the requirements of living.

Rates of employment and mental illness

There are significant levels of unemployment and sickness absence in people with neurotic disorders (Meltzer *et al*, 1995), but unemployment levels are particularly high in people with long-term mental illness and, importantly, this group is much less likely to be economically active than people with physical or sensory impairments (Office for National Statistics, 2000) (Box 19.1).

Figures from the Office for National Statistics survey of adults with psychotic disorders living in the community support these findings (Foster *et al*, 1996). Half the sample of people surveyed were classified as unable to work, one in five was in employment and one in eight was unemployed. These rates do not improve over time. For example, in one London borough, Perkins & Rinaldi (2002) found that unemployment rates for residents with long-term mental illness increased during the 1990s from 80% in 1990 to 92% in 1999. For those with schizophrenia the rates of unemployment

---

Box 19.1 Employment of people with long-term mental illness in Great Britain in spring 2000 (Office for National Statistics, 2000)

- Long-term disabled people with mental health problems as their main difficulty represent 8% of long-term disabled people of working age; 18% of this group were in employment in 2000
- Long-term disabled people with no mental health difficulties at all represent 84% of long-term disabled people of working age; 52% were in employment in 2000

increased from 88% to 96% during the same period. These changes occurred despite an overall fall in unemployment rates during this period.

These low rates of employment should be considered against the facts that 30–40% of people with enduring mental illness are capable of holding down a job (Ekdawi & Conning, 1994) and that many wish to be in some form of employment.

Why is work important?

Work plays a central role in all people's lives. Schneider (1998) proposes the following five main arguments for the promotion of employment for people with mental health problems.

Social and health benefits

Employment provides a monetary reward and is inseparable from economic productivity, with its profits for the employer and its material benefits for society. In addition, employment provides 'latent benefits' – non-financial gains – to the worker. These additional benefits include social identity and status; social contacts and support; a means of structuring and occupying time; activity and involvement; and a sense of personal achievement (Warr, 1987). Work tells us who we are and enables us to tell others who we are; typically, the first questions we ask when we meet someone are 'What is your name?' and 'What do you do?'

Although work is important for everyone, it is particularly crucial for people with mental health problems. People with such difficulties are especially sensitive to the negative effects of unemployment and to the loss of structure, purpose and identity that work brings (Bennett, 1970; Rowland & Perkins, 1988). Consider the additional burden that lack of meaningful activity imposes on those with mental ill health: unemployed people do not exploit the extra time they have available for leisure and social pursuits. Their social networks and social functioning decrease, as do motivation and interest, leading to apathy. Social isolation is often particularly problematic for people who experience mental health problems and work is more effective than occupational therapy in increasing social networks.

Being in work enhances quality of life (Hatfield *et al*, 1992; Hill *et al*, 1996). Work links the individual to society; already socially excluded as a result of their mental health problems, this exclusion is aggravated by unemployment.

Unemployment has been linked with increased general health problems, including premature death (Brenner, 1979; Bartley, 1994). There is a particularly strong relationship between unemployment and mental health difficulties (Warr, 1987; Warner, 1994), with increased use of mental health services (Wilson & Walker, 1993; Warner, 1994) and increased risk of suicide (Platt & Kreitman, 1984).

273

Demand from service users

Despite the high rates of unemployment among people with mental health problems, studies indicate that as many as 90% would like to go back to work (Grove, 1999; Rinaldi & Hill, 2000; Secker *et al*, 2001). There is increasing policy emphasis on the importance of service users' preferences and wishes in the provision of services, and mental health service users clearly say that they want the opportunity to work. Assisting people to gain and sustain employment should be considered a valid 'treatment' in its own right, which assists in achieving many of the targets for mental health services (Posner *et al*, 1996).

The ideological argument: work as a rights issue

The right to work is enshrined in Article 23 of the United Nations Declaration of Human Rights, which states that 'Everyone has the right to work, to free choice of employment, to just and favourable conditions of work and to protection against unemployment' (United Nations, 1948). Yet the majority of people who experience longer-term mental health problems continue to be denied this right.

People with a disability should be valued in the same way as those without, i.e. as entitled to respect, self-determination and empowerment. The disability rights movement has taken this as a cause and promotes empowerment for people with disabilities, including mental health problems.

Discrimination on the part of potential employers is undoubtedly a major obstacle to people with mental health problems gaining work, especially those with diagnoses of schizophrenia (Manning & White, 1995). The Disability Discrimination Act 1995 offers some protection for those with disabilities related to mental illness (Sayce & Boardman, 2003).

Economic argument: work as an economic issue

Enormous amounts of public money in the form of social security payments are spent on supporting people out of work; almost 25% of invalidity payments are paid to people with mental health problems. If some of this resource could be redirected towards enabling people to maintain and/or regain employment, then the social, psychiatric and economic gains are likely to be large (Schneider, 1998).

National policy and the new context of mental healthcare

The run down and closure of the large psychiatric hospitals, which provided most of the work projects in the UK for people with long-term psychiatric disabilities, has placed most mental health services and their users in community settings. Recent government policies have stressed risk minimisation, the containment, monitoring and supervision of people with mental illness, and a mixed economy of care. Some argue that work may provide such non-custodial supervision while at the same time promoting therapeutic ends (Schneider, 1998).

Box 19.2 Barriers to employment facing mental health service users

- Historically, the dependence of the employment of disabled people on economic growth, overall rate of employment and times of labour shortage (Warner, 1994)
- The impact of mental health problems on the individual
- The welfare system's built-in disincentives to returning to work – the so-called 'benefits trap'
- The disadvantages faced by people with a history of mental illness in the open employment market, including stigma, a reluctance to employ them, the risk of failure and the benefits trap
- A tendency for mental health professionals and others to underestimate the capacities and skills of their clients and, possibly, to overestimate the risk to employers – this may extend to general practitioners and employers, some of whom give insufficient attention to helping people return to their jobs
- The dominance of a model of mental illness that emphasises episodes and 'cure', as opposed to one that focuses on the disabilities of people with long-term mental illness. A social model of disability and a rehabilitation philosophy may be more beneficial
- Lack of expertise in business development among mental health professionals
- The limitations of evidence relating to the types of services and approaches that are effective in getting those with mental illness back to work and keeping them in employment

---

Barriers to employment and to the development of employment services

Mental health service users face more significant barriers to work than other disabled people (Box 19.2). Only people with a severe learning disability find it more difficult to get paid work. The high rates of unemployment among people with mental illness, coupled with the desire to obtain work, suggests that work projects that do exist are providing only a limited and restricted service.

Vocational services

History and development

The use of 'constructive occupation' has formed a part of the care for people with mental illness since the development of the mental hospitals. However, vocational rehabilitative and reintegrative efforts have varied historically and this variation is linked to changes in the economic cycle and the availability of employment (Warner, 1994). Mentally ill people have been the marginal elements of the 'Industrial Reserve Army'. High levels of unemployment are associated with limited efforts at rehabilitation and a consequent low recovery rate for those with mental illness.

In the UK in the 1950s and 1960s, there was an increase in employment schemes, mainly based in hospitals. By 1967, 100 out of 122 hospitals surveyed had some form of industrial therapy provision (Wansborough & Miles, 1968). The classic Three Hospitals Study of Wing & Brown (1970) found that at one of the three (Netherne Hospital) there were many fewer cases of severe schizophrenia than in the two less 'active' hospitals. The 'natural history' of schizophrenia, with its decline into inactivity and negativism, thus proved to be highly dependent on the opportunities provided for meaningful activities, and the most malignant element was 'the amount of time doing nothing'.

The Disabled Persons Act 1944 led to the provision of facilities such as industrial rehabilitation units and sheltered employment factories and workshops, and disabled resettlement officers at every employment exchange were responsible for helping disabled people to find work. Local industrial therapy organisations were set up by interested parties. The success of these schemes was limited. They did not lead to many people returning to open employment, and they were not adaptable to changing industrial conditions. Only a small proportion of individuals moved on to open employment. They did, however, succeed in providing a small number of mentally ill people with a 'real job', and many more were offered the opportunity to work, even though the financial rewards might be limited.

As unemployment increased during the 1970s and 1980s, so paid employment opportunities for people with mental illness became limited and schemes that existed were mainly based in or run by hospitals. The bulk of these were based on sheltered work or employment. This period also coincided with the increasing run down of the large mental hospitals. The development of community-based mental health services was not always commensurate with the loss of hospital services, and less emphasis was placed on work schemes, which became fragmentary. The nature of employment also changed, with a loss of manufacturing and a growth in service industries.

An alternative to sheltered work, supported employment (i.e. placing the person in a 'real' employment setting and providing direct support to them and their employer in the workplace), had been espoused in the USA since the 1960s (Newman, 1970). These ideas took force in the 1980s as it was thought that sheltered workshops isolated people from mainstream society (Wehman, 1986). By the late 1980s, supported employment had begun to attract attention in the field of psychiatric rehabilitation (Mellen & Danley, 1987). However, the use of these approaches has been slow to develop in the UK.

During the past two decades there has been an expansion of employment schemes for people with mental illness. These have shifted in location from hospital to community, and are often run by non-statutory agencies. They fall into three broad categories: sheltered employment, 'open' supported employment and social firms (O'Flynn & Craig, 2001).

Work schemes for people with mental illness

Sheltered employment

Traditional sheltered workshops and sheltered employment factories such as those run be Remploy do not provide employment in the open market. They may be of value for those who find open employment difficult and as a means of introducing people to the work situation. They tend to have very low rates of movement into open employment and they often find it difficult to be commercially viable.

Prevocational training

Prevocational training is one way of helping people with severe mental illness return to work. Prevocational training assumes that these individuals require a period of preparation before entering into competitive employment. This preparation includes sheltered workshops, transitional employment (working in a job that is 'owned' by a rehabilitation agency), skills training, work crews and other preparatory activities. Some individuals need to get back into a working regime through programmes of graduated activity; others find it helpful to have short period of confidence-building and developing coping strategies such as offered by PECAN, a community-based organisation set up in Peckham, south London, to address unemployment in the area. These approaches are not ends in themselves.

Supported employment

Supported employment (Box 19.3) places clients in competitive jobs without extended preparation and provides on-the-job support from employment specialists or trained 'job coaches' (Becker *et al*, 1994; Hill & Shepherd, 1997). The concept is simple: a person is hired and paid by

---

Box 19.3 The core principles of supported employment

- The goal is competitive employment in work settings integrated into a community's economy
- Clients are expected to obtain jobs directly, rather than after lengthy pre-employment training
- Rehabilitation is an integral component of treatment of mental illness rather than a separate service
- Services are based on the client's preferences and choices
- Assessment is continuous and based on real work experiences
- Follow-on support is continued indefinitely

a real employer. The job meets both the employee's needs and skills and the employer's requirements. The employee is entitled to the full company benefits and from the beginning employee and employer receive enough help from a support organisation to ensure success.

There are a number of different supported employment programmes, including the assertive community treatment model, transitional employment (e.g., the clubhouse approach) and the job coach model (Bond *et al*, 1997). The model that emerges from the literature as the most promising programme so far is known as individual placement and support (IPS) (Becker *et al*, 1994). In IPS the emphasis is on rapid placement in work with intensive support and training on the job.

The clubhouse model

Clubhouses assist people with long-term mental health problems to address issues such as low self-esteem, low motivation and social isolation (Beard *et al*, 1982; Aquila *et al*, 1999; Macias *et al*, 2001). They promote social inclusion and support people in leading productive and meaningful lives within the community. The clubhouse model is based on principles of meaningful activity and psychosocial rehabilitation, and work is a central factor in its operation.

Social firms

A possible solution to the problem of providing high-quality sheltered work and employment that is being developed in many parts of Europe, including the UK, is the social firm (Grove *et al*, 1997; Grove & Durie, 1999). These are sometimes described as 'modern' versions of sheltered employment, but there are crucial differences that go beyond repackaging and changing the name.

In a social firm, the emphasis is on creating a successful business that can support paid employment. The social firm operates entirely as a business but its methods emphasise participation by employees in all aspects of the enterprise. Although it may offer training on a commercial basis, it is not primarily engaged in 'rehabilitation' and its core staff, whether disabled or not, are paid the going rate for the work. About half the staff will be disabled people, and members of the disabled workforce may be in managerial positions.

Cooperatives can operate like social firms or social enterprises but are owned and managed democratically by the members. A *social enterprise* is a small business that operates semi-commercially, but has a training or rehabilitation function (Grove *et al*, 1997).

Opportunities for volunteering

For many people, making a contribution in a voluntary capacity, particularly to an activity that they regard as socially worthwhile, is a valuable part of their lives. For disabled people there is often added value in volunteering to help others as 'experts by experience'. There are many opportunities for volunteering and many agencies that can act as brokers between the need and the people who can meet it.

The volunteer role, and the process needed to enable disabled people to become volunteers, requires exactly the same kinds of support as paid employment.

Service user employment programmes

The principles of supported employment have been used to great effect in a number of schemes across the UK in which National Health Service (NHS) trusts have committed themselves to the employment of service users. 'Personal experience of mental health problems' will be specified as either a desirable or an essential qualification on specifications for posts.

In these schemes, the first of which was pioneered by South West London and St George's Mental Health NHS Trust, people with mental health problems are employed in existing posts on the same terms and conditions as other employees, and a programme of support for those who need it is built into the normal employment practices of the trust. The effect of the scheme has been interesting on a number of levels, not only creating jobs, but also challenging many of the barriers and misconceptions about employing people with mental health problems (Perkins *et al*, 1997).

Work schemes in the UK

It is not known how many different types of work scheme operate in the UK and how many people are receiving services. Relatively recent surveys of provision estimate that there are at least 135 organisations offering sheltered employment, 77 providing open employment and about 50 social firms (Grove & Durie, 1999; Crowther *et al*, 2001). A survey in the northwest of England found high variation in provision and a poor relationship between the schemes identified and the needs of the areas in which they operated (Crowther & Marshall, 2001). There was a more than 40-fold variation in provision across health authority areas, and the highest level of provision was in the area with the lowest deprivation and unemployment.

Effectiveness of work schemes

Most evidence of effectiveness comes from studies conducted in the USA (Bond *et al*, 2001; Crowther *et al*, 2001). Several randomised controlled trials have compared prevocational training with supported employment. Prevocational training assumes that people with severe mental illness require a period of preparation before going into open employment. Supported employment places people in competitive jobs without extended preparation, and provides on-the-job support from employment specialists or job coaches. In general, supported employment is more effective than prevocational training at helping people with severe mental illness to obtain and keep competitive employment.

More work needs to be done on the effectiveness of such schemes, particularly in the UK. Of particular importance are their cost-effectiveness, their effect on clinical and social outcomes, and job retention.

Successful employment schemes share several critical components:

- the agency providing supported employment is committed to competitive employment as an attainable goal for people with severe mental illness
- supported employment programmes use a rapid job search approach to helping clients find jobs directly (rather than providing lengthy pre-employment assessment, training and counselling)
- staff and clients find individual job placements according to the client's preferences, strengths and work experience
- follow-up support is maintained indefinitely
- supported employment programmes are closely integrated with mental health teams.

Assessing vocational needs

The main components of the assessment and planning process are: whether people really want to work, what their skills are and what they are interested in doing. Once these are established, a programme of support and training can be designed for each individual, which is aimed at achieving their personal goals and ambitions. Three main elements should be considered.

The first is the predictive importance of historical factors. There is a strong relationship between work history and future occupational functioning (Watts, 1983). Detailed work histories are more useful than most clinical measures (e.g. diagnosis) or traditional psychometric testing (e.g. IQ or aptitude tests), which have limited predictive value for occupational performance (Wiggins, 1973).

Second is the importance of personal factors (motivation, confidence and personal objectives). These have consistently been shown to be highly predictive of outcomes and are generally superior to traditional skills or IQ assessments. Thus, if the person really wants to do the job, then they are more likely to succeed.

The third is the setting, the characteristics of the individuals placed in it and the desired outcomes. Outcomes are determined by a combination of historical factors (work history, skills, previous work performance), individual factors (confidence, motivation, personal aims and objectives) and setting factors (such as expectations of staff, opportunities for training and development, links to other programmes). The assessment process must therefore begin by examining these variables. It is important to find out whether an individual wants (or has) a job as early as possible in their contact with health services. Consider both job retention and job placement at this time.

Motivation is contingent and is linked to success, mastery and other factors. Getting a job can change a person's whole outlook and attitude to work, so the premature exclusion of apparently unmotivated individuals may deny them the chance they need to move on in life. Assessment is therefore a highly skilled task and should be considered as an intervention in its own right. It is not a 'one off', but a process that may take time and requires a series of steps or repetition.

The spectrum of occupational and employment services

Employment opportunities cut across several agencies (Box 19.4). The problems that arise are partly a consequence of deinstitutionalisation and the move to community services provided by a mixed economy of care. It has been a constant source of irritation to disabled people that the various agencies in government and the independent sector that provide vocational rehabilitation rarely work together or provide indications of how to get through the system. Developing effective vocational services will require working in partnership, avoiding duplication and enabling individual journeys through the system need to be achieved.

Successful partnerships do exist and they generate real benefits for service users. The possibilities for partnership are almost endless.

The role of health services in the provision of occupation and employment

The provision of employment opportunities for people with psychiatric disabilities inevitably involves working across a variety of different agencies and involves many different agencies and professional groups. For health services the key agencies are general practice, adult general psychiatric services (mainly community mental health teams (CMHTs) and rehabilitation services) and occupational medicine. No one model of service is right for everyone and each approach may help different people

---

Box 19.4   Range of agencies

- Service user/disabled peoples' organisations
- Mental health NHS trusts
- Social services
- Voluntary- and independent-sector providers
- Employers
- Regional disability services
- Training and enterprise councils
- Local authority regeneration departments

at different times in their recovery and reintegration. Ideally, people should have access to a range of work, training and support that is relevant to their changing needs. They should have the opportunity for progression towards paid employment, but they should not be forced to move on to situations of greater stress and responsibility if they do not wish to. Thus, it is generally agreed that a comprehensive local mental health employment service should offer a 'spectrum of opportunities', with possibilities to access this spectrum at any point and to move, or stay, according to individual needs (Grove, 1999).

Such a spectrum is important not just because individuals have different needs: they may also choose different pathways into work. Careful consideration needs to be given to the component parts of this spectrum and their coordination. The consequences of making wrong choices may tie up valuable resources in ineffective services. There will be people whose disabilities are too great to be supported in open employment (or at least for a part of their illness career) regardless of the extent of available support. For these people other approaches to work and structured activity will be needed.

It is adult psychiatric services that are mainly involved with employment issues as they see adults of working age, although specialist services such as those providing for people with drug and alcohol problems also play a role. The key components of mental health services for vocational rehabilitation are:

- CMHTs, which are seen as playing a central role in the delivery of the standards of the National Service Framework, along with crisis teams, assertive outreach teams and services for people with first-onset psychoses (which may have a preventive role)
- in-patient services and associated residential units, which may form an important part of the rehabilitation process following an acute episode of illness (Boardman & Hodgson, 2000)
- day hospitals and day centres: the concept of day care needs to be expanded to provide a range of facilities, all of which have close working links with CMHTs, and provide a range of services, acute and chronic, therapeutic and supportive. They should all have rehabilitation as a central aim and work, activity and employment as central goals. The clubhouse model is one example of this expanded concept.

The care programme approach (CPA) may be of assistance in high-lighting vocational needs in an individual's care plan. All care plans must show plans to secure suitable employment or other occupational activity (Department of Health, 2001).

At present, mental health services place insufficient emphasis on returning people to work and there is no specific provision for work schemes or work liaison schemes in CMHTs. The National Service Framework for Mental Health (Department of Health, 1999) and its associated documents, while implicitly offering opportunities for mental health services to develop employment schemes, does not directly emphasise the development of rehabilitation services. There is a need for all CMHTs to have access to a range of work schemes, and these should be set up along the lines indicated by the available evidence. This central role of CMHTs in local services for people with severe mental illness can be achieved only through the improvement of rehabilitation and day care services in the areas in which they work and by enhancing the skills of team members. There is also a need to identify vocational specialists within the CMHTs (see Department of Health 2006a,b).

Members of CMHTs will need additional training to assist with the delivery of occupational services. This will require the introduction of the concepts of rehabilitation and work in the training of psychiatrists, nurses and others in the multidisciplinary team, as well as skills development, awareness training and information on disability discrimination legislation.

Advice on welfare benefits should be part of the CAP. The Welfare to Work Scheme, for which the lead agency is the local authority social services' department, also requires that benefits advice be integrated with employment assessment. Each CHMT may need to identify a benefit lead and a vocational lead, who would work closely together. The use of welfare and benefits advisors can help service users to obtain the range of benefits available to them and can give appropriate advice on benefits and work.

Although helping service users to make the best of employment opportunities is now fundamental to general community mental health services, in the past this was seen as a role of specialist rehabilitation services, which in some areas still fulfil this function. Indeed, several such services have been given Beacon status as examples to other districts. In addition, specialist rehabilitation services play a particular role in meeting the needs of people with the greatest psychiatric disabilities, including mentally disordered offenders, who have an additional disadvantage in the labour market.

The provision of occupation and employment is a powerful tool in improving social inclusion for people with mental illness and, in a world of limited resources, needs to be assertively championed.

References

Aquila, R., Santos, G., Malahud, T. J., *et al* (1999) The Rehabilitation Alliance in practice: the clubhouse connection. *Psychiatric Rehabilitation Journal*, **23**, 19–23.

Bartley, M. (1994) Unemployment and ill health: understanding the relationships. *Journal of Epidemiology and Community Health*, **48**, 333–337.

Beard, J. H., Propst, R. N. & Malamud, T. J. (1982) The Fountain House model of rehabilitation. *Psychiatric Rehabilitation Journal*, **5**, 47–53.

Becker, D. R., Drake, R. E. & Concord, N. H. (1994) Individual placement and support: a community mental health center approach to rehabilitation. *Community Mental Health Journal*, **30**, 193–206.

Bennett, D. (1970) The value of work in psychiatric rehabilitation. *Social Psychiatry*, **5**, 224–230.

Boardman, A. P. & Hodgson, R. (2000) Community in-patient units and halfway hospitals. *Advances in Psychiatric Treatment*, **6**, 120–127.

Bond, G. R., Drake, R. E., Mueser, K. T., *et al* (1997) An update on supported employment for people with severe mental illness. *Psychiatric Services*, **48**, 335–346.

Bond, G. R., Becker, D. R., Drake, R. E., *et al* (2001) Implementing supported employment as evidence-based practice. *Psychiatric Services*, **52**, 313–322.

Brenner, M. H. (1979) Mortality and the national economy. A review, and the experience of England and Wales. *Lancet*, *ii*, 685–699.

Crowther, R. E. & Marshall, M. (2001) Employment rehabilitation schemes for people with mental health problems in the North West Region: service characteristics and utilisation. *Journal of Mental Health*, **10**, 373–382.

Crowther, R. E, Marshall, M., Bond, G. R., *et al* (2001) Helping people with severe mental illness to obtain work: systematic review. *BMJ*, **322**, 204–208.

Department of Health (1999) *National Service Framework for Mental Health: Modern Standards and Service Models*. London: Department of Health.

Department of Health (2001) *The Mental Health Policy Implementation Guide*. London: Department of Health.

Department of Health (2006*a*) Vocational services for people with severe mental health problems: commissioning guidance. London: Department of Health.

Department of Health (2006*b*) From segregation to inclusion: commissioning guidance on day services for people with mental health problems. London: Department of Health.

Ekdawi, M. & Conning, A. (1994) *Psychiatric Rehabilitation: A Practical Guide*. London: Chapman & Hall.

Foster, K., Meltzer, H., Gill, B., *et al* (1996) *OPCS Surveys of Psychiatric Morbidity in Great Britain. Report No. 8. Adults with a Psychotic Disorder Living in the Community*. London: TSO (The Stationery Office).

Grove, B. (1999) Mental health and employment: shaping a new agenda. *Journal of Mental Health*, **8**, 131–140.

Grove, B. & Durie, S. (1999) *Social Firms – An Instrument for Economic Empowerment and Inclusion*. Redhill: Social Firms UK.

Grove, R., Freudenberg, M., Harding, A., *et al* (1997) *The Social Firm Handbook*. Brighton: Pavilion Publishing.

Hatfield, B., Huxley, P. & Mohamad, H. (1992) Accommodation and employment. A survey into the circumstances and expressed needs of users of mental health services in a northern town. *British Journal of Social Work*, **22**, 60–73.

Hill, R. & Shepherd, G. (1997) Positively transitional or unfortunately permanent? The status of work within clubhouses in the UK. *A Life in the Day*, **1**, 25–30.

Hill, R.G., Hardy, P. & Shepherd, G. (1996) *Perspectives on Manic Depression. A Survey of the Manic Depression Fellowship*. London: Sainsbury Centre for Mental Health.

Macias, C., Barriera, P., Alden, M., *et al* (2001) The ICCD benchmarks for clubhouses: a practical approach to quality improvement in psychiatric rehabilitation. *Psychiatric Services*, **52**, 207–213.

Manning, C. & White, P. D. (1995) Attitudes of employers to the mentally ill. *Psychiatric Bulletin*, **19**, 541–543.

Mellen, V. & Danley, K. (1987) Supported employment for people with severe mental illness. *Psychosocial Rehabilitation Journal*, **9**(2), 1–102.

Meltzer, H., Gill, B., Petticrew, M., *et al* (1995) *OPCS Surveys of Psychiatric Morbidity in Great Britain. Report 3. Economic Activity and Social Functioning of Adults with Psychiatric Disorders*. London: TSO (The Stationery Office).

Newman, L. (1970) Instant placement: a new model for providing rehabilitation services within a community mental health programme. *Community Mental Health Journal*, **6**, 401–410.

Office for National Statistics (2000) *Labour Force Survey. Great Britain, Spring 2000*. London: Office for National Statistics.

Office of the Deputy Prime Minister (2004) *Mental Health and Social Exclusion. Social Exclusion Unit Report*. London: Office of the Deputy Prime Minister.

O'Flynn, D. & Craig, T. (2001) Which way to work? Occupations, vocations and opportunities for mental health service users. *Journal of Mental Health*, **10**, 1–4.

Perkins, R. & Rinaldi, M. (2002) Unemployment rates among patients with long-term mental health problems. A decade of rising unemployment. *Psychiatric Bulletin*, **26**, 295–298.

Perkins, R. E., Buckfield, R. & Choy, D. (1997) Access to employment. *Journal of Mental Health*, **6**, 307–318.

Platt, S. & Kreitman, N. (1984) Trends in parasuicide among unemployed men in Edinburgh 1968–82. *BMJ*, **289**, 1029–1032.

Posner, A., Ng, M., Hammond, J., *et al* (1996) *Working It Out*. Brighton: Pavilion Publishing.

Rinaldi, M. & Hill, R. G. (2000) *Insufficient Concern*. London: Merton Mind.

Rowland L. A. & Perkins, R. E. (1988) 'You can't eat, drink or make love eight hours a day'. The value of work in psychiatry. *Health Trends*, **20**, 75–79.

Sayce, E. & Boardman, J. (2003) The Disability Discrimination Act 1995: implications for psychiatrists. *Advances in Psychiatric Treatment*, **9**, 397–404.

Schneider, J. (1998) Work interventions in mental health care: some arguments and recent evidence. *Journal of Mental Health*, **7**, 81–94.

Secker, J., Grove, B. & Seebohm, P. (2001) *Challenging Barriers to Employment, Training and Education for Mental Health Service Users. The Service Users' Perspective*. London: Institute for Applied Health & Social Policy, King's College London.

United Nations (1948) *Universal Declaration of Human Rights*. http://www.un.org/Overview/rights.html

Wansborough, S. W. & Miles, A. (1968) *Industrial Rehabilitation in Psychiatric Hospitals*. London: King Edwards Hospital Fund.

Warner, R. (1994) *Recovery from Schizophrenia. Psychiatry and Political Economy* (2nd edn). London: Routledge.

Warr, P. (1987) *Work, Unemployment and Mental Health*. Oxford: Oxford University Press.

Watts, F. N. (1983) Employment. In *Theory and Practice of Psychiatric Rehabilitation* (eds F. N. Watts & D. H. Bennett). Chichester: John Wiley & Sons.

Wehman, P. (1986) Supported competitive employment for persons with severe disabilities. *Journal of Applied Rehabilitation Counselling*, **7**, 24–29.

Wiggins, J. S. (1973) *Personality and Prediction: Principles of Personality Assessment*. Reading, MA: Addison-Wesley.

Wilson, S. & Walker, G. (1993) Unemployment and health. A review. *Public Health*, **107**, 153–162.

Wing, J. K. & Brown, G. W. (1970) *Institutionalism and Schizophrenia. A Comparative Study of Three Mental Hospitals. 1960–1968*. Cambridge: Cambridge University Press.

CHAPTER 20

Community support services

Frank Holloway

Most people experiencing severe mental illnesses such as schizophrenia live outside any form of institutional care and a significant proportion remain out of contact with specialist mental health services, receiving treatment from primary care or living without any form of treatment or professional support at all. Community care for people with a mental illness has, at best, a chequered history, with some observers looking back nostalgically to the era of the asylum, when at least individuals' basic needs were met. This chapter reviews the evolution of community support services to people experiencing severe mental illness that may allow them to live valued and fulfilled lives outside a hospital setting. It must be read in conjunction with the chapters describing other vital components of community support, such as residential care and supported housing (see Wolfson, Chapter 17, this volume), and meaningful occupation and employment (see Boardman & Robinson, Chapter 19). The literature on community support services includes a great deal of jargon. Jargon terms that are widely used as abbreviations are defined in Box 20.1.

History

It is salutary to note that the first recorded form of community support for people with a mental illness in England was the right of inmates discharged from the Bethlem in London, until the 18th century the only public institution for the insane in England, to become licensed beggars. Tom O'Bedlam became a well-known figure in early modern England, much imitated by people who sought the benefit of this unique status without having experienced a stay in Bethlem. Local government, at that time based on the parish, provided some relief for those belonging to the parish who were in want: this might include providing funds for people to look after an insane relative.

Over the past 300 years mental health services in Britain have evolved from a state of non-care, where in the early 18th century poor people with severe mental illnesses were managed either at home or, if very disturbed,

Box 20.1 Glossary of common abbreviations

ACT   Assertive community treatment – first elaborated by Stein & Test (1980), later codified by Teague *et al* (1998) in the Dartmouth Assertive Community Treatment Scale

AOT   Assertive outreach team – specialist team identified in the policy implementation guide (PIG) for mental health (Department of Health, 2001), similar to the assertive community treatment

CFT   Community forensic team – a UK initiative to provide community support to offender patients (Judge *et al*, 2004)

CM   Case management – a mechanism for providing community support for people in the era of deinstitutionalisation. Models described include 'brokerage', 'intensive', 'rehabilitation' and 'strengths' (Holloway & Carson, 2001)

CMHT Community mental health team – generic team providing comprehensive secondary mental healthcare in a defined catchment area. Some functions have been taken away by the *Mental Health Policy Implementation Guide* (Department of Health, 2001)

CPA   Care programme approach – neologism coined in 1990 by the Department of Health and regularly redefined ever since. Makes requirements for mental health services to offer a regularly reviewed structured care plan for all service users

CRT   Community rehabilitation team – poorly described but effective service that provides community support to individuals leaving rehabilitation in-patient services (Killaspy *et al*, 2005)

EIP   Early Intervention in psychosis – services required by the mental health policy implementation guide to provide specialist care for people (up to 35 years of age) within 3 years of the onset of their illness (Kuipers *et al*, 2004)

PIG   Policy implementation guide (Department of Health, 2001) – guidance on the implementation of the National Service Framework for Mental Health and the NHS Plan (Department of Health, 1999 & 2000 respectively). Elaboration and updates are available at http://www.dh.gov.uk/PolicyAndGuidance/fs/en

in prisons and Bridewells (houses of correction). People with means could be cared for at home, placed in private 'madhouses' or boarded out with caring families (boarding out being the earliest recorded form of organised community care, dating back to the town of Gheel in 13th-century Belgium (Linn *et al*, 1982)).

From the early part of the 19th century the dominant paradigm for helping 'the insane' was care in the asylum. The initial optimistic expectation was that a 'cure' could be effected if the individual was admitted early enough and appropriate care provided through the medium of 'moral treatment'. Cure would lead to discharge without any requirement for further support, although it was recognised that those who relapsed might require readmission. Discharge rates for the early- to mid-19th-century asylum were impressive. However, in the late 19th century the asylum entered a 'long sleep' that lasted well into the 20th century. This was characterised by massive increase in bed numbers that required an ever-increasing expansion in the asylum system, the espousal of a degeneracy model of lunacy (which rendered the concept of treatment irrelevant) and very low expectations for recovery.

Even during this long sleep there was concern about the needs for the continuing care of people who were discharged from hospital, as evidenced by the founding of the Mental After-care Association (MACA) in 1869 by the Reverend Hawkins, Chaplain of Colney Hatch Asylum (Bennett, 1991). (The MACA remains a significant provider of community care.) Subsequent progress in providing care for people with a mental illness outside hospital was painfully slow and was intimately linked with the development of the welfare state in the UK. The Mental Treatment Act 1930 allowed, for the first time, the voluntary admission of patients to public mental hospitals. It also encouraged, but did not insist on, the development by the local authority of out-patient care and after-care for patients discharged from hospital. A tentative tradition of 'case-work' emerged in the new profession of social work, which involved detailed engagement in the life of someone with a mental illness that attempted to address their health and social care needs and embraced a psychodynamic perspective.

Mental hospital bed numbers in the UK and the USA reached their peak in 1954. They have declined steadily ever since, as the mental hospitals both literally and metaphorically opened their doors. The slogan of the subsequent era has been 'community care'. In fact, hospital admissions increased markedly in the 1950s and have continued to increase subsequently, while average length of stay has steadily fallen: the hospital has always been a vital element of effective community care. Early on, the 'open door' became a 'revolving door' as readmissions become the norm.

There was a slow and very patchy development of services designed to provide community support. In the 1950s social case-work and residential after-care were supplemented by the development of psychiatric day care and sheltered work, an expansion of out-patient clinics and the invention of the community psychiatric nurse (the first nurse working from Warlingham Park Hospital, Croydon). The concept of a comprehensive mental health service based on the local district general hospital rather than a remote mental hospital was described in the 1950s and further elaborated in the 1960s.

By the 1970s commentators in both the UK and the USA were emphasising the failures of community care. A simple system of care based on the mental hospital had been replaced by a complex, confusing and poorly coordinated patchwork of health and social care services. Deinstitutionalisation in the USA, more rapid and more profound than in the UK, was seen to have led to an explosion in the numbers of street-homeless people with severe mental illness and large-scale diversion into the ever-expanding prisons. Community mental health centres, designed to replace the system of state mental hospitals, were increasingly felt to have ignored the needs of people with severe mental illness in favour of a more attractive client group experiencing neurotic illness and problems with living. Careful studies of cohorts of patients discharged from hospital in the UK documented lack of contact with psychiatric professionals, burden on families and poor clinical outcomes.

Many individuals left hospital, even after very long in-patient admissions, without meaningful arrangements for support or follow-up being put in place. The Mental Health Act 1983 (Section 117) placed a specific duty on health and social services to provide after-care for patients discharged from hospital after a compulsory admission. Evidence suggests that this duty was often not well adhered to even into the 1990s. During the 1990s local mental health services were increasingly organised around the community mental health team (CMHT), a multidisciplinary team tasked with providing comprehensive mental health services to a defined catchment area. The inadequacies of the system were graphically illustrated by the Ritchie Report. This report investigated the care provided to Christopher Clunis, a man with ineffectively treated schizophrenia despite multiple contacts with mental health and social care services, who killed Jonathan Zito in 1992 (Ritchie *et al*, 1994). One consequence of this report was a policy move in England and Wales towards compulsory community treatment, an option that has became increasingly available in English-speaking jurisdictions.

After decades of decreasing patient numbers, the majority of the large mental hospitals in England at last closed during the 1990s, to be replaced virtually bed for bed by a network of acute psychiatric in-patient units, residential facilities and longer-term hospital services. This 'virtual asylum' (see Wolfson, Chapter 17, this volume), a metaphorical institution in which most individuals in receipt of long-term high-support care are placed in private-sector accommodation, presents challenges to local services in assuring that people's needs are met and value for money is delivered.

Case management, the care programme approach and care coordination

The concept of case management was developed in the USA in the 1970s specifically to remedy the perceived defects of the 'human services systems' providing care for elderly people and people with learning disabilities or mental illnesses in an era of deinstitutionalisation. These failings can be summarised as fragmentation and consequent absence of continuity of care, lack of accountability for meeting people's needs and inefficiency in the use of scarce resources. However, the core mission of most mental health case management programmes was to prevent rehospitalisation (Holloway & Carson, 2001).

Two distinct models of case management can be identified. In the 'brokerage' model a case manager arranges and coordinates a package of community support for the individual, essentially linking the person to the services they are assessed as requiring. By contrast, 'clinical' case management involves the case manager working directly with the individual in both a practical and therapeutic manner, while also undertaking linking functions to the wider service system and other forms of support. In 'brokerage' models the case-loads tend to be high and the staff to be para-professionals or bureaucrats. Clinical models of case management tend to require professionally trained staff working with lower case-loads. Clinical case management owes much to the model of social case-work initially elaborated in the UK. Varieties of clinical case management have been described which are variations on the clinical theme. These include 'intensive' case management (where case-loads are particularly low); the 'strengths model' (in which the focus is on working with the individual's strengths and wants rather than their professionally defined needs); and the 'rehabilitation' model (where the focus is on attaining rehabilitation goals) (Burns & Firn, 2002).

American case management models began to influence research, policy and practice in the UK during the 1980s. In the face of the escalating costs of community care for all client groups, particularly elderly people, in 1989 the government introduced community care reforms that brought in the concept of the 'care manager', who was responsible for assessing, purchasing, arranging and monitoring care packages funded by social services. The care programme approach (CPA) was introduced into English mental health services in 1990 to address concerns about the poor follow-up of patients discharged from psychiatric hospitals – Scotland, Wales and Northern Ireland remained aloof from this innovation. The CPA required services to develop a care plan for all patients deemed vulnerable and to allocate a keyworker (later renamed care coordinator), who would be responsible for ensuring that the plan was adhered to. Subsequent reworking of national CPA policy and the integration of health and social services has allowed the care manager role, which is a form of brokerage case management, to fade away in mental healthcare.

The CPA care plan is, in theory, the current mechanism by which community support services for people in England with mental health problems are arranged, coordinated, monitored and reviewed. Box 20.2 sets out the headings of the care planning documentation used in one large English mental health trust (a provider unit responsible for the comprehensive mental healthcare of a population of over 1 million people). These headings are strongly reminiscent of the items used in research measures to assess quality of life (e.g. the Manchester Short Assessment of Quality of Life (Priebe et al, 1999)) and patients' treatment and care needs (e.g. the Camberwell Assessment of Need (Phelan et al, 1995)). More recently, in addition to responsibilities for service users, there is now a requirement for the needs of carers to be assessed and, if appropriate, for

---

Box 20.2   Elements of the CPA care plan: South London and Maudsley Trust

- Mental health
- Physical health
- Family and personal relationships
- Daytime activities
- Housing
- Occupation/education
- Finances and welfare benefits
- Risk issues: risks to self and others – including dependent children
- Substance misuse
- Medication
- Contingency and crisis plans

---

them to be offered a formal care plan. The designated care coordinator has an active clinical role for the individual and their carers. The contemporary care coordinator is, in effect, a clinical case manager who works within a multidisciplinary team (see Holloway, Chapter 16, this volume).

Assertive community treatment

In 1980 Stein & Test published their seminal account of a randomised controlled trial of a community treatment programme as an alternative to in-patient admission. Staff who had previously worked within the hospital serving Madison, Wisconsin (a fairly affluent university town), were retrained to provide psychosocially oriented care and tasked with, as far as possible, maintaining people out of hospital. Stein & Test – a psychiatrist and a social worker by profession – based their service model on a set of requirements they believed were necessary to allow individuals with mental illness to maintain tenure in the community (Box 20.3). The study found significant social, clinical and financial gains for patients allocated to the experimental service over a year compared with a control group who were admitted to hospital and offered standard follow-up. Furthermore these gains were lost once the services of the team were withdrawn, which had the rather disturbing implication that the treatment team would need to work with the patient/client over the very long term.

Stein & Test (1980) became the founding text of the expanding industry in the USA of what came to be called assertive community treatment services for people with a severe mental illness. (It is also one of the few published studies relevant to the introduction of home treatment teams as an alternative to hospital admission, which were later to be incorporated in the mandatory policy implementation guide to mental health services in

Box 20.3   Requirements for community tenure of people at risk of hospital admission

Material resources
Food, shelter, clothing, medical care and so on

Coping skills
Budgeting, cooking, using public transport and so on

Motivation
Systems of support to help individuals cope with stress

Freedom from dependent relationships
Aim to break the cycle of dependency

Support and education of community members
To help people in the community to interact appropriately with the individual

Assertive support system
To preclude the tendency to drop out of care

(Stein & Test, 1980)

England (Department of Health, 2001).) Assertive community treatment involves a high-intensity approach to the care of people with severe mental illness at risk of repeated in-patient admissions. Trained staff, working within a whole-team approach, provide assertive community support that includes skills training in the person's own environment, medication management, crisis intervention and attention to the needs of informal carers. The assertive community treatment model has been codified, so that fidelity to the model can be assessed (e.g. by the Dartmouth Assertive Community Treatment Scale (Teague *et al*, 1998), summarised in Box 20.4). Two specific elements of the model deserve special mention: the requirements for expertise in the management of substance misuse and vocational rehabilitation (i.e. placing people in employment or education).

The relationship between assertive community treatment and intensive case management is one of great controversy, the proponents of the former asserting that it is both different and superior. There is abundant evidence that, compared with standard care, assertive community treatment results in fewer days in hospital for people with severe mental illness, whereas careful studies of intensive case management have been less favourable (Ziguras & Stuart, 2000; Holloway & Carson, 2001). A confounding factor is that assertive community treatment studies have tended to be carried out in the USA, where standard community care may be much less assertive and effective than in Europe (where CMHTs are now the norm), whereas intensive case management studies have largely been undertaken in Europe (Burns *et al*, 2001).

Box 20.4 Dartmouth criteria for fidelity to an assertive community treatment (ACT) programme (Teague *et al*, 1998)

Small case-load	1:10
Team approach	Providers function as a team
Programme meeting	Frequent team meetings to review clients
Team leader	Is a practitioner and has a case-load
Continuity of staff	Low staff turnover
Staff capacity	Staff in post
Psychiatrist	Is a member of the ACT team
Nurse	>2 nurses per 100 clients
Work/education	Vocational specialist on team
Programme size	About 100 clients
Admission criteria	Explicit
Intake rate	Low client turnover
Comprehensiveness	ACT team responsible for all aspects of care
Crisis services	ACT team provides 24-h coverage
Hospital admission	ACT team decides
Hospital discharge	ACT team plans discharge
Duration	Time-unlimited services
Treatment	Team works with client in the community
No drop out policy	Clients kept on case-load
Assertive approach	Street outreach and coercive mechanisms used
Service intensity	Prolonged contact time with client
Frequency of contact	Frequent service contact with client
Support system	ACT team works with carers, landlords, employers
Substance misuse	Substance misuse specialist in team
	Individual treatment for substance misuse
	Treatment groups
	Sophisticated treatment model
Consumer role	Clients involved as team members

Assertive outreach teams

By the 1990s the standard form of non-hospital mental healthcare in England was the CMHT, which aimed to meet the treatment and support needs of people referred for secondary mental healthcare. Anyone who has worked within a generic CMHT will attest that these needs are manifold – covering the full range of diagnostic categories, a broad spectrum of disability and individuals at very different stages in their illness career (or, in contemporary jargon, their patient journey). Concern that the generic CMHT cannot effectively meet these very varied demands has led to the elaboration within the mental health policy implementation guide (Department of Health, 2001) of a 'functionally differentiated' model of community provision that involves a number of teams or services. These

293

include, in addition to the CMHT, dedicated services for early-onset psychosis, crisis resolution/home treatment and assertive outreach. The description of the assertive outreach team in the policy implementation guide is highly prescriptive and owes a great deal to fidelity scales for assertive community treatment (Box 20.4). The assertive outreach team is required to be multidisciplinary, including as a minimum psychiatric nurses and psychiatrists but generally also involving the full range of mental health professionals and non-professional support workers. Case-loads are low: typically 1 member of staff to 15 clients.

Burns & Firn (2002) provide a detailed account of the 'whys' and 'hows' of the assertive outreach team that can help practitioners implement the policy implementation guide. They also helpfully discuss the vexed terminological issue of 'patient' or 'client' (opting, as I shall do below, for the term preferred by service users: patient). The concept of the assertive outreach team is an appealing one. A specialist team takes on people from the case-load of the generic CMHTs who present particular difficulties, in terms of poor engagement with services, regular non-adherence with recommended (pharmacological) treatment and recurrent acute hospital admissions – the classic 'revolving-door' patient. Assertive outreach team patients/clients are expected to have psychotic illnesses (the model has not been tested with people who have severe personality disorders) but not to be living in high-support accommodation. On referral to the assertive outreach team many patients/clients will have comorbid substance misuse and most will have been identified as presenting significant risks to themselves or others and been subject to compulsory hospital admission or other coercive interventions. The vast majority will be unemployed and not engaged in meaningful daytime activities. Depending on local morbidity, one assertive outreach team should be serving a borough-wide population of about 300 000, compared with the typical CMHT catchment area of 40 000 total population.

The assertive outreach team should engage and work intensively with the patient/client, addressing their practical 'wants' as well as profession-ally defined 'needs'. There are examples of assertive outreach teams and assertive community treatment teams that successfully employ former service users as support workers, who are in an ideal position to address these practical 'wants'. The assertive outreach team should develop close links with any relevant informal carers (e.g. family, friends and neighbours). In inner-urban areas many assertive outreach team patients/clients will be drawn from ethnic minorities, who are overrepresented in all forms of coercive mental healthcare. Cultural sensitivity is very specifically required of the assertive outreach team (for a useful discussion of the issues see Burns & Firn, 2002: pp. 78–92).

An effective assertive outreach team pays great attention to ensuring adherence to treatment, often to the extent of delivering medication such as clozapine daily to people on the case-load (Burns & Firn, 2002: p. 115). The competent assertive outreach team should, in addition to ensuring optimal psychopharmacological treatment, be able to provide psychoeducation, formal family interventions and psychological treatment for psychosis. Given the propensity to relapse of assertive outreach team patients/clients an important element of the work of the team is to plan for and intervene effectively in crisis. Policy dictates that the success of an assertive outreach or assertive community treatment team is measured by a decrease in admissions and bed-days for its patients/clients.

The aspirations for treatment and care discussed above are, in fact, no different from those of a competent generic CMHT and are completely in accord with the expectations of the CPA. The critical feature of the assertive outreach team is that, given its capped case-load and low staff/patient ratio, staff should have the time to come to a detailed understanding of the needs of the patient/client. Staff in an assertive outreach team must take a long-term view, work closely and effectively with the patient/client and their carers and embrace a philosophy of assertive engagement. Because of the high level of resources required by an assertive outreach team careful attention has to be paid to ensuring that only appropriate individuals come onto the case-load and that there are ready routes back into mainstream services once treatment goals have been met.

Assertive outreach and assertive community treatment share the classic dilemmas of all rehabilitation services. On the one hand these services must strive to promote the autonomy of patients/clients, encouraging them to make their own choices on their individual roads to recovery, constantly seeking to decrease their dependence on the care system. On the other hand, in our current risk-averse age, risks must be managed and adherence to treatment monitored and encouraged. The line between legitimate assertive outreach and unnecessary intrusion in someone's life is a fine one. Assertive outreach and assertive community treatment often, very appropriately, involve paternalistic and coercive practices. However, staff need to be exquisitely sensitive to the ethical dimensions of their work.

Specialist assertive community teams

A number services have been developed that make use of key assertive outreach principles to work with specific client groups. These include: services for early intervention in psychosis; community forensic teams; teams that work with homeless people who are mentally ill (Lehman et al, 1999); and 'dual-diagnosis' teams working with people who have psychosis and comorbid severe mental illness (Drake et al, 1998). In addition, there are teams, usually operating in the voluntary sector, that offer intensive community support to specific disadvantaged minority ethnic groups.

In many areas well-established community rehabilitation teams were providing crisis intervention, assertive outreach and practical support for many years before the publication of the mental health policy implementation guide. Patients on the case-load of the community rehabilitation team will generally have been discharged from specialist rehabilitation units (Killaspy *et al*, 2005) and be characterised by continuing functional deficits requiring direct practical support to maintain independent living or a supported tenancy. A major concern has been that in some areas implementation of assertive outreach has been at the expense of the local community rehabilitation team, which had been working successfully with a less dramatic client group than those seen as requiring assertive outreach. The workings of the community rehabilitation team have been very poorly documented, reflecting the practical orientation of and lack of research in rehabilitation in the UK.

Early-intervention services are discussed in detail by Power *et al* in Chapter 9. They draw on the assertive community treatment model, although many of their clients will, at least initially, have lower levels of disability and disturbance than the norm for people in contact with assertive community treatment and assertive outreach teams. Early-intervention services must take account of the developmental stage of their clients, tailoring their care plans to take account of developmental issues. Psychoeducation is more difficult in the early stages of an illness career, since there will commonly be uncertainty over diagnosis and prognosis. Working with families and managing substance misuse take on an even greater significance than in traditional assertive outreach. Opportunities for maintaining the client in occupation or education are greater than when the illness has become established. The Department of Health vision is of one early-intervention team serving a population of 1 million or so, although model services have been developed to serve populations at the borough level of about 300 000 (Kuipers *et al*, 2004).

Community forensic teams have developed rapidly in England. Although quite heterogeneous in terms of staffing, case-load and functioning, the typical team provides risk assessment and case management to offender patients. Team members carry low case-loads and provide highly assertive outreach, but, in addition to direct care, frequently serve court diversion schemes and offer consultancy and co-working with CMHTs and assertive outreach teams. Many patients on the case-load will be subject to compulsory community treatment via a restriction order. The mean population served by a community forensic team is well over 1 million, although again borough-level services are increasingly common (Judge *et al*, 2004).

Conclusions

High-intensity community support services such as the assertive outreach team are not in themselves effective treatments for severe mental illness. Rather, they are methods for ensuring that people are effectively engaged with the care system, that their needs for treatment and care are assessed and that, as far as possible given existing knowledge, these needs are met.

There is strong evidence that good-quality community support services, backed by effective treatment, can improve outcomes.

The aim of a community support service should be to make itself redundant for a patient/client because they no longer require the level of support, treatment or care that it provides. Services must also be prepared to offer continuing care for those whose needs demand it. The need to balance expectations of recovery with an acknowledgement that for some people long-term support is required for the maintenance of an adequate quality of life remains a dilemma for carers (both formal and informal) working in rehabilitation and continuing care services.

References

Bennett, D. (1991) The drive towards the community. In *150 Years of British Psychiatry* (eds G. E. Berrios & H. Freeman), pp. 321–332. London: Gaskell.

Burns, T. & Firn, M. (2002) *Assertive Outreach in Mental Health*. Oxford: Oxford University Press.

Burns, T., Fioritti, A., Holloway, F., *et al* (2001) Case management and assertive community treatment in Europe. *Psychiatric Services*, **52**, 631–636.

Department of Health (1999) *National Service Framework for Mental Health: Modern Standards and Service Models*. London: Department of Health.

Department of Health (2000) *The NHS Plan. A Plan for Investment, a Plan for Reform*. London: Department of Health.

Department of Health (2001) *The Mental Health Policy Implementation Guide*. London: Department of Health

Drake, R. E., McHugo, G. J., Bebout, R. R., *et al* (1998) Assertive community treatment for patients with co-occurring severe mental illness and substance misuse disorder: a clinical trial. *American Journal of Orthopsychiatry*, **68**, 201–205.

Judge, J., Fahy, T. & Harty, M. A. (2004) Survey of community forensic psychiatry services in England and Wales. *Journal of Forensic Psychiatry and Psychology*, **15**, 244–253.

Holloway, F. & Carson, J. (2001) Case management: an update. *International Journal of Social Psychiatry*, **47**, 21–31.

Killaspy, H., Harden, C., Holloway, F., *et al* (2005) What do mental health rehabilitation services do and what are they for? A national survey in England. *Journal of Mental Health*, **14**, 358–363.

Kuipers, E., Holloway, F., Rabe-Hesketh, S., *et al* (2004) An RCT of early intervention in psychosis: Croydon outreach and assertive support team (COAST). *Social Psychiatry and Psychiatric Epidemiology*, **39**, 358–363.

Lehman, A. F., Dixon, L., Hoch, J. S., *et al* (1999) Cost-effectiveness of assertive community treatment for homeless persons with severe mental illness. *British Journal of Psychiatry*, **174**, 346–352.

Linn, M. W., Klett, C. J. & Caffey, E. M. (1982) Relapse of psychiatric patients in foster care. *American Journal of Psychiatry*, **139**, 778–783.

Phelan, M., Slade, M., Thornicroft, G., *et al* (1995) The Camberwell Assessment of Need: the validity and reliability of an instrument to assess the needs of people with severe mental illness. *British Journal of Psychiatry*, **167**, 589–595.

Priebe, S., Huxley, P., Knight, S., *et al* (1999) Application and results of the Manchester Short Assessment of Quality of Life (MANSA). *International Journal of Social Psychiatry*, **45**, 7–12.

Ritchie, J., Dick, D. & Lingham, R. (1994) *The Report of the Inquiry into the Care and Treatment of Christopher Clunis*. London: TSO (The Stationery Office).

Stein, L. I. & Test, M. A. (1980) Alternative to mental hospital treatment. *Archives of General Psychiatry*, **37**, 392–397.

Teague, C. B., Bond, G. R. & Drake, R. E. (1998) Program fidelity in assertive community treatment: development and use of a measure. *American Journal of Orthopsychiatry*, **68**, 216–232.

Ziguras, S. J. & Stuart, G. W. (2000) A meta-analysis of the effectiveness of mental health case management over 20 years. *Psychiatric Services*, **51**, 1410–1421.

CHAPTER 21

Rolling the stone uphill: leadership, management and longer-term mental healthcare

Tom Harrison

The longer a person remains disabled by illness, the greater is the need for effective leadership of the treatment team. Increasing length and severity of disorder disturbs every domain of a person's life. The consequences of illness require negotiation across many boundaries, including family members, housing providers and employers. To be effective, staff require a wide range of skills as well as encouragement to express differing, even conflicting, views. Plurality is essential to the development of new learning and innovation within any organisation (Heifetz & Laurie, 2001). Diversity increases the resources available to a service or team but capable leadership is needed to ensure that these resources are used effectively.

Rehabilitation staff experience an endless battle for the recognition of the needs of people affected by longer-term mental disorder. Dedicated psychiatric rehabilitation services receive little attention in UK policy and are currently losing out to more 'exciting' developments in early intervention, assertive outreach and crisis resolution. Indeed, some existing rehabilitation teams have been plundered to establish these new services. Staff have to cope with a rapidly changing environment and to maintain an optimistic outlook despite barriers and setbacks. Services are constantly beset by the need to adjust to new policies, managerial changes, paperwork and advances in therapeutic methods.

I will not repeat other management texts (particularly recommended are Onyett (2003) and Øvretveit (2000)) but will pursue an approach, drawing on the psychodynamic insights of Bion and Main, that maximises the effectiveness of staff working with within the multidisciplinary team. My core argument is that everyone involved in the therapeutic endeavour can and should be encouraged to become a leader.

Helicoptering: an overview of the chapter

The first task of anyone in a managerial or leadership role is to take an overview of the situation. Sometimes described as helicoptering, this involves rising above the day-to-day business to survey the broader landscape. Personal conflicts expressed in the microsystem often have their origins at other levels of the organisation. Dealing with these conflicts locally may only attend to the symptoms rather than address root causes. Indeed, rather than being problems, conflicts may provide valuable clues to underlying adaptive changes causing difficulties in the broader system (Heifetz & Laurie, 2001).

This chapter attempts to take such an overview of working in longer-term care services. It emphasises three characteristics of leadership:

- in a complex and dynamic environment the successful leader encourages a flow of flexible, innovative solutions from team members
- to enable the development of longer-term care, teams must feel able and willing to provide and champion solutions: they cannot wait endlessly for 'the management' to recognise their value
- the successful team includes members who directly provide and receive services as leaders.

The words 'management' and 'leadership' are often contrasted. There are clear differences in theory (Box 21.1), but in practice one cannot operate without the other. All actions must accomplish the task in the most productive manner. When the team is functioning well the process will be managed to ensure that it continues that way. If difficulties arise, then encouragement and enterprise are required to resolve them. To avoid repetition I will use the word leadership to encompass both aspects.

Borrill et al (2000) found that the presence of a clear team leader is associated with team effectiveness. Most longer-term care teams have a number of senior individuals who may vie for this role. Potential conflict must be defused at the outset by agreeing who should take this role (Onyett, 2003: p. 171). It is my practice (I am a consultant psychiatrist) to make it explicit that I reserve the right to discuss any decisions but that I will defer to the leadership of the team manager should differences continue. This has rarely, if ever, led to any difficulty, debates being confined to shades of grey rather than polar opposites.

Forms of leadership

There is a tendency to contrast different forms of leadership, for instance 'transformational' against 'transactional' methods. The former is seen as inspirational, visionary, charismatic and considerate towards staff. The latter is viewed as managerial, attending to the day-to-day tasks of the team, using a goal-setting approach, feedback and self-monitoring. This is a false dichotomy. Both approaches have their values, and risks, and should be deployed according to the requirements of the task. The routines of ensuring that patients are seen, receive the appropriate therapy and that their care programmes completed are the foundations of care. Bass (1998), one of the leading advocates of transformational leadership, implicitly acknowledges this in recognising that most leaders have a repertoire of

---

Box 21.1   Management and leadership

Management	*Leadership*
Organising setting procedures	Setting the 'vision'
Creating formal structures	Enthusing/inspiring
Managing/rationing resources	Making the best of what's available
Controlling	Enabling 'ownership'
Discipline	Encouraging people to do more than they thought they could
Staff in an organisation	Partners in an enterprise
Ensuring that there is an infrastructure in which leadership can be effective	Ensuring that people do willingly and well what needs to be done

---

models on which to draw. Corrigan *et al* (2000) found that, in terms of patient satisfaction and quality of life, both approaches are equally effective when compared with laissez faire techniques, which do not work.

Some argue for consensus management, where everyone must agree. This results in the individual who says 'no' wielding the most power. Hours are then wasted in attempting to achieve complete agreement. An alternative style, democracy, requires a leaderless clinical team, giving rise to role confusion, failure to take responsibility and the informal election of implicit leaders whose role is not clearly defined (Øvretveit, 2000).

Understanding leadership

The acquisition of leadership skills is an iterative process, in which the same issues arise repeatedly but in different guises: ideally, each time something new is learnt.

Management or leadership can be viewed as operating at three levels, which are in constant interplay. Self-management is the foundation. Next is the work group. Beyond these lies management outside the team, in a broader context that includes an interconnecting system of care providers. This conception enables each problem to be examined in a systematic manner, and may assist in identifying where difficulties originate, and at which level the solution lies.

The limits of rehabilitation

All people receiving mental healthcare have had their lives disrupted by their experiences but most require little extra support to make the necessary adaptations. The need for specialist services arises in situations where the difficulties are complex, severely affecting the social, psychological and biological aspects of a person's life. What people in this situation need is not the reactive style of acute psychiatric services, but a holistic response, probably paced over a long period of time and aimed at effecting healthy living rather than cure. As Esso Leete expressed it:

'For the past 20 years I have lived with it [schizophrenia] and in spite of it – struggling to come to terms with it without giving in to it... Taking responsibility for my life and developing coping mechanisms has been crucial to my recovery' (Leete, 1989).

Rehabilitation teams

Teams function better when they have a clear remit. Onyett (1999) argues against teams providing interventions for a very broad range of problems, as many current community mental health teams do. Specialist teams, skilled at working over the longer-term, with patience, a holistic approach and the ability to recognise and celebrate small successes, will be more successful at helping people whose needs are complex and persistent.

A major problem in researching psychiatric rehabilitation is the variability in types of service. There is the traditional 'pick and choose' rehabilitation team, to which potentially suitable patients are referred and accepted only if they demonstrate 'motivation'. This approach has the implicit difficulties that those who 'fail' acceptance experience yet another rejection and many with longer-term needs may remain neglected. An alternative is the 'functionalised' approach, in which a range of teams provide comprehensive longer-term care to all those who need it. For example, early-intervention services take people through the first 3–5 years of a psychotic illness. Assertive outreach teams work with patients who have a history of poor engagement with care, often as a result of aversive experiences of the mental health system. Recovery services may seek to support all other patients with complex needs. However, there can be no 'one size fits all' solution. Different geographic areas have differing requirements. It is inappropriate and unwieldy to export a model that works well in the inner city to rural or suburban areas.

Whatever the service model, there should be services for all people who have longer-term disabling disorders. Increasingly there is pressure for services to extend beyond a traditional remit for people with psychotic illnesses to include those who have a primary diagnosis of personality disorder. However, the available evidence suggests that people with severe personality disorder benefit best from specialist care (National Institute for Mental Health in England, 2003). There are similar pressures to provide a response to individuals severely disabled by autistic-spectrum disorders.

Management of the self

Following his experience as a tank commander in the First World War Wilfred Bion (1946) concluded that anybody who had primary ability to consider the needs of others while under stress themselves had the potential to be a leader. This percipient observation introduces some of the counter-intuitive aspects of leadership. Before embarking on a leadership role the individual has to manage and value their own resource. Stress is implicit in any professional or caring role, and although here is not the place to elaborate on this issue, effective leaders should not neglect their own needs or those of their families.

Task organisation

The first task is the need to prioritise overall long-term and intermediate personal objectives. Properly applied, this should achieve a balance between personal, work-task and organisational requirements. Necessarily the exigencies of arriving in the job on the first day lead to potential information (and demand) overload. Bion described this on arriving at Northfield Military Hospital in 1942:

'I was not able to work at this task in an atmosphere of cloistered calm. No sooner was I seated before desk and papers than I was beset with urgent problems posed by importunate patients and others' (Bion, 1961: p. 12).

Mobile telephones, email and other technologies have since further intensified the experience. The expectations of existing staff members are mixed, often tinged with unconscious hopes. The temptation is to respond by 'getting stuck in' immediately. This rapidly leads to the feeling of being overburdened and loss of objectivity. As Bion did, it is important to step back and reflect on what is happening by helicoptering, taking the opportunity to overview, monitor and evaluate how effectively the task is being addressed. It may even be necessary to clarify what the task is. Teams have a tendency to act as if their work is to preserve the dynamics within the team, rather than to change to carry out their allocated task more effectively. Naturally this is not expressed consciously but will be evident in intra-group tensions (Bion, 1961).

Turquet (1974) warns against staying in this role, 'an observer gliding above the fray as a nonparticipant', arguing that the leader would lose contact with vital aspects of the group's activities. It is necessary to remain in contact, enthusing, taking part and engaging in the life of the group.

Rarely will a job description give information that fully clarifies the role. Indeed it might be more harmful than helpful if it did, as effective leadership is about creating an environment where new, previously unconsidered, solutions to old problems are generated.

Once the time to reflect has been gained there are various ways of looking at the job plan. Time management is an essential skill. Effective time management requires the identification of priorities, allocation of appropriate time to each and effective use of this scarce resource (Garratt, 1985).

Personality and leadership

A common approach to finding a team leader is to specify ideal personality traits and argue for recruitment on the basis of these. In identifying the different behaviours of leaders within teams, Belbin (1986) pinpointed a number of types. An example is the 'plant' (rather common among psychiatrists), who is creative, imaginative, unorthodox and able to solve difficult problems. The down side may be that such a person has difficulties in communication and a tendency to ignore details. No team will survive if it consists entirely of 'plants'.

These stereotypes are inappropriate if applied rigidly, but provide an insight into how a person prefers to operate, and the difficulties that arise by sticking to type. Assessing oneself can indicate one's own inherent strengths and the weaknesses that have to be compensated for. A leader must be flexible and willing to act in ways that do not come naturally.

There have been many attempts to identify the inherent qualities of good leaders. The lists generated by this process can be long, contradictory and entirely unrealistic. The leader's primary skill is to ensure that the task is achieved by people acting willingly and effectively.

Expertise

A common misconception is that the leader has to be adept at all the tasks that face a team. This is rarely true as long as other team members have the appropriate expertise. It is the task of the leader to ensure that adequate skills are present or are acquired. Leaders should not be threatened by the expertise of others. The fact that team members produce knowledgeable ideas promotes 'ownership' of the team process and encourages contributions from others.

The working team

No matter how well trained and knowledgeable any individual member of staff is, most longer-term care needs the manifold skills of a multi-disciplinary team. Within this the nature of responsibility is changing. Originally it was argued that the consultant was accountable for every patient. Now all staff have personal responsibility for their actions. Onyett outlines the different forms this takes, identifying employee, professional and legal responsibilities (Onyett, 2003: pp. 171–175).

Even the word 'team' is problematic. The concept tends to suggest a group of people with a single purpose and strictly defined roles, as in a football team. Reality is much more fluid. Indeed the 'multidisciplinary team' usually acts as a resource from which smaller project teams are formed to work with individuals.

In rehabilitation services a number of processes have to progress in order to achieve success. These are primarily the responsibility of everyone who takes a leadership or managerial role, but are shared by all team members to a greater or lesser extent.

Team leadership

Central to the rehabilitation process is the effective integration of staff with varying skills into a coherent team. All members, including recipients of care, have to develop and use leadership skills. Clearly some individuals, by virtue of their knowledge, position and experience, have particular leadership responsibilities for the effective functioning of the overall group, but this is not the exclusive preserve of one profession. The decision as to who takes overall leadership, or managerial, responsibility at any one time has to be determined by the requirements of the task to be completed.

Part of the process of successful rehabilitation is to place the person receiving the service increasingly in the role of leader of their own care. This may be practically demonstrated by chairing their own case conferences, and can extend to gaining confidence to become leaders as advisers within the team and within outside service user organisations. A practical example of the former role is a service user who is a member of an appointment panel interviewing applicants to become new members of staff.

Celebrating complexity

Tom Main, in his pioneering paper on rehabilitation, wrote over half a century ago: 'Health and disease are not things, static or absolute in themselves; both are aspects of the dynamic process of biological adaptation between man and his environment' (Main, 1948: p. 386). The environment and the individual are changing constantly. Rehabilitation was born in the timeless routines of the old psychiatric hospital. Some models still reflect this. Paradoxically, reinventing the wheel is an essential part of rehabilitation. Teaching one person to cook is never the same as teaching another. Each person has a different set of abilities, resources and expectations. The task is to invent the right wheel for the right task at the right time. This means that staff have to be able constantly to face new challenges. There are very few predictable routines, particularly when care is carried out in people's own homes. Present training tends to concentrate on competency. The need in rehabilitation is for capability, not merely competence (Box 21.2). This complexity requires staff in many situations to be empowered to make decisions on the spot, without having to check with others before they can proceed.

A framework for team leadership

One practical framework for conceiving of leadership within the team is provided by Adair (1984). He identifies three interacting core aspects – task, team and individual (Fig. 21.1). Adair's model is useful for analysis:

Box 21.2 Capability and competency

Competency
Traditional training tends to enhance competence, i.e. developing knowledge, skills and attitudes. Competency is usually static and inflexible.

Capability
In a complex world, training should also concentrate on the ability to adapt to changing circumstances, creating new ideas and solutions, and continually improving performance. Capability involves how to carry out skills in varying conditions.

---

if activity within one arena is excessive (or lacking), the leader needs to redress the balance. A team that is solely task driven is likely to burn out if no attention is paid to the coordination of and cooperation between members. The individual needs of team members must also be addressed. In Bion's 'basic assumption' group, pathological unconscious processes predominate, resulting in a preoccupation with team and individual neurotic needs at the expense of the task (Bion, 1961).

Change management

Leadership of change is a popular concept at present. It tends to concentrate on large-scale issues and can fail to recognise that change is a persistent process facing all community teams. The political, social and economic climate is in permanent flux – even chaos. Rather than nostalgically regretting the apparently unchanging past, staff can only welcome the new. Although imposed change carries with it an inevitable burden of destruction of old ways, it provides an endless series of new opportunities.

Reynolds & Thornicroft (1999) discuss the problems of introducing changes to staff at the time when they are well nigh inevitable. It is healthier

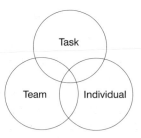

Fig. 21.1 Aspects of leadership within a team (after Adair, 1984; with permission).

Table 21.1 The 'task, team, individual' framework: leadership tasks in team-working

Key actions	Task	Team	Individual
Defining purpose	Define tasks and any difficulties	Share commitment (individual and group) Clarify objectives, gain 'ownership'	
Plan	Collect information: review options, check resources	Consult and encourage ideas, develop suggestions, assess skills, arrange training	
	Decide priorities: time scales, standards	Structure	Allocate jobs, delegate, set targets
Brief	Clarify objectives Describe plan	Explain decisions, listen to and answer questions, enthuse, check understanding	
Monitor support	Assess progress Maintain standards	Coordinate, reconcile conflict Recognise effort – give praise	Advise, assist/ reassure, counsel, discipline
Evaluate	Summarise progress Review objectives Replan if necessary	Recognise and gain from success, learn from mistakes Guide and train – give praise	Appraise performance

(After John Adair, with permission.)

to develop a culture in which innovation is welcomed and encouraged throughout the organisation. The model described here develops this consciousness, and argues that a team should be at the forefront of innovation, rather than dragging its heels behind.

There are different phases in carrying out a task. First, the objectives must be clearly understood and accepted. Then how the job might be executed using the available resources needs to be considered. Once decisions have been made, team members have to be clear about their roles. As the task is carried out, progress must be monitored and contingencies dealt with as they arise. Finally, on completion the process should be evaluated both to recognise success and to learn where there are opportunities for improvement. When the different phases are mapped onto Adair's 'task, team, individual' framework a practical model of leadership actions can be developed (see Table 21.1).

There is no space here to elaborate on this programme of activities. Each stage involves different and easily learnt skills, many of which are already known to mental health professionals, particularly those concerned with the dynamics of group working. Of course, the simplicity of the framework is deceptive. It has to be applied to fluid situations that are not easily divided into boxes and when a number of tasks are being undertaken concurrently. However, apart from its value in training and understanding processes, it provides an effective tool for analysing problematic situations.

Leading in the wider organisation

One of the difficulties that teams face is connecting with other parts of the organisation. A sure sign of how a team is functioning is how it maintains its interfaces with the external world. Leadership is Janus-like, taking account of issues both inside and outside the group (Turquet, 1974). I will enlarge on two aspects here: managing interfaces and championship.

Managing interfaces

A psychiatric rehabilitation service has to engage with a wide range of inter-connecting agencies and individuals. From referral, through collaboration and finally at discharge, the quality of the relationship with other agencies profoundly affects effectiveness. This applies both to organisations external to the service, such as private landlords and the police, and to other parts of the same organisation, such as the nursing hierarchy, other therapeutic teams and support staff. These interfaces bring into play negotiation, conflict resolution and marketing skills.

It is very easy for a team that is experiencing difficulties to blame outsiders for failing to understand. When the culture is to view everything within the group as solely benign and external influences as malign, the team is becoming self-absorbed and losing sight of the task. The work of leadership is to translate this into a recognition of the exigencies of the environment in which the team operates. External organisations have to make savings, impose policies and seek explanations. They frequently fail to understand what is happening in clinical practice, and rarely communicate effectively. Leadership is about interpretation and enthusing the team to address the most significant issues, no matter how distracting they may appear. An innovative approach can take advantage of changes to improve the service.

Championship

Leadership entails publicising the purpose of the longer-term care services, demonstrating their effectiveness, acknowledging difficulties and working on them. Ensuring that members attend other teams' meetings, give advice, talk to managers and other organisations, present papers and research, and welcome students and visitors is part of a continuing offensive to raise the profile, and necessity, of rehabilitation psychiatry. Listening objectively to criticisms provides excellent information on what needs to improve. As with most leadership tasks, every member of the team can participate.

These two aspects of leadership, managing interfaces and championing the cause, recognise that leadership is a '360° operation' requiring management up and down the organisation. It relates not only to the immediate group, but also to other teams and people in management. It recognises that it is pointless blaming others for their poor communication, insensitivity or ignorance. The work involves clarifying others' expectations of the team, arguing for recognition and resources to carry out the task, explaining issues and educating.

Conclusions

Adair's practical approach argues that leadership can, and must, be learnt (Adair, 1984). It is not inborn. It is often counter-intuitive. One aspect of leadership often referred to is the ability to make decisions. However, in real life, successful leadership is assisting others to make decisions and then supporting them in carrying these out.

References

Adair, J. (1984) *The Skills of Leadership*. Aldershot: Gower Publishing.

Bass, B. M. (1998) *Transformational Leadership: Industrial, Military and Educational Impact*. Hillsdale, NJ: Lawrence Ehrlbaum.

Belbin, S. M. (1986) *Management Teams: Why They Succeed or Fail*. London: Heinemann.

Bion, W. R. (1946) The leaderless group project. *Bulletin of the Menninger Clinic*, **10**, 77–81.

Bion, W. R. (1961) *Experiences in Groups*. London: Tavistock Press.

Borrill, C. S., Carletta, J., Carter, A. J., *et al* (2000) *The Effectiveness of Healthcare Teams in the National Health Service.*, Birmingham: Aston University.

Corrigan, P. W., Lickey, S. E., Campion, J., *et al* (2000) Mental health team leadership and consumers' satisfaction and quality of life. *Psychiatric Services*, **51**, 781–785.

Garratt, S. (1985) *Manage your Time*. London: Fontana Collins.

Heifetz, R. A. & Laurie, D. L. (2001) The work of leadership. *Harvard Business Review*, Dec., 131–140.

Leete, E. (1989) How I perceive and manage my illness. *Schizophrenia Bulletin*, **15**, 197–200.

Main, T. F., (1948), Rehabilitation and the individual. In *Modern Trends in Psychological Medicine* (ed. N. G. Harris), pp. 386–411. London: Butterworth.

National Institute for Mental Health in England (2003) *Personality Disorder: No Longer a Diagnosis of Exclusion*. London: Department of Health.

Onyett, S. (1999) Community mental health team working as a socially valued enterprise. *Journal of Mental Health*, **8**, 245–251.

Onyett, S. (2003) *Teamworking in Mental Health*. Basingstoke: Palgrave Macmillan.

Øvretveit, J. (2000) *Co-ordinating Community Care: Multidisciplinary Teams and Care Management*. Milton Keynes: Open University Press.

Reynolds, A. & Thornicroft, G. (1999) *Managing Mental Health Services*. Milton Keynes: Open University Press.

Turquet, P. (1974) Leadership: the individual and the group. In *Analysis of Groups* (eds G.S. Gibbard, J. Hartman & R. D. Mann), pp. 77–87. San Francisco, CA: Josey Bass.

CHAPTER 22

Evaluation of rehabilitation services

Peter Tyrer

The services involved with the care of people with chronic mental illness constitute one of the most complex interventions in medicine. This statement is in danger of being interpreted in another way: 'it is so difficult to evaluate services that there is no point in starting'. I hope to show that this is an inaccurate viewpoint and that, with relatively few resources, it is possible to evaluate rehabilitation services in psychiatry.

What are we evaluating?

This is not self-evident because there are so many different outcomes in mental health. One of the simplest definitions of a successful service is that those 'who receive it recover and do so more rapidly than without it' (World Health Organization, 1991). However, a complication arises when we define the word 'recover' (Table 22.1).

Table 22.1 Possible meanings of the word 'recovery' in chronic mental illness

Measurement	Relevance to recovery
Loss of symptoms	Symptoms are the main 'stuff' of psychiatric illness and if a patient gets better symptoms should improve or disappear
Social functioning and disability	Recovery may be better measured by success in day-to-day living than any other single measure
Quality of life	This is currently the most popular outcome measure for those who are interested in patient-based outcome
Use of hospital services	This is the most important measure for those who plan psychiatric services, as hospital beds are the most-expensive form of mental healthcare. Care in the community is much more cost-effective than repeated readmission

Evaluation of complex interventions

The Medical Research Council has recently summarised the stages of evaluation necessary for a complex intervention (defined as two or more components and their consequent interactions). There are five stages in this evaluation (Fig. 22.1) and all should be considered at some time, but not necessarily in exactly the same order. It is also possible to complete more than one pathway through the evaluation process, depending on the initial results. It is useful to examine each of these stages with regard to rehabilitation and mental health services.

Phase 0 – pre-clinical: theoretical model

Although much of health services research is based on empirical findings and the introduction of new services according to political will and policy rather than theory, the theoretical aspects should never be ignored.

When any new medical service or treatment is being introduced the standard question posed by the general public is 'Does it work?' Unless there is some theoretical basis to the service intervention this question cannot be answered.

Without some form of theoretical basis for the intervention the eight different aims of rehabilitation listed in Table 22.2 can be confused. Sometimes a blunderbuss approach to the measurement of outcome is adopted, which includes measures that address each of these eight aims and often many more. When this number approaches 20 the chances are

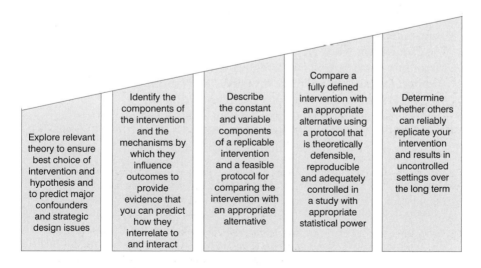

Fig. 22.1 The five phases of a complex intervention. After Campbell *et al* (2000), with permission.

Table 22.2 Possible aims of rehabilitation

Aim	Measure of success
To prolong life	Reduction in mortality
To save money	Patients moved from expensive to less-expensive residential facility
To promote independence	Reduction in the number of people involved in care
To satisfy needs	Greater proportion of needs met after treatment
To improve quality of life	Improvement in quality of life measured by various measures
To reduce burden on others	Reduction in burden on carers and other relevant people
To improve social function	Improvement in general functioning
To improve patient satisfaction	Improvement in general satisfaction

that one will show significant evidence of improvement by chance. There is then a danger that the investigators convince themselves that this is the one measure that they were aiming to improve above all others and therefore that the intervention is an outstanding success. There can often be considerable tension between theory and practice in rehabilitation services. This could happen more readily when the aims of the service deviate from those of the individual patient.

This conflict can be avoided if it is clear in advance what the purpose of the rehabilitation programme is and the type of people more likely to benefit from it. If a programme is set up to promote greater autonomy and independence, then some measure of this needs to be obtained before selecting those who enter the programme. This is very important because a poor mix of participants with respect to this aim will only promote further conflict and dissent and make the operation of the intervention much more difficult than if a homogeneous group was included.

The reason why the theoretical model is usually posed first in evaluating complex interventions is that such a model provides the principles and philosophy of the intervention. It can therefore be called upon to give guidance if difficulties emerge in the administration of an intervention.

As a starting point it is important to try to equate the aims of those requiring rehabilitation with those of the healthy population. A good theoretical model for a healthy population with regard to any form of service intervention is the Jeffersonian aim of 'life, liberty and the pursuit of happiness' in the American Constitution. All services for mental health, whatever their nature, erode some of these principles at times; the task of a good service is to erode them the least for the setting of a good theoretical model.

Phase I – modelling

Many years ago Austin Bradford Hill, the originator of the randomised controlled trial, described such trials as excellent for answering 'a precisely framed question' (Hill, 1962). This is now sometimes forgotten by those who regard the randomised controlled trial as the only form of evaluation that really matters. If the wrong question is being asked, or it is not sufficiently precise, results would be obtained that are misleading.

The main purpose of the modelling phase of a complex intervention is to identify the important components of an intervention and to determine how they interact with each other to yield apparent success. Currently the most-favoured approach for this phase is qualitative analysis. Although it has been criticised, there is little doubt that in health services research there needs to be a careful observational element preceding any controlled investigation (Black, 1996) and without it treatments can become ossified. For example, the 12-step method for the treatment of alcoholism remains a standard approach for intervention but needs to be updated in the light of modern developments and societal changes (Quinn *et al*, 2004). It is likely that not all 12 steps are needed for success of the approach, but such is the dogma and evangelistic fervour surrounding the treatment that adequate studies to probe the interactions between these elements are almost impossible to carry out.

Qualitative analysis is currently the best systematic method of finding out the key elements that are relevant in an intervention and which elements are irrelevant or dependent on others. The investigator should enquire in depth, preferably with relatively few people (usually up to 20), in an open and unbiased manner using methodology that allows as much information to be collected as possible. Information should be separated into chunks that can then be subsequently identified (Rutter, 2006). If the same chunks repeatedly achieve prominence in all the assessments, they are likely to be important and may represent the important constituent of the intervention.

More than one qualitative study may be necessary and further enquiries, including naturalistic cohort studies (i.e. following up a group of people with common characteristics), can help to determine which are the important variables to influence with regard to intervention. Thus if it is established that one outcome (e.g. a symptom such as depression) shows great variation over time but another, such as social function, shows greater stability and is more closely associated with other outcomes, then social function may be regarded as the most-relevant primary outcome in a subsequent controlled study.

Phase II – exploratory trial

The next phase follows naturally from the modelling phase. Once a reasonable guess about the essential parts of the intervention, its duration and time course has been made, the experimental treatment has to be compared with a standard treatment under controlled conditions. This trial is exploratory as it is not known how powerful the effects of the treatment are likely to be (there is always a tendency to overestimate this), how much variability there is likely to be in its effects, and whether it will prove acceptable to patients.

In complex interventions such as those for rehabilitation there is sometimes a tendency to regard the exploratory trial as definitive. When so much effort goes into an evaluation it seems to be devalued by the term 'exploratory', but unfortunately this is the correct word. Time after time exploratory trials demonstrate positive results which are not reproduced when larger studies are performed. The main purposes of the exploratory trial are to set the scene for the larger trial by: (a) determining the 'effect size' of the intervention (the amount it differs from the control treatment allowing for statistical variation) and thereby allowing a power calculation to be made that will determine the sample size of a larger study; (b) determining whether the intervention is feasible in practice (the best way of testing feasibility is to run a small trial); and (c) testing the viability of the control intervention as a comparator.

Other controlled investigations come into this category, including non-randomised controlled trials and quasi-experimental trials in which true randomisation is compromised in some way (Knudsen & Thornicroft, 1996). The more open and transparent these are, the greater will be their value. A new set of guidelines (TREND (Transparent Reporting of Evaluations with Nonrandomized Designs)) has recently been formulated to help this process (Des Jarlais *et al*, 2004).

Phase III – definitive randomised trial

This phase is unfortunately seldom reached in complex interventions in mental health. This is because of the relative expense of definitive randomised trials and their need for considerable resources (most such trials cost around £1 million), their difficulty in execution, and, a less forgivable problem, complacency. Too many people have regarded the exploratory trial as definitive and extrapolate from the findings prematurely.

The reason why this is unwise is because in health services research the small randomised trial, provided that its results are positive, is usually the peak of the intervention's success. Reasons for the differences are summarised in Table 22.3; if these are accepted as valid it would clearly be inappropriate to stop testing an intervention at the phase of the exploratory trial.

Phase IV – long-term implementation

This phase is clearly necessary but not normally within the power of the original research team. However, it is still important to note as without

Table 22.3 Reasons why large (usually multicentre) trials almost invariably show smaller effect sizes than smaller exploratory trials

Small trial (phase 2)	Large definitive trial (phase 3)
Usually promoted and analysed by 'product champions' and therefore prone to bias	Usually analysed independently, preferably by staff who have no involvement with the success or failure of the intervention concerned
Assessments made by staff who are rarely masked adequately with regard to the nature of the intervention	Assessments usually made by independent researchers who have no vested interests in the outcome of the study
Trial enthusiasts ensure that take-up of treatment is maximal	Greater percentage of missing data and drop-out than in small trials and this reduces effect of intervention
Secondary outcomes often converted to primary outcomes if they show significant experimental/control differences	Primary and secondary outcomes usually decided in advance and often published in baseline protocol paper
Intervention given by enthusiasts (often the creators of the treatment) and this degree of expertise cannot be generalised	Intervention given by trained staff who are more likely to be representative of the personnel giving the treatment in practice and therefore results more realistic

it there may be unfortunate delays in the widespread use of effective treatments. An example of such delay is the introduction of lithium for the treatment of bipolar illness by Cade (1949) some 20 years before its efficacy was widely appreciated fully. In contrast, the negative value of debriefing for traumatic stress was reported some 40 years after its recommendation as a therapy (Harrison & Worlock, 1996).

It is also common for phase 3 of evaluation to be missed out if treatments are accepted too readily. Thus insulin coma therapy was widely adopted as a treatment for schizophrenia over two decades without any real evidence of its value until a randomised trial showed that the insulin was irrelevant to its success (Ackner & Oldham, 1962). Evidence of widespread use of a treatment is not necessarily evidence of its efficacy.

Other forms of evaluation

Audit

Audit is the poor man's research methodology. As such it is often undervalued by experienced research workers who are used to working with good resources and no time pressures. However, audit is the best way of ensuring that the benefits of advances in research are not only disseminated into clinical practice but are also maintained. Audit may also be the first stage of useful evaluation. Conventionally, audit cannot be carried out successfully unless there are clear agreed standards in place. Thus, for example, if it is considered necessary for all patients in a rehabilitation setting to have at least one annual review linked to a care programme meeting, then it is relatively easy to carry out an audit of such reviews and to determine the proportion of patients qualifying for the standard. If only 85% qualify, then action needs to be taken to change this and the audit rerun at a later date until the audit cycle is completed when 100% (or very close to 100%) have had their reviews completed in the allotted time.

However, even in the early stages of evaluation audit can be helpful. For example, one of the most important elements of service evaluation is the measurement of satisfaction with services. This may often be regarded as merely a politically correct way of assessing user views, but it probably represents a good proxy measure of quality of care (Shipley *et al*, 2000). In early simple studies it is still important to measure the views of as many respondents as possible. An audit of opinions in which only one in five respond is really of very little use, as the sample size cannot be regarded as representative. There will always be some missing data and it is increasingly recognised that methods of compensating for this are desirable (Everitt, 1995).

Patient preference

Although randomised trials provide the best evidence of efficacy in the comparison of new drugs, patient preference can be important for many psychosocial treatments or when drugs and other treatments are compared. In a consumer society the issue of patient preference with respect to treatment is coming more to the fore. This is particularly true in community settings. One common example is the prescription of antipsychotic drugs in schizophrenia. Although the evidence for the efficacy of these drugs in schizophrenia is overwhelming, there is still a significant minority of people who prefer other forms of treatment, particularly 'alternative therapies' of unproven and doubtful value. In my personal experience the strong personal belief of such patients that these treatments are the only valid ones does have an influence on response to treatment which goes far beyond the simple placebo effect for the preferred treatment and the nocebo effect of the rejected one (Tyrer, 1991).

There is also the possibility that there are important interactions between an individual's preferences and the effects of treatment that are not detected in the standard randomised controlled trial. If these are important the results of the randomised controlled trial may be wrongly attributed to the specific content of the intervention alone (McPherson *et al*, 1997). As a consequence of this there is increasing interest in non-experimental methods in the assessment of efficacy of treatments (Wennberg, 1988) and in different research designs that take account of patients' (or indeed, other people's such as clinicians') preferences. Brewin & Bradley (1989) proposed a partially randomised patient-centred design for the evaluation of psychosocial treatments in which patients who had strong preferences for a particular treatment were allocated to it and those who had no particular preference were randomly allocated in the usual way. The problem with this approach is that in breaks one of the fundamental principles of the randomised controlled trial: ensuring equivalent populations for all factors apart from the treatments under consideration. If, as has been observed, patients who have strong preferences differ from others in their level of education and other potentially important factors (Feine *et al*, 1998), then their results cannot be compared satisfactorily with others. Nevertheless, in practice the differences between patient preference and fully randomised allocation are less than many have predicted (Ward *et al*, 2000).

Special problems in the evaluation of rehabilitation in mental illness

Rehabilitation is a complex intervention spread over a long time period. It offers many different interventions and when one considers that four different interventions offer the possibility of 24 potentially different treatments (taking into account each possible interaction as a new intervention), it is not surprising that few definitive trials have been carried out.

Example of a rehabilitation service evaluation in practice

To examine the difficulties inherent in the evaluation of rehabilitation I will take one example: day hospital therapeutic community treatment for those with personality disorders, a subject that has been mainly studied in Norway, a country with a relatively small population and considerable distance between major centres.

The Norwegian group under the leadership of Per Vaglum was one of the first to attempt to evaluate day hospital therapeutic community treatment. In one of their early papers (Karterud *et al*, 1992) they examined the short-term outcome (6 months) of 97 consecutive patients, 50 of whom had a DSM diagnosis of Cluster A and B personality disorders. The drop-out rate for people with schizotypal and borderline personality disorder was 38%, but less for others. There was a reduction in drug treatment, with 58% of people being drug-free at the time of discharge. There were no suicides during the observational phase.

This information constitutes a low level of evidence at phase 1 of our evaluation hierarchy. There was already a reasonable theoretical model for therapeutic community treatment at day hospitals based on earlier work, but this study, which used a simple cohort design and observational measures, indicated several positive aspects of the intervention. First, it does not seem to have harmed the patients; second, it was largely successful in keeping patients in treatment and, as people with personality often adhere poorly to therapy, this may be a clear advantage; and third, it seems to be associated with a reduction in drug therapy.

The problem is that the study had no control group and we do not know whether the positive results represent part of the natural history of the conditions being treated or whether they are a consequence of the intervention. It is very difficult to obtain good control populations when studying therapeutic communities and hence other attempts have been made to demonstrate their value. These have included showing a favourable change in pathology or cost-offset for those treated at therapeutic communities compared with those who have not had specific treatment (Dolan *et al*, 1996, 1997). However, unless those in the therapeutic community can be regarded as exactly comparable to those who were not (i.e. they were randomised) such comparisons can be invidious and misleading. There is also potential bias because a group reporting findings from its own service might be expected to favour their own treatment.

Bias may not be present but it should be presumed to be. Thus, although there were no suicides reported in the study described (Karterud *et al*, 1992), if two patients had died by suicide just after the period of observation, would they have been reported? From my personal knowledge of this Norwegian group I think they probably would have been, but it is easy to see how such information could be suppressed.

Subsequent studies

In subsequent studies (Wilberg *et al*, 1998*a,b*) further attempts were made to determine the factors influencing the efficacy of the specialised day hospital service for personality disorders. Those without personality disorder, or with Cluster C personality disorders only, were found to have a better outcome, and overall there was reasonable improvement in the group. Hence the service was concluded to be 'promising as a first step towards development of a cost-efficient program for patients with severe personality disorder' (Wilberg *et al*, 1998*b*).

However, although this is a common way of evaluating a rehabilitation programme, the conclusion about cost-effectiveness is premature. This is because all the reported studies to date have made no attempt to compare the components of the intervention (a combination of analytically oriented and cognitive–behavioural group therapy) or to manipulate them in any way. This type of evaluation, commonly described as naturalistic, is much more comfortable for clinicians and researchers, but does not progress beyond phase 1 of our evaluation hierarchy.

When the intervention was compared in a three-site study of three similar programmes, two in England and the original in Ullevål, Norway, a very important difference was found: the severity of pathology was significantly less in the Norwegian patients (Chiesa *et al*, 2002). This is important because without further comparisons of interventions we would be left with only naturalistic pre–post comparisons in which, for a population with mild pathology only, reasonable outcome may have been achieved with much less input and at lower cost.

It is therefore good to report that phase 2 of the complex intervention pathway, an exploratory controlled trial, has recently started in Ullevål, in which the day hospital programme is being compared with specialised out-patient care in a randomised trial (Wilberg *et al*, 2004). There is still the possibility that this will not yield convincing evidence of efficacy as the two programmes may have similar outcomes. This could either mean that both are effective or both ineffective. Only the inclusion of a control minimal treatment intervention could help to decide which was the case.

What is troubling is that after many years of operating a service that all involved would like to believe is effective the possibility remains that it may not be of special value. It therefore takes a certain amount of courage to mount a randomised controlled trial when the outcome is uncertain and even greater courage to allow independent assessors to carry out such a study.

For this reason it is probably wise to move from phase 1 to phases 2 and 3 early rather than late, so that there is less chance for rigidity to influence the therapeutic system. This also encourages others to replicate your work and possibly adopt the intervention. For example, the day hospital programme developed for personality disorders by Bateman & Fonagy (1999) is now being implemented in many other centres because of the positive results of a randomised trial, both in the medium and longer term (Bateman & Fonagy, 1999, 2001). The results of this trial also served to define the treatment more clearly (Bateman & Fonagy, 2004).

Nidotherapy is a new treatment which has been recently introduced into rehabilitation practice and involves the systematic modification of the environment for those with chronic mental illness and/or personality disorder (Tyrer, 2002; Tyrer *et al*, 2003; Tyrer & Bajaj, 2004). Nidotherapy is already being tested in an exploratory trial in phase 2, since without positive feedback from evidence it may not be worthwhile developing it further.

Summary

The seven stages of evaluation of a rehabilitation service are summarised in Table 22.4. It is unlikely that any service will be able to complete all seven. The best example in mental health practice is that of assertive community treatment, which was started in Wisconsin in 1974 and is now adopted in almost all countries worldwide (Stein & Santos, 1998). However, even if only some stages of evaluation are completed, and in the case of specialised services for small numbers (e.g. brain injury services) this will almost always be the case, the exercise is still worthwhile. It should also be

Table 22.4 Recommended stages of evaluation in a rehabilitation service

Stage of evaluation	Tasks to be completed
1. Feasibility and acceptability	Simple audit studies
2. Enquiry	Qualitative and observational studies
3. Outcome	Follow-up of cohorts
4. Intervention dissection	Exploratory trials (case–control and randomised)
5. Confirmation of efficacy in practice	Large randomised controlled trial
6. Audit of standards	Constant monitoring
7. International dissemination	Policy and promotion

remembered that successful rehabilitation is dependent on local context, not just on general principles, and for this reason patient-based evidence can sometimes be regarded as more influential than evidence-based practice in planning for an individual patient.

References

Ackner, B. & Oldham, A. J. (1962) Insulin treatment of schizophrenia 320 – a three-year follow-up of a controlled study. *Lancet*, i, 504–506.

Bateman, A. & Fonagy, P. (1999) Effectiveness of partial hospitalization in the treatment of borderline personality disorder: a randomized controlled trial. *American Journal of Psychiatry*, **156**, 1563–1569.

Bateman, A. W. & Fonagy, P. (2001) Treatment of borderline personality disorder with psychoanalytically oriented partial hospitalisation: an 18-month follow-up. *American Journal of Psychiatry*, **158**, 36–42.

Bateman, A. W. & Fonagy, P. (2004) Mentalisation-based treatment of BPD. *Journal of Personality Disorders*, **18**, 36–51.

Black, N. (1996) Why we need observational studies to evaluate the effectiveness of health care. *BMJ*, **312**, 1215–1218.

Brewin, C. R. & Bradley, C. (1989) Patient preferences and randomised clinical trials. *BMJ*, **299**, 313–315.

Cade, J. F. J. (1949) Lithium salts in the treatment of psychotic excitement. *Medical Journal of Australia*, **2**, 349–352.

Campbell, M., Fitzpatrick, R., Haines, A., et al (2000) A framework for the design and evaluation of complex interventions to improve health. *BMJ*, **321**, 694–696.

Chiesa, M., Bateman, A., Wilberg, T., et al (2002) Patients' characteristics, outcome and cost–benefit of hospital-based treatment for patients with personality disorder: a comparison of three different programmes. *Psychology and Psychotherapy – Theory Research and Practice*, **75**, 381–392.

Des Jarlais, D. C., Lyles, C., Crepaz, N., et al (2004). Improving the reporting quality of nonrandomized evaluations of behavioral and public health interventions: the TREND statement. *American Journal of Public Health*, **94**, 361–366.

Dolan, B. M., Warren, F. M., Menzies, D., et al (1996) Cost-offset following specialist treatment of severe personality disorders. *Psychiatric Bulletin*, **20**, 413–417.

Dolan, B., Warren, F. & Norton, K. (1997) Change in borderline symptoms one year after therapeutic community treatment for severe personality disorder. *British Journal of Psychiatry*, **171**, 274–279.

Everitt, B. S. (1995) The analysis of repeated measures: a practical review with examples. *Statistician*, **44**, 113–135.

Feine, J. S., Awad, M. A. & Lund, J. P. (1998) The impact of patient preference on the design and interpretation of clinical trials. *Community Dental and Oral Epidemiology*, **26**, 70–74.

Harrison, B. & Worlock, P. (1996) A randomised controlled trial of psychological debriefing for victims of road traffic accidents. *BMJ*, **313**, 1438–1439.

Hill, A. B. (1962) The statistician in medicine. *Journal of the Institute of Actuaries*, **88**, 178–191.

Karterud, S., Vaglum, S., Friis, S., *et al* (1992) Day hospital therapeutic-community treatment for patients with personality-disorders – an empirical evaluation of the containment function. *Journal of Nervous and Mental Disease*, **180**, 238–243.

Knudsen, H. C. & Thornicroft, G. (eds) (1996) *Mental Health Service Evaluation*. Cambridge: Cambridge University Press.

McPherson, K., Britton, A. R. & Wennberg, J. E. (1997) Are randomized controlled trials controlled? Patient preferences and unblind trials. *Journal of the Royal Society of Medicine*, **90**, 652–656.

Quinn, J. F., Bodenhamer-Davis, E. & Koch, D. S. (2004) Ideology and the stagnation of AODA treatment modalities in America. *Deviant Behavior*, 25, 109–131.

Rutter, D. (2006) The use of qualitative research methods in psychiatry. In: *Research Methods in Psychiatry: A Beginner's Guide* (3rd edn) (eds C. Freeman & P. Tyrer). London: Gaskell.

Shipley, K., Hilborn, B., Hansell, A. *et al* (2000) Patient satisfaction: a valid index of quality of care in a psychiatric service. *Acta Psychiatrica Scandinavica*, **101**, 330–333.

Stein, L. I. & Santos, A. B. (1998) *Assertive Community Treatment of Persons with Severe Mental Illness*. London/New York: Norton.

Tyrer, P. (1991) The nocebo effect – poorly known but getting stronger. In *Side Effects of Drugs Annual 15* (eds M. N. G. Dukes & J. K. Aronson), pp. 19–25. Amsterdam: Elsevier.

Tyrer, P. (2002) Nidotherapy: a new approach to the treatment of personality disorder. *Acta Psychiatrica Scandinavica*, **105**, 469–471.

Tyrer, P. & Bajaj, P. (2004) Nidotherapy: making the environment do the therapeutic work. *Advances in Psychiatric Treatment*, 11, 232–238.

Tyrer, P., Sensky, T. & Mitchard, S. (2003) The principles of nidotherapy in the treatment of persistent mental and personality disorders. *Psychotherapy and Psychosomatics*, **72**, 350–356.

Ward, E., King, M., Lloyd, M., *et al* (2000) Randomised controlled trial of non-directive counselling, cognitive-behaviour therapy, and usual general practitioner care for patients with depression. I: Clinical effectiveness. *BMJ*, **321**, 1383–1388.

Wennberg, J. E. (1988) Non-experimental methods in the assessment of efficacy. *Medical Decision Making*, **8**, 175–176.

Wilberg, T., Friis, S., Karterud, S., *et al* (1998*a*) Patterns of short-term course in patients treated in a day unit for personality disorders. *Comprehensive Psychiatry*, **39**, 75–84.

Wilberg, T., Karterud, S., Urnes, O., *et al* (1998*b*) Outcomes of poorly functioning patients with personality disorders in a day treatment program. *Psychiatric Services*, **49**, 462–1467.

Wilberg, W., Karterud, S., Pedersen, G., *et al* (2004) Short-term day hospital treatment and outpatient continuation treatment for patients with personality disorders. *Proceedings of the Vth European Congress of the International Society for the Study of Personality Disorders*. Zaragoza: ISSPD.

World Health Organization (1991) *Evaluation of Methods for the Treatment of Mental Disorders* (WHO Technical Report Series no. 812). Geneva: World Health Organization.

Part 4

Special considerations

CHAPTER 23

Acquired brain injury

Matthew Allin and Simon Fleminger

Many patients in psychiatric rehabilitation settings will have suffered a brain injury. Indeed one or two neuropsychiatric brain injury units in the UK were originally set up because it was evident that a significant minority of long-stay patients in mental health hospitals had suffered brain damage of one sort or other. Those patients who have had both a mental illness, such as schizophrenia, and overt brain injury are particularly likely to develop chronic disability and therefore come to the attention of psychiatric rehabilitation services. The assessment of these patients is complicated by the fact that the symptoms of brain injury may overlap with those of chronic severe mental illness; general psychiatrists need to be aware of the potential confusion.

The methods used in brain injury rehabilitation to manage cognitive and behavioural symptoms will be of interest to psychiatric rehabilitation services looking after patients with different diagnoses but with similar problems.

In this chapter we survey the neuropsychiatric sequelae of acquired brain injury and the rehabilitation principles and practices at different stages. The common causes of brain injury include trauma (as a result of road traffic accidents, assaults and falls), anoxia or hypoglycaemia, subarachnoid haemorrhage, alcohol, encephalitis and meningitis (Teasdale, 1995). Cognitive impairments in the domains of memory and executive function tend to dominate. Behavioural and psychiatric symptoms are common and tend to be more disabling than neurophysical problems; patients may have quite severe cognitive and behavioural problems and yet be fully mobile.

Understanding disability following acquired brain injury

The International Classification of Impairment, Disability and Handicap (ICIDH; World Health Organization, 1980) is a useful model for considering how rehabilitation may improve quality of life after a brain injury (see Box 23.1).

Box 23.1 International Classification of Impairment, Disability and Handicap (ICIDH)

- Impairments – measurable limitations in function as a direct consequence of damage; e.g. the limited power or reduced speed of movement of a limb following a stroke or memory impairment seen after temporal lobe damage.
- Disability – consequence of impairment on ability to function, particularly in activities of daily living in everyday life. The Barthel Disability Scale (Mahoney & Barthel, 1965) rates ability to perform simple tasks, e.g. putting an electric plug into a socket or brushing teeth. Measures of disability owing to cognitive or memory impairment would look at the ability to plan and carry out a shopping task or evidence of a need for help in remembering and getting to appointments.
- Handicap – consequences of the injury on the ability to engage in activities and return to their normal social role. Thus left hemiplegia will have a much greater effects on the handicap of a violinist than a sports commentator.

Physical impairments may be improved by rehabilitation such as physiotherapy, but it is generally accepted that the ability of cognitive rehabilitation to improve cognitive impairment is very limited. For example, memory exercises probably do not improve memory. However, cognitive rehabilitation can improve disability. This often involves enabling the person to use alternative strategies or aids to get around what may be a fairly fixed impairment. Thus memory rehabilitation will concentrate on enabling the person to use memory aids, such as a palm organiser, 'Post It' notes and an alarm watch to prompt them to perform certain activities, such as taking their medication.

Rehabilitation targeted at handicap should look at ways of improving access to the community to engage in social activities or to overcome hurdles in the way of return to work. As a general rule, interventions early after injury tend to address impairments and disability, whereas later interventions tend to concentrate on disability and handicap.

There have been moves recently to change the names from impairment, disability and handicap to impairment, activity and participation to reflect a more-positive approach to rehabilitation.

Understanding the injury

Planning rehabilitation for somebody who has suffered an acquired brain injury depends heavily on a proper understanding of the nature and severity of the injury. For non-focal injuries, the depth of unconsciousness, measured using the Glasgow Coma Scale (GCS; 3 = completely unresponsive coma, 15 = normal conscious level, <9 = unconscious; Teasdale & Jennett, 1974), duration of unconsciousness, and duration of post-traumatic amnesia are used to predict the severity of brain injury. The duration of post-traumatic amnesia is the period from the brain injury until there is return of continuous day-to-day memory and is the best predictor of prognosis. The advantage of using post-traumatic amnesia as a measure of the severity of brain injury is that it can usually be measured fairly accurately retrospectively, by asking the patient what he remembers of the immediate aftermath of the injury. As a rule of thumb those with amnesia of less than 1 week will usually do reasonably well, whereas those in which it lasts longer than a month are unlikely to return to work (Bishara *et al*, 1992). Although symptoms after even a mild head injury, defined as a GCS of 13–15 and loss of consciousness for no more than a few minutes, may last several weeks or months, most people with a mild head injury will have fully recovered by 3 months post-injury.

In a closed head injury definite neurological sequelae, indicating focal damage, suggest significant generalised brain injury. Closed head injury results in two intracerebral processes: localised contusions and diffuse axonal injury. The latter produces damage in the white matter which may be manifested by small haemorrhages.

Contusions often occur at the bone–brain interface, particularly in medial orbitofrontal and anterior temporal regions (see Fig. 23.1). Damage in these areas probably explains why problems with social interactions, behaviour, executive function and memory are particularly troublesome after brain injury.

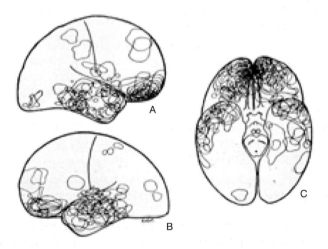

Fig. 23.1 A composite of the contusions from 50 people who died as a result of head injury. Reproduced with permission from Courville, C. B. (1945) *Pathology of the Central Nervous System.* Mountain View, CA: Pacific Press.

Magnetic resonance imaging (MRI) is the preferred investigation to identify these changes. It is generally more sensitive than computed tomography, especially at the bone–brain interface where computed tomographic scans tend to produce artefacts. The most-sensitive imaging for diffuse axonal injury is a combination of a fluid-attenuated inversion recovery (FLAIR) MRI sequence, which is sensitive to white matter damage, alongside gradient echo sequences, which are good at identifying old haemorrhages. However, the extent of the brain injury visible on structural brain imaging may not be a good predictor of the amount of damage present; for example, profound dementia may be seen after anoxic brain injury in somebody with almost no evidence of brain atrophy on computed tomography or MRI.

Mental illness as a predisposing factor

Those who have a mental illness antedating their brain injury are particularly likely to develop subsequent behavioural and other neuropsychiatric problems. One factor is the person's constitutional vulnerability. Another factor is that some individuals suffer their brain injury as a result of deliberate self-harm and it is probably particularly difficult for a person to adjust to their disability when it is self-inflicted. Alcohol and substance misuse are strongly associated with risk of brain injury, and are likely to complicate any post-injury rehabilitation (Neiman, 1998). In patients with schizophrenia it is likely that the cognitive impairments associated with brain injury aggravate negative schizophrenic symptoms. Patients with antisocial personality disorder are at risk of head injury through assault and risk-taking behaviour, and are also more likely to demonstrate aggressive behaviour post-injury. A prior head injury, particularly if accompanied by behavioural disinhibition or cognitive impairment, makes a further head injury more likely (Teasdale & Engberg, 1997).

Outcome after acquired brain injury

Neuropsychological impairment

Cognitive impairments associated with acquired brain injury improve rapidly over the first year after injury, but after 2 years improvements in disability and handicap will usually be the result of the employment of more-effective coping strategies. Non-specific impairments such as slowness and reduced concentration are commonly reported after brain injury. Assessment of neuropsychological functioning may be done at the bedside using the Mini-Mental State Examination (Folstein *et al*, 1975), perhaps supplemented by the Frontal Assessment Battery (Dubois *et al*, 2000). Such tests are useful as a baseline assessment and for subsequently monitoring progress. For many patients a full neuropsychological assessment will also be required. However, it is important to remember that it is possible for a person to score in the normal range on many neuropsychological tests after a brain injury yet be quite disabled by cognitive impairment, particularly of memory and executive function.

Deficits of executive function

Frontal lobe damage, particularly to the medial orbitofrontal cortex, gives rise to a loss of the normal abilities to plan, schedule, monitor and inhibit activity, and tends to lead to rigid 'concrete' patterns of thinking and behaviour. Such a 'dysexecutive syndrome' can result in significant disability which tends to be more evident in everyday life than in the structured setting of hospital care or a residential unit (Shallice & Burgess, 1991). The patient's disability may not be evident on standard neuropsychological testing because they tend to do better with structured tasks with clear instructions. Patients with a dysexecutive syndrome often lack insight and may not cooperate with rehabilitation.

Memory

This is the most-common neuropsychological impairment after brain injury. The enduring difficulty with new leaning is known as anterograde amnesia. In most patients damage to several areas combines to produce the impairment. Frontal lobe injury may be implicated – as it affects the 'executive' processes that are responsible for accessing memories. Implicit (including procedural) memory for example, motor skills such as the ability to ride a bike – is usually preserved.

Communication

Brain injury tends to produce difficulties in higher level communication – for example, understanding metaphor or sarcasm – and difficulties complying with conversational rules, such as turn-taking. Although not easy to identify, such problems may have significant effects on relationships and probably contribute to the problems experienced by people with brain injury in maintaining a good social network. Difficulties in finding words are also very common.

Personality change

Personality change after brain injury can be catastrophic – resulting in marital breakdown, loss of employment and social isolation. Magnetic resonance imaging may reveal associated brain lesions. For example, lesions of the lateral frontal cortex (also known as the 'convexity') are associated with impairment of drive, whereas orbitofrontal lesions are associated with disordered social behaviour. After brain injury pre-existing personality traits are often exacerbated. The changes in personality may include apathy and lack of motivation, impulsivity, reduced ability to tolerate frustration and inability to take decisions. Sexual disinhibition may occur – ranging in severity from inappropriate comments to sexual assault. Fortunately, although sexual disinhibition is not infrequently observed soon after injury, it often improves. Antisocial personality traits are often associated with a dysexecutive syndrome.

Confabulation and psychosis

As the patient recovers from the confusional period after brain injury, confabulation, false memories which are usually short lived, and delusions (including delusional misidentification) are not infrequently observed. Most such symptoms which occur early after injury remit spontaneously.

Later, when the acute phase of the illness has resolved, a psychosis that is clinically very similar to schizophrenia may occur, although it can be difficult to know whether or not the illness is a result of the head injury (Corcoran & Malaspina, 2001). Some people with schizophrenia go on to suffer brain injury, for example as a result of falls or suicide attempts. In these people anecdotal evidence suggests that the psychotic illness may become more treatment resistant and negative symptoms more prominent. It is noteworthy that the impairments of concentration, memory, psychomotor speed and executive function seen in patients with schizophrenia without brain injury are rather similar to those seen after acquired brain injury.

Mood disorders

Not surprisingly depression is common after brain injury – 20–40% of people experience depression in the first year and 50% at some time following the injury. However, the symptoms of depression have significant overlap with those of acquired brain injury. For example, tiredness, frustration and poor concentration, and even anhedonia, may be a direct consequence of the brain injury. In diagnosing depression after brain injury it is therefore essential to elicit depressed mood, although symptoms such as guilt and self-deprecation are also helpful. There is no good evidence that the location of the lesions can predict which people with brain injury will become depressed. Depression can exacerbate cognitive impairments (Fleminger et al, 2003).

Significant brain injury is associated with an increased risk of suicide, which has been estimated to be around three times that of the general population. Part of this excess risk may reflect pre-injury characteristics that also predispose to acquiring a brain injury. The assessment of the risk of suicide and self-harm is an essential part of the psychiatric assessment in acquired brain injury.

Mania may follow brain injury and be mistaken for the disinhibition and childlike behaviour that can occur after severe frontal lobe injury. Mania may be a cause of aggressive behaviour.

Anxiety disorders

These are common following brain injury – occurring in about 30% of patients. Anxiety symptoms develop as frequently after mild head injury as after moderate or severe injuries. Obsessive–compulsive disorder may also be seen.

Aggression

Generalised disturbance of brain function commonly gives rise to agitation and aggression in the acute period after the injury. This usually remits spontaneously. It is possible for complex partial seizures to be associated with aggression and where there is doubt about the aetiology or there are suspicious clinical features (e.g. stereotypic episodic aggression, starting instantaneously without an obvious trigger, followed by periods of increased confusion) an electroencephalogram is indicated. Early agitation may be followed by chronic aggressive behaviour, which is more likely in the presence of pre-existing antisocial behaviour. Agitation and aggression may also be associated with psychotic symptoms, such as persecutory delusions, and mood disturbance.

Management of neuropsychiatric sequelae

Management rests on an understanding of the cause of the patient's current difficulties; this needs to be set into the context of what the patient was doing before the injury, their current social supports and future prospects and ambitions (e.g. whether or not they may have a job to return to).

Medical issues need to be dealt with – it is not uncommon for there to be loose ends which need following up; for example, ensuring that a patient with anoxic brain injury as a result of a cardiac arrest has a follow-up with a cardiologist. Referral to specialist medical and neurological rehabilitation teams may be required. The psychiatrist must be vigilant on behalf of the patient to the possibility that medical problems, infection, pain, constipation, etc. may be exacerbating any psychiatric symptoms. This is particularly relevant for patients who are confused or have dementia. Prescribed drugs may have to be rationalised.

Post-traumatic epilepsy needs vigorous treatment since epilepsy contributes to behavioural problems after injury. However, there is no evidence that anticonvulsants are useful as a prophylactic measure to prevent post-traumatic epilepsy.

One can then plan cognitive, behavioural and psychiatric rehabilitation. Members of the rehabilitation team need to work together to produce concerted goal plans, guided as much as is feasible by the wishes of the patient and their family and carers. Most of the rehabilitation programmes for patients after brain injury are led by therapists, particularly occupational therapists. Psychologists play an important role both in defining the neuropsychological impairments that are present and setting up appropriate cognitive–behavioural programmes.

Neuropsychiatric input is likely to be needed for the more-complex cases, particularly if there is evidence of significant depression, psychosis, dementia or behavioural problems. The neuropsychiatrist will advise on psychotropic medication, risk management and assessment of capacity, in particular with regard to consenting to treatment. Patients with a history of psychiatric illness or whose injury is a result of self-harm should have access to a psychiatric assessment reasonably promptly.

Drug treatment

The psychiatrist should be a little less ready to prescribe medication for a psychiatric symptom in somebody recovering from a brain injury, particularly early post-injury. The patient is likely to be sensitive to the side-effects of medication and not infrequently the symptom will resolve spontaneously. Anecdotal evidence, backed up by a little empirical evidence, suggests that medication may be less effective in the presence of brain injury. Nevertheless if there are treatable psychiatric symptoms, then suitable medication should be offered following some general prescribing principles. It is sensible to start with a low dose, to increase gradually and to avoid giving more than one psychotropic at a time. It is also desirable to choose drugs that have less potential for central nervous system toxicity or side-effects (see Box 23.2).

In general, less-frequent dosing with longer-acting preparations is preferred, as this is less likely to cause withdrawal effects or addiction and to reinforce unwanted behaviours.

Agitation and aggression

Anticonvulsant therapy, with carbamazepine or sodium valproate, is often used to treat agitation and aggression. This may be helpful in about one-third of cases and has the advantage of being anti-epileptic and mood stabilising. During the early phase of recovery, benzodiazepines may be

---

Box 23.2 Potential side-effects of psychotropic medication

- Lowering seizure threshold (e.g. clozapine, chlorpromazine)
- Anticholinergic activity causing or exacerbating confusion (e.g. amitriptyline)
- Extrapyramidal side-effects (e.g. 'conventional' neuroleptics such as halo-peridol)
- Drug interactions/enzyme induction
- Cardiac effects

used, although they may increase confusion and can cause disinhibition and paradoxical agitation in people with brain injury. Benzodiazepines also have considerable potential for misuse and addiction and the reinforcement of unwanted behaviour. For this reason their longer-term use should be avoided.

Psychosis

The drug treatment of psychosis after brain injury is essentially similar to the treatment of psychosis in other clinical settings, although there is little in the way of an evidence base to guide treatment. Again it is important to take into account the vulnerability of those with brain injury to side-effects.

Mood disorders

The choice of antidepressant is essentially the same as for depression without brain injury, except that antidepressants with anticholinergic side-effects should be avoided if there is evidence of confusion. A pragmatic approach would be to start with a selective serotonin reuptake inhibitor. If a sedative antidepressant is desired, trazodone may be appropriate. The presence of brain injury may make depression more resistant to treatment.

Apathy

Apathy and lack of motivation may reflect untreated depression – in which case, antidepressant therapy may be effective. If depression has been excluded, the dopaminergic agent bromocriptine may be useful, but should not be used when psychosis is present.

Rehabilitation programmes

Most symptoms that are manifested early after brain injury improve with time, and it has not been easy to demonstrate that rehabilitation has much to offer over and above spontaneous recovery. Nevertheless there is evidence that in those with severe injury early rehabilitation results in better outcome. There is conflicting evidence as to whether those with moderate cognitive impairments do better on an in-patient rehabilitation unit or treatment at home.

Increasing activities at home

For those with mild-to-moderate impairments (e.g. somebody with a post-traumatic amnesia lasting about 1 week who is likely to be capable of looking after themselves at home within a few weeks and is likely to be able to return to some employment), rehabilitation will focus on ensuring a safe discharge home and a graded return to activities. Early symptoms are likely to include fatigue, poor concentration and memory, headaches (particularly if stressed) and dizziness or difficulties with vision. There may be musculoskeletal injuries to recover from.

The guiding principle is to offer realistic optimism, recognising that it is difficult to predict outcome early after injury. The doctor should be wary of reading too much into the results of neuropsychological tests. Some patients do far worse than predicted: presumably the tests failed to pick up their subtle but severely disabling executive problems. Other patients confound predictions of poor outcome by successfully returning to their old job despite evidence of significant cognitive impairments. Poor insight is a worrying sign; the patient often refuses all offers of help and it may only be when they fail to return to work that they are able to accept/realise that there is a problem that needs to be addressed.

Time is needed to make a good recovery. Patients may do well while at home with few demands made on them, but when challenged with employment latent impairments may become apparent. Only then may they become aware of difficulties with multitasking which slow them down at work, or find that their sensitivity to hustle and bustle has made commuting much more stressful. Anxiety is likely to increase, which may aggravate all symptoms including cognitive impairments. Clear guidance on returning to work is likely to be helpful (see Box 23.3).

Some people will require help from a vocational rehabilitation programme to return to work. A job coach may be allocated who will initially work with the person at the place of work.

Rehabilitation for patients with moderate-to-severe impairments

Many people with acquired brain injury may benefit from cognitive rehabilitation, which is usually carried out by psychologists in specialist

---

Box 23.3 Guidelines for return to work

- Agree more time off sick than you are likely to need, rather than less
- Set up a meeting between your employers and your rehabilitation team to educate your employers about your problems
- Start part-time, a few hours a day
- Try and arrange an initial period of returning to/starting work where you don't actively engage in work, e.g. shadowing a colleague
- Undertake only one job at a time
- Start with small, easily achievable tasks to gain confidence
- Carve work up into doable chunks
- Give yourself more time to complete tasks
- Plan your week so that demanding days are followed by quiet days
- Write down important information
- Monitor how much you do, and how quickly you increase your activities, against your symptoms; if symptoms such as headache or fatigue are increasing this a sign that you are doing too much
- Get regular feedback from your employer about progress

units. Cognitive rehabilitation focuses on minimising the disability and handicap that result from cognitive impairments.

Cognitive rehabilitation relies heavily on identifying clear functional targets for improving independence, e.g. for the patient to find their way to and from their local shops, or to manage the computer software that is needed at work. Guided by an understanding of the patient's cognitive impairments a programme of activities is put into place, and progress reviewed at subsequent goal-planning/review meetings. The neuropsychological assessment will not only document the severity of any impairments but will also identify unexpected cognitive strengths or weakness. Cognitive rehabilitation that relies merely on describing the disability and which does not attempt to diagnose the psychological impairments is in danger of missing the point. For example, one occasional sequel of anoxic brain injury is visual agnosia, a failure to comprehend what is being seen. This will result in numerous problems in activities of daily living and until it is recognised a lot of effort may be expended by both therapists and patient without any benefit.

Memory impairment is common after brain injury. Rehabilitation based on memory exercises does not work, but programmes based on facilitating procedural memory may have some success. For example it may be possible to help somebody learn a new route by repeatedly taking them over the route, gradually reducing the amount of support they are given until they are able to make the journey independently. Error-less learning is an important principle (Wilson & Evans, 1996) for improving learning in those with a moderate-to-severe memory impairment; errors made while learning a new task are difficult to eradicate. Electronic devices, for example pagers or personal digital aids are playing an increasing role in helping the patient with amnesia. The patient wears or carries the aid, which is programmed to bleep when a task needs to be performed. These aids increase independence not just in those with amnesia but also those with apathy.

Specialist cognitive rehabilitation is usually part of multidisciplinary goal-planning. Measurable, achievable and relevant functional goals are set and where possible are negotiated with the patient. Progress should be reviewed at regular intervals, with new goals added as necessary. Progress with achieving goals may be used as an outcome measure.

Behaviour modification

In general, implicit memory is relatively preserved after brain injury compared with explicit memory. The relative preservation of procedural memory, for example the ability to learn a new motor skill, which is one form of implicit memory, can be used to facilitate independence. This is done using behaviour modification, which involves increasing a useful behaviour and/or decreasing an unwanted behaviour (see Box 23.4).

Examples of useful behaviours include getting dressed independently or finding one's way to the local shops and back. Increasing such behaviours

> **Box 23.4** Behaviour modification
>
> Increasing a useful behaviour may be facilitated by:
> - reinforcement
> - modelling
> - repetition
>
> Reducing an unwanted behaviour is based on analysis of:
> - antecedents
> - the behaviour itself
> - consequences of the behaviour
>
> and can be achieved by:
> - differential reinforcement of other behaviour
> - 'time out on the spot'

may be facilitated by reinforcement, modelling, usually with diminishing cues, or simply repetition. Reinforcement will reward the wanted behaviour and may be done using a token economy or star chart. In modelling with diminishing cues the patient is shown what to do and then helped to build up the whole sequence of the task with numerous cues, before finally slowly reducing the number of cues needed to get them to complete the task. For example, for a preparation of a simple meal the therapist will first show what is done, then get the patient to carry out the task using a sufficient number of cues/prompts, before finally reducing the number of prompts required to enable the patient to carry out the task independently. This whole process may take many sessions over several weeks.

Sexual disinhibition is an example of an unwanted behaviour. Reducing such unwanted behaviours will involve a programme based on an assessment of the behaviour, concentrating on antecedents, the behaviour itself and the consequences of the behaviour. This analysis should help identify what triggers the behaviour and what may reinforce it, which will then be the target of the behaviour programme. It is not acceptable to help the patient reduce unwanted behaviours using any method that may be considered punitive. Extinction of unwanted behaviour must therefore be based on removal of rewards; that is, unwanted behaviour results in less reward. This behaviour modification usually runs alongside a programme of rewarding appropriate behaviour. This is known as differential reinforcement of other behaviour (DRO). A token economy or star-chart system can be used. Another technique that is commonly used in neurobehavioural units is 'time out on the spot' (TOOTS). Social interaction thought to reinforce unacceptable behaviour is removed after unwanted behaviour.

Most behaviour modification techniques demand a consistent approach across all staff, who must therefore be trained. As such they are difficult to implement anywhere except on a specialist unit.

Long-term rehabilitation

People with severe disability are likely to need lifelong supported hostel/ nursing home accommodation. Nevertheless it is important that these placements maintain a therapeutic environment. This is usually best achieved if the unit has a philosophy of long-term rehabilitation rather than simply providing care. Residents are likely to need structure to the day and an activity programme that promotes independence and minimises boredom. Many of the skills necessary for the long-term care of people with brain injury are very similar to those needed in hostels for those with chronic severe mental illness.

Planning after-care for discharge from an in-patient unit

Even people with brain injury who have no significant psychiatric illness are likely to need coordinated after-care plans similar to those of the care programme approach. Various services will usually need to work together to ensure that social, mental health and physical rehabilitation needs are met. It is useful to identify a named keyworker.

For those with mental health problems early liaison with the community mental health team (CMHT) and other services is good practice, although this can be difficult when the address to which the patient is to be discharged is only known shortly before discharge.

Not infrequently there are concerns about how the person will manage on discharge from hospital. This may be because of a history of alcohol/drug misuse, or because they have been expressing some depressive ideation, or because their safety in the home is of concern as a result of poor judgement. A risk assessment will need to address a variety of potential risks (see Box 23.5).

Box 23.5 Risk assessment

- Self-harm
- Aggression/violence to others
- Sexually inappropriate behaviour
- Wandering and getting lost
- Poor memory – fire risk, risk of leaving front door open
- Ability to self-medicate safely
- Alcohol/drug misuse
- Road safety and awareness of other dangers
- Falls
- Choking
- Vulnerability to exploitation
- Ability to manage finances and affairs
- Risk to dependents – in particular children

Outcome measurement

It is very difficult to identify one outcome measure to cover the very hetero-geneous problems that follow brain injury. Improvement of individual problems can be assessed using goal attainment measures. Various outcome measures focus on either physical disability or neurobehavioural problems. Particular scales may be needed, such as the Overt Aggression Scale (Yudofsky *et al*, 1986). The Health of the Nation Outcome Scales, adapted for patients with acquired brain injury (HoNOS-ABI; http://www.rcpsych. ac.uk/crtu/healthofthenation/acquiredbraininjury.aspx), may be a useful global outcome scale, particularly in relation to neuropsychiatric disability following brain injury.

Service provision

After-care for head injury is best delivered in the context of a multi-disciplinary team – including speech and language therapy, occupational therapy, psychology and psychiatry. There is unfortunately still a lack of services for those with brain injury and insufficient funding and provision of rehabilitation facilities.

In-patient care

In-patient units tend to deliver more-specialist programmes, with those focusing on neurophysical rehabilitation, often led by a neurological/medical rehabilitation physician, separate from units providing cognitive, behavioural and psychiatric treatment. These latter are led by psychiatrists or psychologists. However, even within these latter units there are issues because patients with cognitive impairment alone are unlikely to feel comfortable on a unit with patients with significant challenging behaviour.

Units looking after patients with cognitive–behavioural problems need to be capable of being locked and of detaining patients under the Mental Health Act 1983. A significant proportion of patients are likely to lack capacity to consent to treatment and wander off or demand to leave, yet not be safe to leave the unit; those patients that actively resist staying on the unit may need to be detained.

Community care

Community rehabilitation teams for patients with physical disability need to have psychology and occupational therapy input, so that they have the comprehensive skills to manage the range of physical and neurobehavioural impairments seen after brain injury. Nevertheless such teams usually lack the skills to deal with many of the neuropsychiatric issues that can arise, particularly if there are concerns about risk management. They therefore can benefit from establishing good working relationships with the local CMHT or neuropsychiatric service.

Voluntary sector

In the UK Headway, a charitable organisation set up by families and carers of people with a brain injury, provides much of the longer-term care and support for people with a brain injury. They provide local groups offering information and support, particularly to family and carers. Headway houses are day centres which offer much needed long-term support under the banner 'a head injury is for life'.

Social services

Longer-term care tends to be funded by social services. Every person with a severe brain injury needs a social worker allocated early in the course of their recovery to ensure that services and support are available in a timely manner. Carers/family will also need a carers' assessment. Some social workers are able to act as care managers, coordinating care, support and rehabilitation as needed.

Funding

Most healthcare for people with brain injuries in England and Wales is funded by the 'physical disability' stream of funding, which is separate from mental health funding. This split of funding streams is often not advantageous for people with brain injury who have both mental health and physical disability needs. This is particularly evident for those whose injury arose from a mental health problem such as self-harm or long-term alcohol misuse.

Mental health services

Local CMHTs do have something to offer many people who have suffered a brain injury. A Royal College of Psychiatrists Working Party (Barrett et al, 1991) recommended that every health district had a named consultant psychiatrist to act as the liaison psychiatrist for people with brain injury. However, because of the pressures on CMHTs, this ideal is rarely achieved.

Conclusions

Rehabilitation strategies for people with acquired brain injury have much in common with those for chronic severe mental illness. This common ground is underlined by the observation that many with brain injury also have psychiatric illness. Psychiatric rehabilitation teams and CMHTs have much to offer these patients.

References

Barrett, K., Fenton, G., Lishman, A., *et al* (1991) Services for brain injured adults – Report of a Working Group of the Research Committee of the Royal College of Psychiatrists, 1990. *Psychiatric Bulletin*, **15**, 513–518.

Bishara, S. N., Partridge, F. M., Godfrey, H. P., *et al* (1992) Post-traumatic amnesia and Glasgow Coma Scale related to outcome in survivors in a consecutive series of patients with severe closed-head injury. *Brain Injury*, **6**, 373–380.

Corcoran, C. & Malaspina, D. (2001) Traumatic brain injury and risk for schizophrenia. *International Journal of Mental Health*, **30**, 17–32.

Dubois, B., Slachevsky, A., Litvan, I., *et al* (2000) The FAB: a Frontal Assessment Battery at bedside. *Neurology*, **55**, 1621–1626.

Fleminger, S., Oliver, D. L., Williams, H. W., *et al* (2003) The neuropsychiatry of depression after brain injury. *Neuropsychological Rehabilitation*, **13**, 65–87.

Folstein, M. F., Folstein, S. E. & McHugh, P. R. (1975) "Mini-mental state". A practical method for grading the cognitive state of patients for the clinician. *Journal of Psychiatric Research*, **12**, 189–198.

Mahoney, F. I. & Barthel, D. (1965) Functional evaluation: the Barthel Index. *Maryland State Medical Journal*, **14**, 56–61.

Neiman, J. (1998) Alcohol as a risk factor for brain damage: neurologic aspects. *Alcoholism: Clinical and Experimental Research*, **22** (suppl. 7), 346s–351s.

Shallice, T. & Burgess, P. W. (1991) Deficits in strategy application following frontal lobe damage in man. *Brain*, **114**, 727–741.

Teasdale, G. M. (1995) Head injury. *Journal of Neurology, Neurosurgery and Psychiatry*, **58**, 526–539.

Teasdale, T. W. & Engberg, A. (1997) Duration of cognitive dysfunction after concussion and cognitive dysfunction as a risk factor: a population study of young men. *BMJ*, **315**, 569–572.

Teasdale, G. & Jennett, B. (1974) Assessment of coma and impaired consciousness. *Lancet*, **2**, 81–84.

Wilson, B. A. & Evans, J. J. (1996) Error-free learning in the rehabilitation of people with memory impairments. *Journal of Head Trauma Rehabilitation*, **11**, 54–64.

World Health Organization (1980) *International Classification of Impairments, Disabilities and Handicaps*. Geneva: World Health Organization.

Yudofsky, S. C., Silver, J. M., Jackson, W., *et al* (1986) *Overt Aggression Scale*. New York: Endicott & Williams.

CHAPTER 24

Psychiatric rehabilitation for people with learning disability

Neill Simpson

People with learning disabilities are susceptible to mental illness (NHS Health Scotland, 2004). There has recently been a great increase in published information about the detection and diagnosis of illness in people with learning disability. Most publications about mental health services for people with learning disability focus on assessment and (short-term) treatment. Less has been written about providing services for people who have enduring mental health needs in addition to developmental disabilities. Textbooks about learning disability often fail to address acquired persistent disability and those about enduring mental illness often refer to developmental disabilities only in relation to differential diagnosis.

Coexistence of developmental and acquired disabilities

Epidemiological studies in this field are difficult. There are problems in defining and measuring developmental disability, in defining, identifying and diagnosing additional psychiatric disorders, case-finding, obtaining consent for research, in addition to numerous other problems.

At present, it is not possible to compare the prevalence of mental illness in people with learning disability directly with that in the general population. The methods used in the general population are not valid for people with severe intellectual impairment, and there have been no calibration studies in the general population using methods that may have general validity. Expert consensus is that several disorders occur more frequently in association with developmental disabilities, but some may occur less frequently (Table 24.1).

Diagnostic classification systems have been designed to incorporate multiple coexisting disorders. DSM–IV treats multiple conditions as 'comorbidity' (American Psychiatric Association, 1994). ICD–10 has a multi-axial version for use in this field (World Health Organization, Division of Mental Health and Prevention of Substance Abuse, 1996). The International Classification of Functioning, Disability and Health has been

Table 24.1 Psychiatric disorders in people with learning disability

	Type of disorder	Comment
Disorders seen uncommonly in general adult psychiatry services	Tourette's syndrome Asperger syndrome Attention-deficit hyperactivity disorder/hyperkinetic disorder Epilepsy-related disorders: • recurrent delirium • complex partial seizures • non-epileptic seizures	Established before adulthood. Often associated with educational problems, even if intellect is unimpaired
Disorders seen in learning disability services more frequently than in general psychiatry	Early-onset schizophrenia (and related disorders) Anxiety disorders (including PTSD) Adjustment and stress disorders Personality disorders	May result in educational problems before adulthood, resulting in difficulty measuring intellectual function
Disorders seen in both learning disability services and general psychiatry services	Persistent affective disorders Acquired cognitive impairment (brain injury)	In the absence of rehabilitation services for acquired disorders, people with persistent disorders of any type may be referred to learning disability services
Disorders seen uncommonly in learning disability services	Alcohol and substance misuse	

PTSD, post-traumatic stress disorder.

developed to examine the social consequences of disability (formerly called 'handicap', now referred to as 'participation restriction') as a component of health. None of these systems is designed to take account of the patho-plastic effects of ageing and development. Diagnostic criteria for psychiatric disorders for use with adults with learning disabilities/mental retardation (DC–LD; Royal College of Psychiatrists, 2001) were designed to classify developmental disorders and their causes as dimensions independent of acquired disorders, and are intended for use with this population.

Variation in referral patterns to specialist services is not entirely dependent on the epidemiology. People who have persistent mental disorders are sometimes referred to learning disability services whether or not the developmental history shows that the person had intellectual impairment causing social impairment. The service model offered by general adult psychiatry services may be deemed inappropriate to the needs of a person with persistent disabilities, and a developmental history may not be available to identify the person's premorbid functioning.

Consequently, people who could benefit from a rehabilitative approach may instead be offered a service more suitable for developmental disabilities. Service users of both populations can experience difficulties with access to relevant services because of a variety of exclusion criteria, including age, personality disorder and substance misuse. The criteria for rehabilitation services include evidence of severe mental illness but should not exclude comorbid problems.

A frequent (but inappropriate) reason for referral to a learning disability service is that the person had special educational needs in childhood arising for reasons other than intellectual impairment. Examples include sensory impairments such as deafness, motor impairments such as cerebral palsy, specific cognitive impairments such as developmental dyslexia, communication problems, and emotional, behavioural or health problems affecting schooling, such as hyperkinetic disorder. It is not surprising that general practitioners, seeking any service to meet the needs of their patients, sometimes translate 'special educational need' (via 'learning difficulty') into 'learning disability'. Specialist services should not perpetuate the error, which might result in significant discrimination, by failing to assess the source of difficulty and hence to ensure an appropriate service response.

Assessment

The assessment of individuals with learning disabilities has been described elsewhere (Cooper, 2003). In summary, there should be a diagnostic assessment of the person's level of learning disability, the cause of the intellectual impairment, identification of any other developmental disorders, and identification of acquired disorders. Acquired mental and physical disorders should be diagnosed, with investigation of aetiology. Emotional and behavioural consequences of illness should be identified. There should be an assessment of risk, related to the person's behaviour and their social situation, which should include consideration of the person's vulnerability to harm from other people and severe self-neglect. These two areas of risk are often not assessed as thoroughly in general psychiatry, where the focus is more on risk of harm to others and self-harm. For learning disability and rehabilitation services self-neglect and vulnerability are often the two areas of risk that are of greatest concern. There should be an assessment of the person's decision-making capacity in the context of ensuring a safe, effective and sustainable service.

These assessments should lead to the construction of a care plan, with consideration of whether it is necessary to invoke the powers or protection of legal provision (such as the Mental Health Act 1983 or the Adults with Incapacity (Scotland) Act 2000) or other formal procedures, such as protection of vulnerable adults (POVA) guidance (available as a free download at http://www.dh.gov.uk/PolicyAndGuidance/HealthAndSocialCareTopics/SocialCare/POVA/fs/en). The multidisciplinary care plan should build on the strengths of the individual to ensure that they can live in the least-restrictive environment and maximise the quality of life, a philosophy shared by learning disability and rehabilitation services.

Standardised tools for assessment of ability are desirable but have limits to their validity. An important example is the Wechsler Adult Intelligence Scale (Wechsler, 1981), which is the standard psychometric tool for assessing intellectual function in the general population. Some of the sub-scales are timed and require cooperation and concentration. Therefore a person who is poorly motivated, easily distracted or whose responses are slow because of mental illness will score lower than their potential. The alternative approach to assessing the ability of a person with intellectual impairment is to obtain information about the person's skills and adaptive behaviour, for example by using the Vineland Adaptive Behavior Scales (Sparrow et al, 1984). If the informant does not know about the person's abilities before the onset of illness, it may be impossible to distinguish between developmental disability and disability acquired through illness.

Tools to assist the assessment of additional disorders include the mini-Psychiatric Assessment Schedule for Adults with Developmental Disabilities (Mini PAS–ADD; Prosser et al, 1998), which allows an initial assessment of psychiatric features, and the Developmental Behaviour Checklist (DBC; Einfeld & Tonge, 1995), which is designed for young people with developmental disabilities. Risk assessment tools have been devised that may be useful for some groups (such as offenders with mild learning disability), but there is insufficient research to permit any tool to be recommended.

Instruments have been devised to measure outcome. Some have a broad spectrum of relevance, such as the Health of the Nation Outcome Scale for People with Learning Disabilities (HoNOS–LD; Roy et al, 2002), whereas others have a restricted scope, such as the Aberrant Behavior Checklist (ABC; Aman et al, 1995), which is designed to be sensitive to change of hyperactive behaviour during treatment. However, none is widely used yet. There are great problems in devising scales that can be used across the whole range of heterogeneous abilities while being sensitive to change. This problem is also experienced by rehabilitation services, where there is a need to measure changes in overall quality of life rather than symptom control or the number of days spent in hospital. Alternative approaches have been proposed, such as goal attainment scaling (Ottenbacher & Cusick, 1990), which depends on service staff defining expected outcomes and deter-mining the extent to which they are achieved. Systematic evaluation of consumer satisfaction has not been undertaken yet.

Types of disability

Secondary and tertiary disability are the impaired performance that is not directly attributable to intellectual impairment or mental illness but follows from frequent consequences (such as unemployment) or reactions.

Common social consequences of learning disability and severe mental illness include dependency on a carer, unemployment, poverty, lack of roles and relationships, and experiencing the consequences of the low expectations of other people. Psychological consequences include low self-esteem, lack of identity, loneliness and boredom. In the general population, many of these issues are risk factors for mental illness, and it is assumed that they are also risk factors for people with learning disability (NHS Health Scotland, 2004).

Consequences of mental illness affect social and psychological adjustment. Frequently, families that have coped with inadequate support for a long time cease to cope when the disabled member of the family becomes ill. This is an important contributor to the problem of delayed discharge from in-patient assessment and treatment units.

Tertiary disability, the disabling consequences of the way people treat a person who has an impairment, is often observed as avoidant behaviour. A person who repeatedly experiences demands that they cannot meet will learn methods that result in avoiding those demands. A person with learning disability may turn away from an interviewer and ask a carer to give information that they are capable of giving themselves. Interviewers may find themselves interviewing the carer when the patient could answer. For people with severe learning disability, 'challenging behaviour' often has the function of avoiding demands. People served by rehabilitation services, whose disabilities are acquired as a consequence of mental illness, may also show avoidance.

Comorbidity is a frequent problem. The prevalence of autistic-spectrum disorder, personality disorder, hyperkinetic disorders and epilepsy are all inversely related to intelligence, and each of these conditions is a risk factor for depressive disorder. Autistic-spectrum disorders, which include Asperger syndrome, are a complex group of developmental disorders that often have comorbid psychiatric illness (Royal College of Psychiatrists, 2006). Barriers emerge when this group of patients leave child and adolescent services, especially if the degree of intellectual impairment is less than the eligibility criterion for learning disability services. There is often diagnostic uncertainty. Diagnosis involves a multidisciplinary assessment of cognitive, educational, social and communication abilities. Multidisciplinary teams in rehabilitation and learning disability have expertise in these areas. There is also an emerging role for early intervention teams, with the emphasis on differential diagnosis for acute psychosis and for the management of vulnerable adults in the community by home treatment/crisis services. It is not uncommon to encounter a person with two or three developmental disorders, who may also have epilepsy, who then acquires a mental illness.

It is important to realise that identifying a behaviour problem is not a substitute for diagnosis. People who have severe communication problems may have a limited means for showing distress. Challenging behaviour may represent a final common path for expression of pain or of emotional distress. The cause may be a response to a life event such as bereavement, fear of abuse, or it may be a response to a symptom of illness. For this reason, DC–LD avoids the term 'behaviour disorder', preferring 'behaviour problem'.

There are special problems concerning rehabilitation of offenders with learning disability, among whom convictions for sexual offences and fire-setting occur more frequently than in the general population.

Prognosis

There is little research on the outcome of psychiatric disorders in people with learning disability and people who have severe mental illness with complex needs. Too often, continued use of services is used as a proxy for outcome. Extended hospital admission is frequently reported but is an unsatisfactory measure of outcome. Admission to hospital depends on factors that may include the availability of carers willing to continue to provide care during an episode of illness and the availability of a hospital place. Discharge from hospital depends on the availability of community services capable of delivering a safe, effective and sustainable care plan. Hospitals that are remote from family and other carers have difficulty in testing elements of the discharge plan, and therefore the plan may have to be 'all or nothing'. There is a massive increase in expenditure on these out-of-area placements (Ryan *et al*, 2004), which have emerged because of the lack of capacity of local services to care for this group of people with complex needs.

Methods of risk assessment are poorly developed for this group. In the general population, clinical assessment incorporates self-report about intention, which is often not possible to elicit from people with learning disability. If the consequences of the identified risk are serious for others, involving violence or sexual offences, lack of information for a risk assessment often results in delayed progress.

In the absence of research, specialists believe that the outcome of severe mental illness in people with learning disability is worse than for the rest of the population. For some conditions, such as Alzheimer's disease in people with Down's syndrome, it seems that the biological processes of the disorder cause accelerated decline. For schizophrenia, poor premorbid functioning is associated with worse outcome. Anxiety disorders are largely unrecognised and untreated.

Service models

Service funding in the UK, as in the USA, is usually partitioned between services for people with mental health needs and services for people with developmental disabilities (including intellectual disability). People with both disabilities may seek care from one or the other service, but tend to encounter barriers, or even to be rejected by both. The phrase 'dual diagnosis' was introduced in the USA to draw attention to the needs of people with mental retardation who have mental illness (Stark *et al*, 1988). The largest organisation in the USA for professionals interested in the mental health of people with learning disability is the National Association for the Dually Diagnosed (NADD). The term has been criticised (Szymanski, 1988) and recently confusion has arisen because of the use of the same term to describe people with mental illness who misuse substances.

One consequence of this separation of services has been that practitioners and researchers use different language to describe phenomena that may be more similar than is apparent from the literature. An example is the use of 'self-injurious behaviour' as a subtype of 'challenging behaviour' of people with learning disability. The research on this topic makes virtually no links with the literature on 'deliberate self-harm' in people with enduring mental health needs.

Specialist services for people with learning disability in the UK have undergone radical reshaping, with closure of most long-stay hospitals. Almost all services have increased the range of options for supported housing, employment and other daytime activities. Most have also developed local specialist health services, capable of responding to complex health needs (including mental illness) that are temporary and moderate in intensity.

Specialist community-based services for people who have severe enduring mental illness and learning disability are rarely well-developed, and many services are currently experiencing problems because of the lack of capacity. The consequences include overburdened carers, exclusion from community services and delayed discharge from in-patient care.

Effective models of rehabilitation for people with learning disability and severe enduring mental illness require recognition that these individuals need support for personal development because of their developmental disability, and they need treatment of episodes of illness, prevention of recurrences and rehabilitation because of their illness. The rate of change in each area varies between individuals, and it is usually necessary to use multiple models. Some staff of learning disability and mental health services find this difficult. Some learning disability nurses and social workers have expertise in working with people with mental illness whereas others have very little. It should be borne in mind that the current training of non-medical staff specialising in learning disability includes very little about mental health.

The process of rehabilitation typically requires completion of an assessment and implementation of a care plan. The service required to deliver the care plan is then specified; a service specification will usually include the characteristics of the physical and interpersonal environment required to promote safe, effective and sustainable support (Box 24.1). 'Effective' implies that the aims of the care plan should be explicit. The psychiatric aims usually include reducing symptoms as much as possible (or to a level that the person can tolerate), minimising adverse effects of

Box 24.1 Specification of service required to deliver the care plan

Statement of service aims as they apply to the individual
- Health: physical and mental
- Emotional well-being
- Quality of life
- O'Brien's five service accomplishments:
  - community presence
  - encouraging valued social roles
  - promoting choice
  - supporting contribution
  - community participation
- Protection
- Taking account of the person's wishes and decision-making capacity (perhaps supported by advocacy or legal protection)
- Consultation with other people with an interest in the person's welfare, such as family (perhaps supported by family advocacy)

Residential service
- Setting: environmental and social requirements (space, garden, noise, traffic, neighbours)
- Building – special adaptations or constraints required for access, privacy or safety:
  - ramps
  - gates on stairs/all one level
  - safety glass
  - sensors to alert staff
- Domestic equipment: any special arrangements for toilet, bath, shower, etc.
- Staffing level – day and night (waking or sleepover) with explanation of reasons for specified minimum level of staffing
- Staff characteristics – special skills or other characteristics required, including qualifications, gender, build, responsiveness to specific client characteristics
- Client numbers – maximum and minimum numbers of residents the person can live with, and explanation for these specifications
- Client mix – issues that affect compatibility
- Risk management – any special arrangements required to respond to risk assessment, including legal protection, procedures, skills, supervision arrangements, etc.
- Other factors such as contact with family, continuity of other relationships, transport, or anything specifically needed to promote service aims

Day activities
- Same list of considerations, adapted for activities such as:
  - employment and vocational activity
  - education and training
  - social, recreational and leisure activities
  - therapeutic activities

Visiting services
- Determined by individual assessment

treatment, and achieving and maintaining stability of mental health. The service specification should be written in such a way that the service will expect some ongoing mental health problems, and will continue to support the person's development with sustainable levels of input from community-based health services and realistic availability of additional services such as hospital admission.

A common error of inexperienced services is to rely on the continuous availability of a component of additional service that is not, in fact, provided. High expectations lead to burnout of the staff, who feel they have to respond; and if the expectations are not met, confidence in the service will be lost. It is more successful to plan for the expectation that the person will continue to have unstable mental health and to continue to present the risks that have previously been assessed. If the person subsequently turns out to have less need for support, the care plan can be reviewed and unnecessary levels of support phased out.

A highly individualised, flexible approach requires staff who have advanced skills in assessing and managing developmental disabilities, mental illness and behavioural problems, evaluating risk and decision-making capacity, and working with patients, families, health and social care organisations, and other agencies, sharing information but at the same time respecting confidentiality. Health policy in the UK expects this to be done by supporting people in accessing ordinary services where possible, and with additional services where necessary. There has been no research on this topic, but I am not aware of any service that achieves this without teams of specialist staff.

In some areas, service commissioners seem to believe that people with such needs do not exist. In the absence of planned services, there has been an expansion of residential provision in the independent sector to meet these needs when they arise and to provide continuing care. The effect has been to move some people with learning disability and severe mental illness who have the most complex health needs into unplanned long-term institutional care, remote from their families and at relatively high expense. I am not aware of evidence that such services provide rehabilitation. Many of the factors that adversely affect the quality of life of people with learning disabilities will be familiar to psychiatrists working in rehabilitation services, because they also affect people with enduring mental illness. There needs to be a sustained effort to campaign for high-quality services for this group of people who do not demand a service for themselves, but could have a better quality of life with adequate service provision.

References

Aman, M. G., Burrow, W. H. & Wolford, P. L. (1995) The Aberrant Behavior Checklist–Community: factor validity and effect of subject variables for adults in group homes. *American Journal of Mental Retardation*, **100**, 283–292.

American Psychiatric Association (1994) *Diagnostic and Statistical Manual of Mental Disorders* (4th edn) (DSM–IV). Washington, DC: APA.

Cooper, S.-A. (2003) Classification and assessment of psychiatric disorders in adults with learning disabilities. *Psychiatry*, **2**, 12–16.

Einfeld, S. L. & Tonge, B. J. (1995) The Developmental Behaviour Checklist: the development and validation of an instrument to assess behavioural and emotional disturbance in children and adolescents with mental retardation. *Journal of Autism and Developmental Disorders*, **25**, 81–104.

NHS Health Scotland (2004) *People with Learning Disabilities in Scotland (Health Needs Assessment Report)*. Glasgow: NHS Health Scotland.

Ottenbacher, K. & Cusick, A. (1990) Goal attainment scaling as a method of clinical service evaluation. *American Journal of Occupational Therapy*, **44**, 519–525.

Prosser, H., Moss, S. C., Costello, H., *et al* (1998) Reliability and validity of the Mini PAS–ADD for assessing psychiatric disorders in adults with intellectual disability. *Journal of Intellectual Disability Research*, **42**, 264–272.

Roy, A., Matthews, H., Clifford, P., *et al* (2002) Health of the Nation Outcome Scales for People with Learning Disabilities (HoNOS–LD). *British Journal of Psychiatry*, **180**, 61–66.

Royal College of Psychiatrists (2001) *Diagnostic Criteria for Psychiatric Disorders for Use with Adults with Learning Disabilities/Mental Retardation* (Occasional Paper OP48). London: Gaskell.

Royal College of Psychiatrists (2006) *Psychiatric Services for Adolescents and Adults with Asperger Syndrome and Other Autistic-spectrum Disorders* (CR136). London: Royal College of Psychiatrists. (http://www.rcpsych.ac.uk/publications/collegereports/cr/cr136.aspx)

Ryan, T., Pearsall, A., Hatfield, B., *et al* (2004) Long term care for serious mental illness outside the NHS. A study of out of area placements. *Journal of Mental Health*, **13**, 425–429.

Sparrow, S. S., Balla, D. A. & Cichetti, D. V. (1984) *Vineland Adaptive Behavior Scales*. Lisse: Swets & Zeitlinger.

Stark, J., Menolascino, F., Albourelli, M., *et al* (eds) (1988) *Mental Retardation and Mental Health: Classification, Diagnosis, Treatment, Services*. Berlin: Springer-Verlag.

Szymanski, L. S. (1988) Integrative approach to diagnosis of mental disorders in retarded persons. In *Mental Retardation and Mental Health: Classification, Diagnosis, Treatment, Services* (eds J. Stark, F. Menolascino, M. Albourelli, *et al*), pp. 124–139. Berlin: Springer-Verlag.

Wechsler, D. (1981) *Wechsler Adult Intelligence Scale–Revised*. New York: Psychological Corporation.

World Health Organization, Division of Mental Health and Prevention of Substance Abuse (1996) *ICD–10 Guide for Mental Retardation*. Geneva: World Health Organization.

CHAPTER 25

Forensic rehabilitation

Steffan Davies and Pat Abbott

There is increasing recognition of the importance of rehabilitation skills within forensic services. This has been brought into focus recently by the development of longer-term medium secure services in the National Health Service (NHS) as part of the process of reducing the size of the high-security hospitals. Rehabilitation services, which have always included a proportion of people discharged from secure services, seem to be dealing with a group who require greater forensic skills. This chapter provides an overview of the development of forensic rehabilitation services and their underlying principles, and a description of patient groups and of some intervention strategies. It concentrates on secure psychiatric services, particularly high and medium secure services for men, and concludes with a brief discussion of possible future developments in forensic rehabilitation services.

Background

The three English high-security hospitals (Ashworth, Broadmoor and Rampton) historically had large numbers of beds (over 1000 each) and a significant population of long-stay patients, often with stays of over 20 years. Many patients with severe psychotic illness and learning disabilities received limited therapeutic input except for a wide variety of day care activities and well-equipped workshops and extensive gardens. A large proportion did not require high security as highlighted by a number of studies (e.g. Maden, *et al*, 1995). The development of regional secure units with an 18- to 24-month time frame for admissions did little to help this patient group. As regional secure units developed it also became clear that a proportion of their population required much longer stays than 2 years. This paralleled the development of a new long-stay population in general adult psychiatry following the asylum closure programme of the 1980s and 1990s (Abbott, 2002). Although the numbers of these patients were often small, their very protracted lengths of stay accounted for a large percentage of bed occupancy and reduced the ability of regional secure units to carry out their primary task of assessment and shorter-term treatment. Regional secure units were therefore very reluctant to accept patients from high-security facilities if they were unlikely to move on within 2 years. They also lacked the extensive facilities of the high-security hospitals, which limited the quality of life of long-stay patients. The independent sector initially filled several of these gaps, with charitable hospitals and private sector facilities developing longer-term secure services, single-gender services for women and learning disability services. At one stage they provided around half the medium secure beds in England. Longer-term low secure services usually developed out of locked wards in the old asylums that were retained in some parts of the country when the main hospitals shut down. They were usually part of local rehabilitation services, forming part of a spectrum of provision from longer-term low security through varying levels of NHS in-patient care to hostels and supported community placements.

The 'Tilt Report' (Department of Health, 2000) recommended substantial upgrading of the physical and procedural security of the high-security hospitals and also set specific targets for reducing the number of patients who no longer required high security by the end of 2004. The accelerated discharge programme it set in motion increased the rate of reduction in the high-security population, with bed numbers across three hospitals predicted to fall to a total of around 900 by 2006 (Abbott et al, 2005). Many of the former NHS regions responded by developing their own longer-term medium secure facilities, whereas others placed all longer-term patients in the independent sector. There are a variety of approaches being used for the development of NHS longer-term services, ranging from tacking a few rooms on to an existing regional secure unit, conversion of old asylum wards (which with a little imagination can provide spacious and attractive accommodation) to purpose-built services. A joint working party of the Faculties of Forensic Psychiatry and Rehabilitation and Social Psychiatry has made recommendations about the key elements of forensic rehabilitation medium secure services, which include greater allocation of physical space than in traditional regional secure units, access to fresh air and exercise within the secure perimeter, a range of therapeutic and occupational activities and managing the therapeutic environment (A. O'Hallorhan, personal communication, 2004). Another joint working party has made recommendations on the training required for forensic rehabilitation, emphasising the need for a combination of skills from both disciplines (T. Tattan, personal communication, 2004).

The reduction in numbers of patients in high-security facilities has been paralleled by an increase in therapeutic resources with case-loads for consultants falling dramatically and with greatly improved consultant recruitment. There have also been increases in the numbers of psychologists, occupational therapists and other therapists (for example arts therapists), along with improved training for nursing staff. Some of the consultant psychiatrists recruited have been trained in rehabilitation (including the authors). This has spurred the development of dedicated forensic rehabilitation services for those with severe enduring mental illness at Ashworth (Davies, 2004*a*) and Rampton (Davies, 2004*b*; Davies & Mooney, 2004). These services have worked closely with the developing NHS forensic rehabilitation medium secure services and the independent sector to move patients out of high-security facilities. The development of forensic rehabilitation services has occurred alongside greater specialisation within the high secure estate; for example, the development of national high secure deaf, learning disability and women's services at Rampton, dedicated personality disorder services at Ashworth and Rampton, and most recently dangerous and severe personality disorder services at Rampton and Broadmoor.

The very welcome development of forensic rehabilitation medium secure services and the discharge from high-security hospitals of patients who no longer require these services is, however, likely to create a further bottleneck between forensic rehabilitation and local services. The long-term, often lifelong, nature of the psychiatric disabilities of this population, and the risks they continue to pose, mean that they require a different style of service to that traditionally provided by community forensic and general psychiatry. Movement out of forensic rehabilitation medium secure services is likely to be through local long-term low secure facilities, open rehabilitation and continuing care facilities, and eventually into supported accommodation. The patient group is likely to need high levels of support rather than assertive follow-up, and many will be subjected to Home Office restrictions imposed at sentencing or because they are sentenced prisoners transferred to hospital. The diversion of resources from many rehabilitation services into assertive outreach teams and the closure of many long-term NHS in-patient units are likely to exacerbate this bottleneck.

Patient groups

Male patients served by current forensic rehabilitation services are characterised by treatment-resistant psychotic illness and remain symptomatic, with severe positive and/or negative symptoms, despite drug treatment. Patients will usually have severe deficits in social skills and activities of daily living, and often be unable to participate in the usual therapeutic and occupational groups. There is either a history of serious offending, violence, sexual offences, arson or of similar behaviours that have proved unmanageable in less-secure settings but have not led to conviction. Comorbidity is the rule, with high rates of personality disorder, substance misuse, low IQ and physical problems.

Two subgroups are clinically apparent. First those with serious offences who have been unable to engage in offence-related treatment programmes, but who rarely, if ever, exhibit risk behaviours in hospital settings. Many of this group were among the first patients to move on as the accelerated discharge programme started. Anecdotally a substantial proportion are already moving into lower-grade secure local services after 2 or 3 years. For this group with chronic psychosis but settled behaviour the question is often one of the minimum level of external support and control needed to maintain safety while maximising autonomy and quality of life. In spite of continued psychotic symptoms there are often numerous general factors which reduce risks to others: medication and psychological interventions may make symptoms less distressing and less likely to be acted upon; patients will be older (strongly correlated with reduced offending in the general population); better support supervision and social stability (e.g. accommodation and finances) than at the time of the index offence; good therapeutic relationships and understanding of previous risk behaviour. These factors need to be included in the risk equation, as well as ongoing psychotic symptoms and a failure to complete a formal offence-related programme such as sex offender treatment programmes. Rehabilitation for this group will need to be slow, carefully graduated and with acknowledgement that a point may be reached beyond which progress into a community placement is not safe. Long-term supervision is essential, especially in less-supported community placements, as risk may re-emerge with destabilising influences such as relapse of illness, loss of accommodation or substance misuse, even after many years of stability.

The second group is one that continues to exhibit disturbed behaviour such as verbal aggression, minor assaults, property damage, but not serious violence. The key question for risk management is whether this behaviour is a precursor of more-serious violence that is only prevented by the level of security they are managed in or whether this is the level of disturbance that needs to be managed long term. Developing an understanding of triggers of problem behaviours (bullying and victimisation by more-able patients are surprisingly common) is essential. For this chronically disturbed group, management needs to concentrate on: optimising drug treatment, particularly reducing levels of arousal, which are often related to affective symptoms, anxiety and akathisia; engagement in a programme of meaningful activities to provide structure and enhanced quality of life; management of the environment to reduce overstimulation (noise, crowding); avoiding flash points such as medication and meal times. For this group the key aspects of security, in addition to a detailed understanding and good therapeutic relationship, involve limiting access to potential weapons through controlling the environment and searching. This group requires more active day-to-day management and more detailed work on care packages to maintain safety and hence has been slower to leave high-security settings, but is beginning to do so. This often requires extensive liaison with the units they move onto, including numerous visits and staff from the receiving unit spending time with the patient to familiarise themselves with management approaches before transfer.

Black service users in secure settings

The influence of ethnicity upon patterns of service usage is complex and research is sparse and fraught with methodological problems. It has been clear for a number of years that Black men are over-represented in secure services. Murray (1996) noted that there was a higher than expected proportion of African–Caribbean males in secure facilities. Coid *et al* (2001) reported that a higher than expected proportion of Black patients in forensic settings were diagnosed as suffering from psychosis and that there was a lower than expected rate of diagnosis of personality disorder in this group. The pathways into mental healthcare for Black men have been shown to be more complex, with increased involvement of the police, increased rates of compulsory detention and a lower rate of specialist referral from primary care (Bhui *et al*, 2003). The David (Rocky) Bennett Inquiry Report (Blofeld, 2003) highlighted a range of problems for Black patients in forensic services. These include experiences of isolation and alienation, which may result from being placed in secure units far from home without an appropriately diverse ethnic mix of patients or staff. This report has a number of recommendations to improve the services for this patient group and a Department of Health (2005) action plan was developed in response to this Inquiry and other documents, including: *Breaking the Circles of Fear* by the Sainsbury's Centre for Mental Health (2002); *Inside Outside: Improving Mental Health Services for Black and Minority Ethnic Communities in England* (National Institute for Mental Health in England, 2003); and *Delivering Race Equality: A Framework for Action* (Department of Health, 2003).

It is important that the cultural needs of each individual are assessed and a care plan is drawn up to meet these needs. Services need a range of structures in place to ensure these needs can be met, including access to interpreters, community groups, cultural activities and spiritual care. This is in addition to meeting basic needs such as dietary requirements and specialist hairdressing. Raising staff awareness and increasing their sensitivity to the needs of Black patients are very important. Further work is required to look at specific interventions which may improve recovery outcome for this group.

Principles

Forensic rehabilitation requires a combination of skills from forensic and rehabilitation psychiatry. The detailed assessment of risk and management through the use of security are traditional forensic skills. The reduction of risk through successful treatment of psychotic illness and the provision of psychological programmes aimed at reducing future risk (e.g. sex offender treatment programmes) are, however, less applicable to this group. Rehabilitation approaches, which concentrate on improving social and functional skills and providing more individualised support and service packages, are essential for this patient group. The concentration on individual needs and the management of risks rather than fitting patients into existing services and programmes will play an increasing role in the future. Important considerations include: quality of life; an acceptance of disability; realistic long-term goals while maintaining therapeutic optimism; a constant awareness of risk issues.

The development of forensic rehabilitation services at Ashworth and Rampton illustrates some of these points. A common feature of these units is the provision of a dedicated service on a single ward for a more diagnostically and functionally homogeneous patient group. In the past patients with severe mental illness were spread over a number of wards, which tried to cater for a wide range of patients, precluding the development of a therapeutic programme specifically for their needs. Concentrating similar patients together has a number of advantages including: development of expertise in managing complex medication regimes; the ability to provide flexible, accessible and functionally appropriate therapeutic activities, which are often ward based; concentrating on engaging an often institutionalised group with severe negative symptoms in therapeutic relationships and psychological interventions; developing a more appropriate security regime, concentrating more on relational aspects rather than physical security. There is a focus on the ward social environment as a key part of therapy using a psychosocial intervention model (Ashworth; Davies, 2004a) and a therapeutic community approach (Rampton; Davies, 2004b; Davies & Mooney, 2004).

Interventions

Medication

Patients in forensic rehabilitation services are treatment resistant in many ways. They often have many predictors of poor outcome of psychosis: poor premorbid adjustment; long duration of untreated illness, often in prison; poor or inconsistent adherence to or delivery of treatment; comorbid personality disorder and substance misuse. It is therefore not surprising that even clozapine treatment often produces only partial responses. Treatment with clozapine has been demonstrated (Swinton & Haddock, 2000) to correlate with discharge from high-security settings. It is important to maximise the benefit of prescribing clozapine by including regular monitoring of plasma levels. These can change over time and there are multiple potential interactions of clozapine with other psychotropic and physical medications. Plasma levels also help to monitor adherence. Augmentation with other antipsychotics is often beneficial and individual patients can show very different responses to augmentation with different atypicals. Affective symptoms are common and often inadequately treated. Mood stabilisers, particularly sodium valproate and increasingly lamotrigine, play an important role. Managing side-effects of clozapine, particularly constipation and hypersalivation, is also important for patients' quality of life. A significant proportion of patients should not be prescribed clozapine owing to previous side-effects, failure to benefit, or refusal to cooperate. For some, high doses or combinations of antipsychotics can sometimes produce benefits (Freudenreich & Goff, 2002; Stahl, 2002). This has to be undertaken with caution, with monitoring of benefits and side-effects, and with well-documented consent or explicit support of the appropriate regulatory body. This is an area with a very small evidence base, owing in part to small patient numbers, lack of capacity to consent and little commercial interest in funding research.

Daytime activities

The provision of structured daytime activities is an essential aspect of forensic rehabilitation services. Although lacking an 'evidence base' in formal terms, they have been advocated at least since Tuke's description of moral treatment (Tuke, 1813). Patients and carers frequently identify the lack of daytime activities on acute wards as a deficit. The UK government's social inclusion agenda requires mental health social services to assist people with mental health problems back into the workforce (see Shepherd, Chapter 6, this volume). For patients detained for extended periods in secure psychiatric services, the provision of daytime recreational, occupational and therapeutic activities seems a basic human right. For the difficult-to-engage forensic rehabilitation population it is essential that dedicated occupational therapy sessions are provided on the ward in a flexible manner, with maximum patient participation in planning and delivery. Reliance on hospital- or unit-wide programmes that often cater for a more-able population is not sufficient; previous experience has shown failure of these to engage this patient group or patients to receive little benefit. The occupational therapist is a vital member of the multidisciplinary team and this should be reflected in their job plan. Occupational therapists should attend team meetings, as well as ward management and community meetings.

Psychological interventions

The evidence base for psychological interventions for psychotic disorders is expanding rapidly and they have become recommended core interventions for schizophrenia (National Institute for Clinical Excellence, 2002). Unfortunately again there is little, if any, specific evidence for psychological therapies in the forensic rehabilitation patient group. Very few are able to engage, at least initially, in more-formal structured therapies such as cognitive–behavioural therapy (CBT). For many the initial task is to engage in any therapeutic relationship with any member of the multidisciplinary team, irrespective of the modality. Non-specific factors in the therapeutic alliance have been demonstrated as beneficial in other groups, as shown by some of the trials of CBT *v.* befriending (Sensky *et al*, 2000). However, the long-term aim would be engagement in more-formal therapy. This is also a group with multiple needs for psychological interventions; often these other problems may have more effect on patients lives than psychotic symptoms. For example, treatment of a needle phobia may allow a trial of clozapine or addressing the anxiety about working with female staff could open up more therapeutic opportunities. A wide range of psychological therapies should be available, but with an acknowledgement that these will need to be made accessible and delivered over a much longer time frame than is usual. Creative therapies in particular are highly valued by patients. Their use of non-verbal communication as a primary tool often makes these therapies more accessible and less threatening. Anecdotal experience has found art therapy a particularly good way of encouraging initial engagement with a very withdrawn, institutionalised patient group. Material generated in art therapy can also be extremely informative for risk assessment and monitoring.

Risk management and therapeutic security

The management and reduction of risk is the primary task for forensic psychiatric services. The need for security and the importance of relational security has long been recognised.

'In the construction of [asylums], cure and comfort ought to be as much considered as security, and I have no hesitation in declaring that a system which, by limiting the power of the attendant, obliges him not to neglect his duty, and makes his interest to obtain the good opinion of those under his care, provides more effectively for the safety of the keeper, as well as for the patient, than all the apparatus of chains, darkness and anodynes' (Tuke, 1813: p. 107).

In simplistic terms, traditional NHS forensic services operate by admitting someone to a level of security at which they can be safely contained, treating the mental disorder, addressing offence-related issues and providing ongoing treatment and supervision through lower levels of security into the community. This model informed the 18- to 24-month time scale during the development of regional secure units. Although effective for many individuals, the forensic rehabilitation population, by definition, does not fit into this model well. The effects of treatment-resistant psychotic illness, often compounded by other deficits such as low IQ, adverse early life experiences and disruptive attachments, exclude patients from offence-focused programmes. Ongoing positive and negative symptoms contribute to continuing risks related to mental illness, and other areas such as substance misuse, personality disorder and deviant sexual interests are likely to remain unaddressed. Patients are therefore unlikely to complete the risk reduction work required to move through generic forensic services, and require a different approach. This will involve a much more-detailed assessment of security needs than the traditional high, medium and low security of the past.

The level of security a patient requires is often the subject of intense debate between clinicians. There are many reasons for this: decisions are complex, difficult and with no gold standard to compare against; there maybe a reluctance to admit long-term patients who may 'bed block'; poor definitions of security, resulting in a lack of common language. Security has traditionally been divided into physical, procedural and relational domains (Collins & Davies, 2005; Box 25.1).

There have not been standardised definitions of security in the past but the implementation of the 'Tilt Report' has led to a much greater standardisation of security in the high-security hospitals. Clinicians generally regard the relational aspect of security to be the most important for their work as it is intimately linked to therapeutic activity. Procedural aspects, for example searching, often have the greatest impact on patients' lives and have the potential to cause conflict. Security levels also vary within units. For example, within high-security settings there may be a highly staffed, very restrictive intensive care unit and a pre-discharge villa with low staffing levels and a much more-relaxed regime. Much of what goes wrong with security is related to failure in relational and procedural security rather than physical deficits, for example problems identified by the Fallon Inquiry into the Ashworth Personality Disorder Unit (Fallon et al, 1999; Department of Health, 2000). There are also aspects of the therapeutic regime, patient mix and the security regime that interact in a

---

Box 25.1 The three domains of security (after Collins & Davies, 2005)

Physical. This is the domain that most people are familiar with and includes perimeter fences, doors, locks and other physical elements.

Procedural. This domain covers the variety of procedures that take place within the physical elements to maintain security integrity. Examples include the restriction of certain items within a unit and searching of patients and the environment.

Relational. This domain is more complex but in general refers to a detailed understanding of those receiving secure care and their management, including the management of violence and aggression. For example, a competent forensic nurse will have a full knowledge of a patient, including their history and potential risk behaviours, and also a relationship with the patient that exists within an open acknowledgement of the level and potential for dangerous behaviour in any number of given situations.

positive or negative way. These may be more important than the overall level of security, certainly of physical security.

Recent research has investigated the development of a security needs assessment profile which divides security into 22 domains, each rated from 0 (no need), through 1 (low level) and 2 (medium) to 3 (high level of need; Collins *et al*, 2003). This allows the production of a patient security profile, which can be used to inform management or placement decisions. The terms high, medium, low (or open) do not sufficiently define a care setting, whereas a security needs assessment profile specifically defines the patient's security needs and can assist placement in the increasing variety of specialist provision within secure services. For example, a patient in high security who has a history of chronic assaults and whose assaults are driven by over arousal and poor impulse control, who does not plan or sustain assaults or who rarely uses weapons and then only those easily to hand, will need a regime concentrating on high levels of supervision, a medium level of restriction of weapons in the environment and an ability to respond rapidly to incidents but without a requirement for protective equipment such as body armour and shields. They would not require a high-security perimeter, sophisticated security intelligence, monitoring of external communications, and high levels of searching which are currently provided in high-security units. In the past an assessment from a local regional secure unit would often ask for a period of settled behaviour before they would consider the person for transfer. Although such a patient would not fit easily into a traditional medium secure unit, designing a suitable treatment regime in medium security would be a matter of having a sufficient patient group to ensure a viable service rather than overcoming any great technical obstacles. The use of more-detailed assessments of security needs and matching placements to these needs should enable placements in more-appropriate security regimes than are currently available.

Therapeutic environments

With the development of community services and the asylum closures of the past three decades there has been a relative neglect of in-patient environments. There has been a renewed interest in in-patient environments of late, partly because of a realisation of how awful some acute wards have become. A large impetus for this has come from user/carer organisations (McCann 2004; Ruane 2004). There is little recent literature about the beneficial aspects of therapeutic environments. Some of the earlier literature such as the 'Three Hospital Study' (Wing & Brown, 1970) and Tuke's (1813) description of 'The Retreat' remain relevant. Borthwick *et al* (2001) discusses the relevance of Tuke's moral treatment to contemporary mental healthcare. Smith (2000) conducted a systematic review of papers on therapeutic environments and schizophrenia between 1978 and 1998. She concludes:

> **Box 25.2** Key features of a therapeutic community environment
>
> - Highly supportive environment
> - Emphasis on relationships
> - Relaxed non-restrictive approach
> - Opportunities for user involvement

'In brief such an environment should be highly supportive, with an emphasis on relationships and orientated toward individual needs. There should be little expression of anger and aggression, a relaxed, non-restrictive regime of care and opportunities for user involvement.'

Smith argued that 'a therapeutic community model, modified to provide high levels of emotional support and individual care, may help such patients'. Key features identified were: a highly supportive environment; an emphasis on relationships; orientated towards individual needs; relaxed; non-restrictive; with opportunities for user involvement (Box 25.2). These are similar both to Tuke's moral treatment and the features identified by users and carers as being important in an in-patient environment (McCann 2004; Quirk & Lelliott, 2004; Ruane 2004).

In forensic rehabilitation services the majority of activity currently takes place in an in-patient setting. Much of the work can be seen to parallel that of the earlier resettlement services as asylums ran down, albeit with a group of patients with higher risk (Abbott, 2002). The therapeutic features of in-patient environments identified above are often at variance with some of the requirements of security regimes. The balancing of observation, searching, restricting potential weapons, monitoring communications, controlling disturbed behaviour and maintaining therapeutic relationships is an extremely skilled task.

The therapeutic environment needs to be consciously addressed and managed as much as any other aspect of care, such as medication or treatment groups. Nursing staff are the primary providers of the therapeutic environment, but this task can be greatly aided or undermined by other disciplines, particularly consultant medical staff. Taking an interest in the therapeutic environment, having a lead consultant for the ward (as recommended by the acute in-patient policy implementation guide; Department of Health, 2002), discussion of the milieu by the multi-disciplinary team, attending ward community meetings are practical steps medical staff can take. Other professions can make important contributions. Kinderman (2004) describes the positive contribution of a well-supervised assistant psychologist in improving psychological perspectives of the ward and individuals' treatment in an acute setting. Social workers can play an important part in developing and maintaining links with the outside world. Occupational therapists can provide appropriate therapeutic and recreational activities on the ward and can facilitate access to off-ward activities and promote social interaction. Arts therapies (art, drama, music) are valued highly by patients and contribute greatly to the milieu and physical environments. Other issues such as cultural sensitivity, a commitment to working with the patient group and the provision of staff support and supervision are also important.

Although complex, the ward atmosphere can be measured (Timko & Moos, 2004) and the results used to target areas for improvement. The most commonly used instrument is the Ward Atmosphere Scale (Moos, 1996). This is rather complex to administer and analyse. An updated version designed for psychotic populations and a brief (5-item) Good Milieu Index have been developed more recently in Scandinavia (Rossberg & Friis, 2003a,b). Ward atmosphere has been shown to correlate with patient's satisfaction, staff morale (Middelboe et al, 2001; Rossberg & Friis, 2004) and patient outcomes (Davies et al, 2005). Regular measurement of the milieu and feedback to the team can assist in the development of a more-therapeutic environment.

Forensic rehabilitation in the community

There is evidence that the majority of forensic service users who move on from high and medium security are supported by adult and rehabilitation services rather than forensic services in the long term. This is not surprising considering that this population has a high incidence of treatment-resistant psychosis and comorbid conditions. Many of these people will require either high-intensity community support or 24-h staffed accommodation, neither of which have been common features of forensic community teams, which generally are used to supporting patients who have responded to antipsychotic treatment but have ongoing risk issues relating to substance misuse and personality disorder but are capable of independent living.

The principles behind intensive case management models of care would appear to be as applicable to the population with treatment-resistant mental illness who have been users of forensic services as those within adult services. There is evidence that the focus should be upon the delivery of evidence-based interventions rather than increased frequency of contact per se in order to reduce readmission (Burns et al, 1999). The value of 'sensitive anticipatory action' in terms of reducing psychiatric emergencies was identified as part of the UK700 trial (Weaver et al, 2003). This encompassed promoting engagement, patient-centred review of medication, assessing and responding to social care needs and developing robust crisis care plans. There is need for ongoing social care, such as supported accommodation, and a long-term perspective on their care which ensures that risk issues are not lost sight of even after periods of sustained stability. The importance of very good multidisciplinary teamworking cannot be overstated in terms of supporting a high-risk patient population in the community.

Future trends

When the accelerated discharge programme is completed the flow of patients from high-security hospitals into forensic rehabilitation medium secure services will reduce but continue. Many of the patients that are new to forensic rehabilitation medium secure services will come from existing NHS medium secure services, with fewer moving into independent sector facilities in the future. The prison population represents a source of referral to forensic rehabilitation medium secure services and is likely to contain substantial numbers who could benefit from the forensic rehabilitation approach, particularly in the long-term dispersal population (i.e. those patients with sentences of many years to life managed in long-term rather than local prisons) (Royal College of Psychiatrists, 2006). Rates of psychosis among male sentenced prisoners have been estimated at 7% by the Office of National Statistics (Singleton *et al*, 1997). Many will be receiving treatment in prison and not cross the current threshold for diversion into NHS in-patient services. Pressure on medium secure beds means a patient has to demonstrate a high level of need to warrant transfer: usually being floridly psychotic, refusing medication and actively dangerous. Many patients with partially controlled psychosis or those who are 'quietly mad' are receiving sub-optimal treatment, both in terms of drug therapy (particularly clozapine which is rarely prescribed in prisons) and psychological and psychosocial interventions. The cognitive, motivational and social deficits caused by psychotic illness also make it much less likely that this group will complete offence-related programmes. Mentally disordered offenders are therefore also disadvantaged by spending longer periods in higher-security prisons and receiving fewer opportunities for rehabilitation before release. For life sentence prisoners their time in custody will be prolonged as, without completing offence-related programmes, they are much less likely to be judged suitable for release by the parole board or discretionary lifer panel. With the transfer of responsibility for prison healthcare to the NHS and a commitment to provide an equivalent service for prisoners, there should be provision of services equivalent to community rehabilitation teams within the longer-term prisons. This is in contrast to the in-reach model of assessment, short-term treatment and diversion, which is very appropriately provided to local remand prisoners with a high turnover and more acute psychiatric problems. There should also be integration of sentence planning and offence-related work with the care programme approach (CPA) to ensure such work takes place, risks are properly assessed and not overestimated and that transfer to NHS services, possibly for more-active rehabilitation or adapted offence-related programmes, takes place as necessary.

The development of forensic rehabilitation medium secure services is also creating a bottleneck with local long-term low secure services, open in-patient rehabilitation and continuing care facilities. The ability of community rehabilitation teams to provide intensive support and monitoring to an increasingly difficult and risky population in the community is also being stretched. Although this group have always been cared for by rehabilitation services, with good results according to the little evidence available (Pullen, 1998), their number and complexity is likely to increase as forensic rehabilitation services develop in parallel with existing forensic services.

Conclusions

Recent years have seen an increased acknowledgment of the need for a combination of forensic and rehabilitation skills, and the development of specialist services to serve the population with treatment-resistant psychoses and high-risk behaviours. Although these services have tended to develop in high-security hospitals and the independent sector, the need for low secure, open and community services able to provide this combination of skills is becoming apparent. In the future there will be an increasing need for such skills within the prison service as well as in the health sector.

References

Abbott, P. (2002) Reconfiguration of the high security hospitals: some lessons from the mental hospital retraction and reprovision programme in the United Kingdom. *Journal of Forensic Psychiatry*, **13**, 107–122.

Abbott, P., Davenport, S., Davies, S., *et al* (2005) Potential effects of retraction of the high-security hospitals. *Psychiatric Bulletin*, **29**, 403–406.

Bhui, K., Stansfeld, S., Hull, S., *et al* (2003) Ethnic variations in pathways to and use of specialist mental health services in the UK: systematic review. *British Journal of Psychiatry*, **182**, 105–116.

Blofeld, J. (2003) *Independent Inquiry into the Death of David Bennett*. London: Department of Health.

Borthwick, A., Holman, C., Kennard, D., *et al* (2001) The relevance of moral treatment to contemporary mental health care. *Journal of Mental Health*, **10**, 427–439.

Burns, T., Creed, F. & Fahy, T. (1999) Intensive versus standard case management for severe psychotic illness: a randomised trial. *Lancet*, **353**, 2185–2189.

Coid, J., Kahtan, N., Gault, S., *et al* (2001) Medium secure forensic psychiatry services: comparison of seven English health regions. *British Journal of Psychiatry*, **178**, 55–61.

Collins, C. & Davies, S. (2005) Measuring security needs: a multidimensional approach. *International Journal of Forensic Mental Health*, **4**, 39–52.

Collins, M., Davies, S. & Ashwell, C. (2003) Meeting patients' needs in secure forensic psychiatric units. *Nursing Standard*, **17**, 33–34.

Davies, S. (2004a) Toxic institutions. In *From Toxic Institutions to Therapeutic Environments: Residential Settings in Mental Health Services* (eds P. Campling, S. Davies & G. Farquarson), pp. 20–31. London: Gaskell.

Davies, S. (2004b) Secure psychiatric services. In *From Toxic Institutions to Therapeutic Environments: Residential Settings in Mental Health Services* (eds P. Campling, S. Davies & G. Farquarson), pp. 233–243. London: Gaskell.

Davies, S. & Mooney, P. (2004) The birthing pains of Cedars Community: developing a therapeutic community for patients with schizophrenia in a high security hospital. *Therapeutic Communities*, **25**, 5–15.

Davies, S., Bennion, L., McPhee, D., *et al* (2005) Cedars Community: using a therapeutic community approach in a high security hospital. *Therapeutic Communities*, **26**, 139–149.

Department of Health (2000) *Report of the Review of Security at High Security Hospitals.* London: Department of Health.

Department of Health (2002) *Mental Health Policy Implementation Guide: Adult Inpatient Care Provision.* London: Department of Health.

Department of Health (2003) *Delivering Race Equality: A Framework for Action.* London: Department of Health. http://www.dh.gov.uk/assetRoot/04/06/72/29/04067229.pdf

Department of Health (2005) *Delivering Race Equality in Mental Health Care.* London: Department of Health.

Fallon, P., Bluglass, R., Edwards, B., *et al* (1999) *Report of the Committee of Inquiry into the Personality Disorder Unit, Ashworth Special Hospital.* London: TSO (The Stationery Office).

Freudenreich, O. & Goff, D. C. (2002) Antipsychotic combination therapy in schizophrenia. A review of efficacy and risks of current combinations. *Acta Psychiatrica Scandinavica*, **106**, 323–330.

Kinderman, P. (2004) Delivering psychological therapies in acute inpatient settings. In *From Toxic Institutions to Therapeutic Environments: Residential Settings in Mental Health Services* (eds P. Campling, S. Davies & G. Farquarson), pp. 197–207. London: Gaskell.

Maden, A., Curle, C., Meux, C., *et al* (1995) *Treatment and Security Needs of Special Hospital Patients.* London: Whurr.

McCann, J. (2004) What users want. In *From Toxic Institutions to Therapeutic Environments: Residential Settings in Mental Health Services* (eds P. Campling, S. Davies & G. Farquarson), pp. 159–165. London: Gaskell.

Middelboe, T., Schjodt, T., Byrsting, K., *et al* (2001) Ward atmosphere in acute psychiatric inpatient care; patients perceptions, ideals and satisfactions. *Acta Psychiatrica Scandinavica*, **103**, 212–219.

Moos, R. H. (1996) *Ward Atmosphere Scale* (3rd edn). Redwood City, CA: Mind Garden.

Murray, K. (1996) Use of beds in NHS medium secure units in England. *Journal of Forensic Psychiatry*, **7**, 504–524.

National Institute for Clinical Excellence (2002) *Schizophrenia: Core Interventions in the Treatment and Management of Schizophrenia in Primary and Secondary Care.* London: NICE.

National Institute for Mental Health in England (2003) *Inside Outside: Improving Mental Health Services for Black and Minority Ethnic Communities in England.* London: Department of Health. http://www.dh.gov.uk/assetRoot/04/01/94/52/04019452.pdf

Pullen, G. (1998) Special hospital transfers. *Journal of Forensic Psychiatry*, **9**, 241–244.

Quirk, A. & Lelliott, P. (2004) Users' experience of inpatient services. In *From Toxic Institutions to Therapeutic Environments: Residential Settings in Mental Health Services* (eds P. Campling, S. Davies & G. Farquarson), pp. 45–54. London: Gaskell.

Rossberg, J. I. & Friis, S. (2003a) A suggested revision of the Ward Atmosphere Scale. *Acta Psychiatrica Scandinavica*, **108**, 374–380.

Rossberg, J. I. & Friis, S. (2003b) Do the Spontaneity and Anger and Aggression subscales of the Ward Atmosphere Scale form homogeneous dimensions? A cross section study of 54 wards for psychotic patients. *Acta Psychiatrica Scandinavica*, **107**, 118–123.

Rossberg, J. I. & Friis, S. (2004) Patients' and staff's perceptions of the psychiatric ward environment. *Psychiatric Services*, **55**, 798–803.

Royal College of Psychiatrists (2006) *Prison Psychiatry: Adult Prisons in England and Wales.* Council Report (CR141). London: Royal College of Psychiatrists. In press.

Ruane, P. (2004) A carer's perception of the therapeutic value of inpatient settings. In *From Toxic Institutions to Therapeutic Environments: Residential Settings in Mental Health Services* (eds P. Campling, S. Davies & G. Farquarson), pp. 166–173. London: Gaskell.

Sainsbury's Centre for Mental Health (2002) *Breaking the Circles of Fear*. http://www.scmh. org.uk/80256FBD004F3555/vWeb/flPCHN6FMJZP/$file/breaking+the+circles_on-screen+version.pdf

Sensky, T., Turkington, D., Kingdon, D., *et al* (2000) A randomised controlled trial of cognitive–behavioural therapy for persistent symptoms in schizophrenia resistant to medication. *Archives of General Psychiatry*, **57**, 165–172.

Singleton, N., Meltzer, H. & Gatwood, R. (1997) *Psychiatric Morbidity Amongst Prisoners*. London: Office for National Statistics.

Smith, J. (2000) The healing elements of an environment for those with chronic psychosis. *Therapeutic Communities*, **21**, 37–46.

Stahl, S. (2002) Anti-psychotic polypharmacy: evidence based or eminence based? *Acta Psychiatrica Scandinavica*, **106**, 321–322.

Swinton, M. & Haddock, A. (2000) Clozapine in special hospital: a retrospective case controlled study. *Journal of Forensic Psychiatry*, **11**, 587–596.

Timko, C. & Moos, R. H. (2004) Measuring the therapeutic environment. In *From Toxic Institutions to Therapeutic Environments: Residential Settings in Mental Health Services* (eds P. Campling, S. Davies & G. Farquarson), pp. 143–156. London: Gaskell.

Tuke, S. (1813) *Practical Hints on the Construction and Economy of Pauper Lunatic Asylums*. York: Alexander. Reprinted in 1996 by Process Press Ltd: London.

Weaver, T., Tyrer, P., Ritchie, J., *et al* (2003) Assessing the value of assertive outreach: qualitative study of process and outcome in the UK700 trial. *British Journal of Psychiatry*, **183**, 437–445.

Wing, J.K. & Brown, G. W. (1970) *Institutionalism and Schizophrenia: A Comparative Study of Three Mental Hospitals 1960–1968*. Cambridge: Cambridge University Press.

Part 5

Where are we going?

CHAPTER 26

Rehabilitation and recovery in the 21st century

Sarah Davenport, Frank Holloway, Glenn Roberts
and Theresa Tattan

This book, with its many voices, perspectives and styles, is in the best sense eclectic. In bringing together in a single volume a diverse and rich group of contributions the editors have sought to inspire, challenge and perhaps at times provoke or irritate the reader. The aim has been to support practice and practitioners and stimulate dialogue and debate about the future shape of rehabilitation, recovery and continuing care services. So, looking ahead, what should this dialogue be about and who are the important participants in the debate?

The centrality of user and carer experience

A key issue for contemporary health and social services is how to put the experience of the user (sometimes misleadingly called the consumer or customer) at the heart of the way the service is organised. If this is to be achieved, then professionals need to improve the quality of their dialogue and partnership with service users and their carers. 'Dialogue' (according to the *Oxford English Dictionary*) is essentially a conversation, a listening to and a hearing of the thoughts and opinions of two equal participants. The challenge here is to find the way towards reciprocal conversation with service users and carers, rather than the uneasy tokenism that can often prevail. The challenges are particularly daunting when working with people with a severe mental illness, whose treatment has been characterised more by suppression than expression and who have historically been marginalised, without an articulate voice. That these challenges can be overcome is vividly demonstrated within the field of learning disability.

The Faculty of Rehabilitation and Social Psychiatry was the first within the Royal College of Psychiatrists to invite service users and carers onto its Executive Committee as full participant members in 2003. The Executive have tried hard to listen and to hear what these members have brought to the table, but the task is not always straightforward. The apparently 'necessary business' of a committee within a professional organisation (which can seem devoid of personal meaning) may overwhelm users and carers, or merely be rather boring. Committee members may in turn feel overwhelmed when they actually hear from users and carers about the gap between the care that is on offer and the experience of what is actually needed. There may be parallels between the function of the Rehabilitation Faculty Executive Committee and a care programme approach review, where there is a struggle to promote equal participation rather than pursuing a patronising, professionally dominated agenda. Perhaps we should keep this in mind to help us do better in both settings. Thanks are due here and now to the Rethink representatives who have been patient enough to stay with the committee during the early development of partnership working; their tenacity and vivacity has helped us begin to explore the breadth, depth and some of the tensions within a meaningful partnership.

The dialectics of rehabilitation

Perhaps it is some of these creative tensions that suggest that we need to extend our developmental dialogue into a dialectic. The *Oxford English Dictionary* provides a particularly helpful definition of dialectic as both adjective and noun: 'logical, of disputation; (person) skilled in critical inquiry by discussion'.

Our dialogue with service users, carers and other partners in care should be guided through respectful and reciprocal conversation to the point where real differences of opinion, attitude and aspiration can be honestly explored through dialectic.

There has, of course, long been a dialectic within rehabilitation services. In the past the disputes were held between different professional groups and individual staff members. These disputes were only in part a result of competing conceptual models of severe mental illness. Good rehabilitation practice has always thrown up dilemmas for which there are no ready answers, such as balancing the duty of care held towards a vulnerable individual who may lack capacity with the promotion of individual autonomy (Box 26.1). These dilemmas are just that: issues that lack an easy or obvious solution. A core competence for individual practitioners and teams has always been to respond sensitively and appropriately to each challenging situation as it emerges. What is new is the requirement to involve users and carers as equal partners in the discussion, which demands a significant change in attitude within rehabilitation and recovery services over the next decade. This will include honestly facing the many inequalities present in the room each time we meet, and through understanding and accepting these, overcoming them.

It is important to emphasise that professionals (who come from many differing backgrounds), users, carers and families all have perspectives to offer within the dialectic or dialogue: no actor has the monopoly of wisdom and all have access to important information that the others lack. However, in any specific situation not all stories are of equal value. A key issue then

---

Box 26.1 Some common dilemmas in rehabilitation and recovery practice

Assessment
- Whose view of needs should prevail – the professional, carers or the service user?

Diagnosis
- Is it best to name disorders, and if so how?
- What is the difference between a label and a badge?

Information sharing
- How do we involve carers when the patient refuses?
- When is it justified to break confidentiality?
- What views or values guide selecting information to share?

Treatment and care
- When is compulsory treatment justified?
- What does 'choice' mean for people with impaired insight and judgement?
- How do we make treatment judgements for people who lack decision-making capacity?
- Can we allow people to 'rot with their rights on'?
- Is there a role for 'benign paternalism?'
- When is it justified to force people to live in a particular setting not of their choice?
- What justifies taking control of people's finances?

Risk management
- How do we promote autonomy in a risk-averse world?
- How do we balance potential harms with potential benefits?
- How do we develop skills and confidence in 'creative risk-taking'?

Lifestyle choices
- What about sex and the single psychotic?
- Whose responsibility is it to pursue healthy living?
- How should we think about recreational drug taking?

---

becomes how to resolve leadership and decision-making dilemmas, both in general terms and in specific situations.

The time is now clearly right to be exploring and experimenting with ways of involving service users and carers meaningfully in the process of delivering, monitoring, evaluating and commissioning services for people with complex long-term disorders. We do now have the professional commitment. We also have the national policy to back the necessary cultural change towards truly user- and family-centred services. Readers of this book will be painfully aware that this process of collaborative working and risk-sharing is being promoted in parallel with contradictory policy trends that link mental health services with a public protection agenda and explicitly encourage coercive approaches towards mental healthcare.

Exploring values in rehabilitation practice

There are cultural factors that influence learning. Many of these are value-based. Values have been defined as: 'Deeply held views that act as guiding principles for individuals and organisations'. Pendleton & King (2002) go on to say that:

'When values are declared, they are the basis of trust. When they are left unstated, they are inferred from observable behaviour. When they are stated and not followed, trust is broken'.

Value-based cultural attitudes held by an institution and those working within it can impede or accelerate the acquisition of appropriate new ways of working. Where the underlying value has become historically implicit within training and no longer accessible to reflection or revision, there is a risk that this historical value becomes embedded in the 'hidden curriculum' and subverts the intended learning objective. For example, the historical assumption that the doctor is 'in charge' may translate into values around leadership and decision-making which conflict with balanced collaboration and risk-sharing with other professionals and service users. In such circumstances the 'hidden curriculum' subverts the aspiration of the overt new curriculum to train doctors who can work in teams and in partnership with service users and their families (Hafferty & Frank, 1994).

Training for the new services

It is impossible to overemphasise the importance of training. *Rehabilitation and Recovery Now* (Royal College of Psychiatrists, 2004) sets out a vision for the recovery-oriented user-focused rehabilitation service of the future. Paying attention to the culture and the values of rehabilitation and recovery practice and providing high-quality training will be crucial to bringing about changes in the ways services work.

One of the challenges and satisfactions of rehabilitation practice is the requirement to simultaneously access a deeply humanitarian concern for the patient as a fellow human being, while applying a considerable body of knowledge though professional skills. We inevitably fall short in all departments at times but gain much from living with the requirement to juggle these dimensions and their impact on our personal and professional development.

The *Ten Essential Shared Capabilities* framework has a potential role to play here (Box 26.2). The framework was developed by the Department of Health, the National Institute for Mental Health in England and the Sainsbury Centre, as a set of generic skills to underpin new roles and ways of working in mental health (Hope, 2004). These essential capabilities are radical in their breadth and perspective. It is clearly possible to incorporate them into a programme of audit and review to provide

Box 26.2 The Ten Essential Shared Capabilities

1 Working in partnership: Developing and maintaining constructive working relationships with service users, carers, families, colleagues, lay people and wider community networks. Working positively with any tensions created by conflicts of interest or aspiration that may arise between partners in care.

2 Respecting diversity: Working in partnership with service users, carers, families and colleagues to provide care and interventions that not only make a positive difference but also do so in ways that respect and value diversity.

3 Practising ethically: Recognising the rights and aspirations of service users and their families, acknowledging power differentials and minimising them whenever possible. Providing treatment and care that is accountable to service users and their carers within the boundaries prescribed by national (professional) legal and local codes of ethical practice.

4 Challenging inequality: Addressing the causes and consequences of stigma, discrimination, social inequality and exclusion on service users, carers and mental health services. Creating, developing or maintaining valued social roles for people in the communities they come from.

5 Promoting recovery: Working in partnership to provide care and treatment that enables service users and carers to tackle mental health problems with hope and optimism and to work towards a valued lifestyle within and beyond any mental health problem.

6 Identifying people's needs and strengths: Working in partnership to gather information to agree health and social care needs in the context of the preferred lifestyle and aspirations of service users, their families, carers and friends.

7 Providing service user-centred care: Negotiating achievable and meaningful goals, primarily from the perspective of service users and their families. Influencing and seeking the means to achieve these goals and clarifying the responsibilities of the people who will provide any help that is needed, including systematically evaluating outcomes and achievements.

8 Making a difference: Facilitating access to and delivering the best quality evidence-based, values-based health and social care interventions to meet the needs and aspirations of service users and their families.

9 Promoting safety and positive risk-taking: Empowering the person to decide the level of risk they are prepared to take with their health and safety. This includes working with the tension between promoting safety and positive risk-taking, including assessing and dealing with possible risks for service users, carers, family members and the wider public.

10 Personal development and learning: Keeping up to date with changes in practice and participating in lifelong learning, personal and professional development for one's self and colleagues through supervision, appraisal and reflective practice.

quality monitoring. *New Ways of Working* (Department of Health, 2005) requires this framework to be implemented in our training and continuing professional development.

The ten capabilities include qualities central to rehabilitation practice such as 'promoting recovery' and 'practising ethically'. Finding an appropriate individual solution to the multiple dilemmas faced by rehabilitation practitioners requires both sensitivity to the issues being raised and, at some level, the capacity to draw on the fundamental ethical principles underlying health and social care (Beauchamp, 1999). For psychiatrists there is a particular difficulty in balancing the overtly paternalistic approach demanded by their role as responsible medical officer within the Mental Health Act 1983 and the ethical imperative of promoting the autonomy of the service user. This difficulty is compounded by the policy requirements on mental health services to assure public protection from harm and to take account of the views and needs of carers. The user and carer views by no means invariably coincide, resulting in yet another common dilemma for mental health services (see Box 26.1).

What might it take to achieve the type of mutually respectful partnerships that will promote this user- and family-centred longer-term care? We need to think carefully about training in rehabilitation and recovery services, to ensure that service users and carers are involved in our training in a manner that would make it truly service user-centred and responsive. There is an associated need in advanced user/professional collaborations for service user colleagues to grow in understanding of the constraints, compromises and responsibilities carried by psychiatrists.

The Royal College of Psychiatrists has recently implemented a requirement for service users and carers to be involved in the training programmes organised for junior psychiatrists. It can be argued that medical education, which has traditionally promulgated paternalistic values, needs radical revision of the curriculum to take account of the philosophy of working 'with' service users rather than working 'on' them. However, the reality of severe mental illness is such that psychiatrists will need at times to choose, and be prepared to justify, the right time and right way to employ paternalistic, and at times compulsory, interventions, which risk being experienced as coercive. Rehabilitation and recovery practitioners also need to be prepared to make mistakes and reflect on them, to learn from service users and their families and to make changes in their approach. New patterns of training experience could arise where qualified staff, service users and carers train together, learn together and model the mutually respectful styles of practice that we aspire to.

The generic skills outlined in the 'ten capabilities' include a perhaps somewhat grudging recognition that practitioners require not only appropriate attitudes towards service users and carers and good communication skills but also a high degree of technical competence appropriate to their role. Reading a book does not automatically result in technical competence. Modern mental health services need to ensure that an adequate framework of supervised practice and lifelong skills-based training is in place. Multidisciplinary teamworking allows for much informal transfer of skills between people from different professional backgrounds (and no professional background at all).

Rehabilitation and recovery services and the new functional teams

A major aim of this book has been to promote debate, primarily about where and how rehabilitation and recovery services might sit within the comprehensive range of secondary mental health services. Adult mental healthcare is going through a period of unparalleled change, probably even more profound than the mental hospital closure programme, which was the end product of a steady decrease in in-patient psychiatric beds over 50 years. We have seen the rapid introduction of new functional teams: assertive outreach teams, early intervention teams and crisis resolution/home treatment teams (Department of Health, 2001). Many of the skills required within assertive outreach and early intervention teams in particular are, or should be, core competencies of rehabilitation practitioners and visa versa. There are sound reasons for these teams to join the local rehabilitation services in a family of psychosis services (Holloway, 2005). However, the targets set by the *NHS Plan* (Department of Health, 2000) have driven some providers to prioritise the establishment of the new functional teams at the expense of well-established rehabilitation services. (A recent survey identified 20 out of 186 assertive outreach teams in England as being renamed rehabilitation teams taking on a new client group.) Some people who would benefit from a rehabilitation and recovery model of care appear to have lost out in the modernised mental health service. These individuals are excluded by their chronicity from being prioritised for care by community mental health teams (CMHTs), by their age and length of disorder from early intervention teams, by their dependency and history of previous engagement with services from assertive outreach teams and by their lack of dangerousness from community forensic teams. They have indeed become the 'forgotten generation' (Rethink, 2004).

The virtual mental hospital

As the mental hospitals closed, many people moved into supported accommodation, registered residential and nursing homes and, more recently, private hospitals, which in effect form a local 'virtual asylum' of roughly the same size as the original hospital. These services are generally provided by the private-for-profit and voluntary sectors. Although there are regulatory agencies responsible for overseeing the quality of this care (currently the local Supporting People function, the Commission for Social Care Inspection and the Care Services Improvement Partnership), engagement with statutory mental health services is very patchy. A significant number of people fall out of effective sight of local mental health services when they move into the 'virtual asylum'.

In part this is because some individuals have such complex long-term needs that their needs cannot be met within their own health and social care economies. They are consequently managed as out-of-area placements. Placements are often remote from families and social networks and are not always subject to appropriate monitoring. The barriers to social inclusion these people face are often insuperable (Ryan *et al*, 2004). There have been two large-scale surveys of out-of-area treatments (placements funded by the National Health Service in hospital settings) purchased in the North-West and West Midlands regions. These have identified a worrying variability in the quality of care and have underlined the enormous cost to local health economies. This expenditure is obviously not available for the development of more appropriate local rehabilitation and recovery services. Local rehabilitation and recovery services should respond to the challenge of those service users and their families experiencing problems with out-of-area placements, to gain the opportunity to develop socially inclusive alternatives (Davies *et al*, 2005).

The situation with out-of-area placements replicates developments in the field of forensic psychiatry. In areas where demand for in-patient forensic care exceeds supply, notably in London, dedicated teams that work with out-of-area placements have been developed with a specific remit to drive people through the care system towards less restrictive (and cheaper) forms of care. In many areas forensic and rehabilitation services are becoming closer and we have, of course, seen the development of a specialty of forensic rehabilitation, and the growth of non-forensic low secure settings. This could go some way to overcoming the significant problem in managing the step-down transition from often geographically remote services to local rehabilitation and recovery services. Timely access to such provision could close the gap involved in such moves, which otherwise provides a reason for considerable delays.

Rehabilitation and recovery services in the 21st century

We need to think not only about incorporating new guiding values into practice and providing evidence-based interventions but also about the service structures that will deliver the best quality treatment and care. There are a number of important and difficult questions that lack fully authoritative answers.[1] As editors we have both posed the questions and provided our view of the answers *(in parentheses)*.

---

1. The Rehabilitation and Social Psychiatry Faculty of the Royal College of Psychiatrists has published a position statement that elaborates on the ideas presented here (see Holloway, 2005).

- Is a specific service for rehabilitation and continuing care an unnecessary and outmoded concept? *(Definitely not: the need has not gone away.)*
- When should rehabilitation begin? *(As an attitude and approach – at first contact, but resources seldom permit in-reach or appropriate training.)*
- Is 'rehabilitation' the best term to define our practice? *(Possibly not, but no better term has yet emerged.)*
- Should a modern rehabilitation and recovery service be part of a CMHT, in which particular team members are trained in rehabilitation and have protected smaller case-loads to provide flexible support to those whose recovery is likely to take place over an extended time period? *(Unlikely to succeed in helping the most disabled individuals and perpetuates the risk of displacement of such needs by acute priorities.)*
- Should there be specialised rehabilitation and recovery teams providing assessment, advice and support for persons referred from other parts of the service? *(Yes, if resources allow.)*
- Should local rehabilitation and recovery services focus on those who are consigned to the 'virtual mental hospital' of supported accommodation, residential and nursing home care or are at risk of placement? *(Perhaps, but only as a first step.)*
- Is high-support provision best provided within the statutory or private and voluntary sectors? *(There is no published evidence, although local monitoring of non-statutory care is essential on the grounds of clinical and financial governance.)*
- Is it possible to pursue recovery-based practice with patients detained under the Mental Health Act 1983? *(Yes, but the necessary mobilisation of choice within an individualised patient-centred approach combined with compulsory treatment needs particular care and attention.)*
- Should there be an extended family of specialist psychosis services that includes assertive outreach teams, early intervention teams, a recovery, rehabilitation and continuing care team, and dedicated in-patient resources? *(Yes: it is very difficult to find arguments against this proposition.)*
- In each case how should we define who receives a specialist service and who receives care from a generic CMHT or general practitioner? *(Really difficult to answer in the absence of any data.)*

Despite the apparent confidence of our views as editors, the evidence base currently offers no clear answers to these questions. To compound the difficulty, even where evidence exists it can be confusing and contradictory and will be subject to change over time. On occasion, evidence as most people understand it is irrelevant to large-scale service change, and is generally limited when it comes to complex choices with individuals. As an example, the move towards non-statutory providers of long-term residential and hospital care depends upon policy trends that transcend any evidence from within mental health services. These relate to complex macroeconomic discussions about accounting for capital developments (private sector good

– public sector bad) rather than a comparison of the quality of care and value for money of different forms of provision. Given these constraints on the availability and relevance of a robust evidence base, it is appropriate that local needs and partnerships determine which of the possible models of care is the most suited to local circumstances. Whatever arrangements are put in place need to be regularly reviewed and critically evaluated both in the light of local experience and the evolving evidence base.

Conclusions

Despite the uncertainties surrounding the way forward for rehabilitation, recovery and continuing care services one thing is clear: the promotion of social inclusion should be an essential guiding principle for local service development. As we have seen, potential users of rehabilitation and recovery services are characterised not only by particular diagnostic labels (notably that of schizophrenia) and the consequent stigma, but also by multiple indices of social exclusion: they tend to be poor, socially isolated, inadequately housed, unemployed and at risk of victimisation. People from minority ethnic groups are over-represented, although there is good evidence that their special needs have been systematically overlooked by mental health services. Those who are most excluded are individuals experiencing the most severe forms of disability and those presenting challenging behaviours, which may in turn result in contact with the criminal justice system.

We have already noted that a society can be judged by how it treats those of its members who are most in need of its care and compassion. As a community of professionals and collaborators we too can be judged by how we treat those who are most in need of our care and support. There is very good evidence from the literature on the hospital closure programme that people who have been written off as 'untreatable' for decades can be offered the opportunity for a better life, and we are also well aware of the associated concerns. This book provides much experience and many useful suggestions of steps that services and practitioners can take towards making a reality of community care. It also offers suggestions and support for how rehabilitation services can progress towards supporting recovery of citizenship for people disenfranchised by severe mental illness.

We have gathered an authoritative account of how far we have come and where we have got to, but the journey we are taking together with service users and carers continues. Current reviews of what it takes to provide a good mental health service (Boardman & Parsonage, 2005) continue to underline how far there is yet to go before the ambitions of the National Service Framework for Mental Health (Department of Health, 1999) are fulfilled. We hope that this present volume has offered some guidance on the preservation and opening of routes to recovery and that as we embark on 'new ways of working', this is emphatically 'not the end of the story'.

References

Beauchamp, T. L. (1999) The philosophical basis of psychiatric ethics. In *Psychiatric Ethics* (eds S. Bloch, P. Chodoff & S. A. Green), pp. 25–48. Oxford: Oxford University Press.

Boardman, J. & Parsonage, M. (2005) *Defining a Good Mental Health Service*. London: The Sainsbury Centre for Mental Health.

Davies, S., Mitchell, S., Mountain, D., *et al* (2005) *Out of Area Treatments for Working Age Adults with Complex and Severe Psychiatric Disorders: Review of Current Situation and Recommendations for Good Practice*. London: Faculty of Rehabilitation and Social Psychiatry, Royal College of Psychiatrists. http://www.rcpsych.ac.uk/PDF/Reccomendations05.pdf

Department of Health (1999) *National Service Framework for Mental Health: Modern Standards and Service Models*. London: Department of Health. http://www.dh.gov.uk/assetRoot/04/07/72/09/04077209.pdf

Department of Health (2000) *The NHS Plan: A Plan For Investment, A Plan For Reform*. London: Department of Health.

Department of Health (2001) *Mental Health Policy Implementation Guide*. London: Department of Health.

Department of Health (2005) *New Ways of Working for Psychiatrists: Enhancing Effective, Person-Centred Services Through New Ways of Working in Multidisciplinary and Multiagency Contexts*. London: Department of Health. http://www.dh.gov.uk/assetRoot/04/12/23/43/04122343.pdf

Hafferty, F. & Frank, R. (1994) The hidden curriculum, ethics teaching and the structure of medical education. *Academic Medicine*, **69**, 861–871

Holloway, F. (2005) *The Forgotten Need for Rehabilitation in Contemporary Mental Health Services*. London: Faculty of Rehabilitation and Social Psychiatry, Royal College of Psychiatrists. http://www.rcpsych.ac.uk/pdf/frankholloway_oct05.pdf

Hope, R. (2004) *The Ten Essential Shared Capabilities: A Framework for the Whole of the Mental Health Workforce*. London: Department of Health. http://www.dh.gov.uk/assetRoot/04/08/71/70/04087170.pdf

Pendleton, D. & King, J. (2002) Values and leadership. *BMJ*, **325**, 1352–1355.

Rethink (2004) *Lost and Found. Voices from the Forgotten Generation*. http://www.rethink.org/how_we_can_help/publications/lost_and_found.html

Royal College of Psychiatrists (2004) *Rehabilitation and Recovery Now*. (Council Report CR121). London: Royal College of Psychiatrists.

Ryan, T., Pearsall, A., Hatfield, B., *et al* (2004) Long term care for serious mental illness outside the NHS: A study of out of area placements. *Journal of Mental Health*, **13**, 425–429.

Rating scales

Lindsey Kemp and Theresa Tattan

This appendix lists a selection of basic rating scales and tools to be used in the psychiatric rehabilitation of people with severe mental illness. At present there is no clear guidance on what are 'the best' for any particular service. Reviews across rehabilitation services find a very wide range of tools in use, and many that use none at all. Very few services use the same selection. At present it remains a matter of local choice. Developing reliable and comparable outcome indicators will be an important issue for the future, in particular as services become more oriented towards enabling recovery and sensitive to how this may be defined quite differently by different service users. Further scales can be found in *Psychiatric Instruments and Rating Scales: A Select Bibliography* (Royal College of Psychiatrists, 1994, Occasional Paper OP23).

Abnormal Involuntary Movements (AIMS)
Wojcik, J. D., Gelenberg, A. J., Labrier, R. A., *et al* (1980) Prevalence of tardive dyskinesia in an outpatient population. *Comprehensive Psychiatry*, **21**, 370–380.

Auditory Hallucination Rating Scale
Haddock, G., Benthall, R. P. & Slade, P. (1996) Psychological treatments for auditory hallucinations, focussing or distraction? In *Cognitive–Behavioural interventions with Psychotic Disorders* (eds G. Haddock & P. Slade), pp. 45–71. London: Routledge.

Beck Anxiety Inventory (BAI)
Beck, AT., Epstein, N., Brown, G. (1988) An inventory for measuring clinical anxiety: psychometric properties. *Journal of Consulting and Clinical Psychology*, **56**, 893–897.

Beck Depression Inventory (BDI)
Beck, A. T., Ward, C. H., Mendelson, M., *et al* (1961) A self-rated inventory for measuring depression. *Archives of General Psychiatry*, **4**, 561–571.

Beliefs About Voices Questionnaire – Revised
Chadwick, P., Lees, S. & Birchwood, M. (2000) The revised Beliefs About Voices Questionnaire (BAVQ–R). *British Journal of Psychiatry*, **177**, 229–232.

Beliefs and Convictions Scale
Brett-Jones, J., Garety, P. & Hemsley, D. (1987) Measuring delusional experiences: a method and its application. *British Journal of Clinical Psychology*, **26**, 257–265.

Brief Psychiatric Rating Scale (BPRS)

Overall, J. E. & Gorham, D. R. (1962) The Brief Psychiatric Rating Scale. *Psychological Reports*, **10**, 799–812.

Brief Scale for Predicting the Rehospitalization of Former Psychiatric Patients

Willer, B. & Miller, G. A. (1977) A brief scale for predicting the rehospitalization of former psychiatric patients. *Canadian Psychiatric Association Journal*, **22**, 77–81.

Calgary Depression Scale

Addington, D., Addington, J. & Maticka-Tyndale, E. (1993) Assessing depression in schizophrenia: the Calgary Depression Scale. *British Journal of Psychiatry*, **163** (suppl. 22), 39–44.

Camberwell Assessment of Need (CAN)

Slade, M., Thornicroft, G., Loftus, L., *et al* (1999) *CAN: The Camberwell Assessment of Need. A Comprehensive Needs Assessment Tool for People with Severe Mental Illness.* London: Gaskell.

Community Placement Questionnaire (CPQ)

Clifford, P., Charman, A. & Webb, Y. (1991) Planning for community care: the Community Placement Questionnaire (CPQ). *British Journal of Clinical Psychology*, **30**, 193–211.

Comprehensive Assessment of Symptoms and History (CASH)

Andreasen, N. C. (1987) *The Comprehensive Assessment of Symptoms and History.* Iowa City, IA: University of Iowa College of Medicine.

Andreasen, N. C., Flaum, M. & Arndt, S. (1992) The Comprehensive Assessment of Symptoms and History (CASH). *Archives of General Psychiatry*, **49**, 615–623.

Delusions Rating Scale

Haddock, G. (1994) *Delusions Rating Scale.* Manchester: University of Manchester. Can be downloaded from http://www.mentalhealthnurse.co.uk/more_info.asp?current_id=85

Drug Attitude Inventory

Hogan, T. P., Awad, A. G. & Eastwood, R. (1983) A self-report scale predictive of drug compliance in schizophrenics: reliability and discriminative validity. *Psychological Medicine*, **13**, 177–183.

Early Signs Scale

Birchwood, M. J., Smith, J. Macmillan, F., *et al* (1989) Predicting relapse in schizophrenia: the development and implementation of an early signs monitoring system using patients and families as observers. *Psychological Medicine*, **19**, 649–656.

Family Questionnaire (FQ)

Barrowclough, C. & Tarrier, N. (1987) A behavioural family intervention with a schizophrenic patient: a case study. *Behavioural Psychotherapy*, **15**, 252–271.

General Health Questionnaire (GHQ)

Goldberg, D. P. (1972) *The Detection of Psychiatric Illness by Questionnaire (GHQ)* (Maudsley Monograph 21). London: Oxford University Press.

Hall Engagement Scale

Hall, M., Meaden, A., Smith, J., *et al* (2001). The development of an observer-rated measure of engagement with mental health services. *Journal of Mental Health*, **10**, 457–465.

Health of the Nations Outcome Scales (HoNOS)

Wing, J., Curtis, R. & Beevor, A. S. (1996) *Health of the Nations Outcome Scales (HoNOS).* London: Royal College of Psychiatrists' Research Unit.

High Royds Evaluation of Negativity (HEN)
Mortimer, A. M., McKenna, P. J., Lund, C. E., *et al* (1989) Rating of negative symptoms using the High Royds Evaluation of Negativity (HEN) scale. *British Journal of Psychiatry*, **155** (suppl. 7), 89–92.

Knowledge about Schizophrenia (KASI)
Barrowclough, C., Tarrier, N., Watts, S., *et al* (1987). Assessing the functional value of relatives' knowledge about schizophrenia : a preliminary report. *British Journal of Psychiatry*, **151**, 1–8.

Lancashire Quality of Life Profile – European Version
Gaite, L. Vazquez-Barquero, J. L., Oliver, J., *et al* (2006) The Lancashire Quality of Life Profile – European Version. In *International Outcome Measures in Mental Health: Quality of Life, Needs, Service Satisfaction, Costs and Impact on Carers* (G. Thornicroft, T. Becker, M. Knapp, *et al*), pp. 130–138. London: Gaskell.

Life Skills Profile (LSP)
Parker, G., Rosen, A., Emdur, N., *et al* (1991) The Life Skills Profile. Psychometric properties of a measure assessing function and disability in schizophrenia. *Acta Psychiatrica Scandinavica*, **83**, 145–152.

Liverpool University Neuroleptic Side Effect Rating Scale (LUNSERS)
Day, J. C., Wood, G., Dewey, M., *et al* (1995) A self-rating scale for measuring neuroleptic side-effects. Validation in a group of schizophrenic patients. *British Journal of Psychiatry*, **166**, 650–653.

Manchester Scale (Rating of negative symptoms)
Krawiecka, M., Goldberg, D. & Vaughan, M. (1977) A standardised psychiatric assessment scale for rating chronic psychotic patients. *Acta Psychiatrica Scandinavica*, **55**, 299–308.

Manchester Short Assessment of Quality of Life
Priebe, S., Huxley, P., Knight, S., *et al* (1999) Application and results of the Manchester Short Assessment of Quality of Life (MANSA). *International Journal of Social Psychiatry*, **45**, 7–12.

Mini-Mental State Examination (MMSE)
Folstein, M. F., Folstein, S. E. & McHugh (1975) 'Mini-mental State': a practical method for grading the cognitive state of patients for the clinician. *Journal of Psychiatric Research*, **12**, 189–198.

Morningside Rehabilitation Status Scales (MRSS)
Affleck, J. W. & McGuire, R. J. (1984) The measurement of psychiatric rehabilitation status. A review of the needs and a new scale. *British Journal of Psychiatry*, **145**, 517–525.

Neurological Rating Scale for Extrapyramidal Effects
Simpson, G. M. & Angus, J. W. S. (1970) A rating scale for extrapyramidal side effects. *Acta Psychiatrica Scandinavica, Supplementum*, **212**, 11–19.

Personal Beliefs About Illness Questionnaire
Birchwood, M., Mason, R., Macmillan, F., *et al* (1993) Depression, demoralization and control over psychotic illness: a comparison of depressed and non-depressed patients with a chronic psychosis. *Psychological Medicine*, **23**, 1–9.

Personal Functioning Scales (PFS)

Barrowclough, C. & Tarrier, N. (1990) Social functioning in schizophrenic patients. The effects of expressed emotion and family intervention. *Social Psychiatry and Psychiatric Epidemiology*, **25**, 125–129.

Positive and Negative Syndrome Scale (PANSS)

Kay, S. R., Opler, L. A. & Lindenmayer, J.-P. (1987) The Positive and Negative Syndrome Scale (PANSS): rationale and standardisation. *British Journal of Psychiatry*, **155** (suppl. 7), 59–67.

Psychotic symptom rating scale (PSYRATS)

Haddock, G., McCarron, J., Tarrier, N., *et al* (1999) Scales to measure dimensions of hallucinations and delusions: the Psychotic Symptom Rating Scales (PSYRATS). *Psychological Medicine*, **29**, 879–889.

Quality of Life Scale (QoLS)

Heinrichs, D. W., Hanlon, T. E. & Carpenter, W. T. (1984) The Quality of Life Scale: an instrument for rating the schizophrenic deficit syndrome. *Schizophrenia Bulletin*, **10**, 388–398.

Rating Scale for Drug-induced Akathisia

Barnes, T. R. (1989) A rating scale for drug-induced akathisia. *British Journal of Psychiatry*, **154**, 672–676.

Recovery Style Questionnaire

Drayton, M., Birchwood, M. & Trower, P. (1998) Early attachment experience and recovery from psychosis. *British Journal of Clinical Psychology*, **37**, 269–284.

Rehabilitation Evaluation Hall and Baker (REHAB)

Baker, R. & Hall, J. N. (1988) REHAB: a new assessment instrument for chronic psychiatric patients. *Schizophrenia Bulletin*, **14**, 97–111.

Relative Assessment Interview (RAI)

Barrowclough, C. & Tarrier, N. (1992) *Families of Schizophrenic Patients: Cognitive Behavioural Intervention*. London: Chapman & Hall.

Scale for Assessment of Thought, Language and Communication

Andreasen, N. C. (1979) Thought, language and communication disorders. I: Clinical assessment, definition of terms and assessment of their reliability. *Archives of General Psychiatry*, **36**, 1315–1321.

Scale for the Assessment of Negative Symptoms (SANS)

Andreasen, N. C. (1982) Negative symptoms in schizophrenia. *Archives of General Psychiatry*, **39**, 784–788.

Andreasen, N. C. (1982) *The Scale for the Assessment of Negative Symptoms (SANS)*. Iowa, IA: University of Iowa College of Medicine.

Scale for the Assessment of Positive Symptoms (SAPS)

Andreasen, N. C. (1984) *The Scale for the Assessment of Positive Symptoms (SAPS)*. Iowa, IA: University of Iowa College of Medicine.

Social Functioning Scale (SFS)

Birchwood, M., Smith, J., Cochrane, R., *et al* (1990) The Social Functioning Scale. The development and validation of a scale of social adjustment for use in family intervention programmes with schizophrenic patients. *British Journal of Psychiatry*, **157**, 853–859.

Support Needs Questionnaire (SNQ)

Davis, F. A., Burns, J., Lindley, P., *et al* (2002) Evaluation: assessing individual needs using the Support Needs Questionnaire. In *Working for Inclusion* (ed. P. Bates). London: Sainsbury Centre for Mental Health.

Yale–Brown Obsessive–Compulsive Scale (Y–BOCS)

Goodman, W. K., Price, L. H. & Rasmussen, S. (1989) The Yale-Brown Obsessive Compulsive Scale. I. Development, use, and reliability. *Archives of General Psychiatry*, **46**, 1006–1016.

Young Compensation Inventory

Young, J. E. (1995) *Young Compensation Inventory*. New York: Cognitive Therapy Centre of New York.

Young Parenting Inventory

Young, J. E. (1994) *Young Parenting Inventory*. New York: Cognitive Therapy Centre of New York.

Young–Rygh Avoidance Inventory

Young, J. E. & Rygh, J. (1994) *Young–Rygh Avoidance Inventory*. New York: Cognitive Therapy Centre of New York.

Young's Schema Questionnaire

Young, J. E. & Brown, G. (1990) *Young Schema Questionnaire*. New York: Cognitive Therapy Centre of New York.

Useful websites

Lindsey Kemp and Theresa Tattan

BBC Online: Mental Health

http://www.bbc.co.uk/health/conditions/mental_health/index.shtml

BBC website providing accessible, comprehensive information on a wide range of mental health conditions, as well as resources for getting help and treatment.

Department of Health

http://www.dh.gov.uk   Tel: 0207 210 4850

Department of Health website providing health and social care policy, guidance and publications.

International Journal of Psychosocial Rehabilitation

http://www.psychosocial.com

Online journal with a variety of articles from around the world. Posted on the web in a variety of languages and available in printed form if required.

International Society for the Psychological Treatments of the Schizophrenias and Other Psychoses (ISPS)

http://www.isps.org

This is the largest active interest group on psychological approaches to psychosis in the UK. It is part of an international network which organises conferences and produces books and newsletters. Membership is open to all.

National Electronic Library for Mental Health

http://www.nelmh.org/index.asp

This specialist library sits within the National Electronic Library for Health and aims to provide access to the best available evidence to answer mental health questions. It is for mental health professionals, service users and carers.

National Institute for Health and Clinical Excellence (NICE)
http://www.nice.org.uk   Tel: 0207 067 5800

NICE makes recommendations on treatments and care using the best available evidence.

National Institute for Mental Health in England (NIMHE)
http://nimhe.csip.org.uk   Tel: 0113 254 5127

NIMHE supports local communities to improve mental health and the quality of services for people affected by mental health problems.

Royal College of Psychiatrists
http://www.rcpsych.ac.uk   Tel: 0207 235 2351

The website of the Royal College of Psychiatrists, which provides up-to-date information for service users and professionals and access to journal articles and College publications. Information concerning the Faculty of Rehabilitation and Social Psychiatry, including current and past newsletters, at: http://www.rcpsych.ac.uk/college/faculties/rehabilitationandsocial. aspx

Sainsbury Centre for Mental Health
http://www.scmh.org.uk   Tel: 0207 827 8300

This is a charity that works to improve the quality of life for people with severe mental health problems. It carries out research, development and training work to influence policy and practice in health and social care.

SANE (Schizophrenia: A National Emergency)
http://www.sane.org.uk   Tel: 0845 767 8000

This is a national campaigning charity providing advice, literature and a national helpline (Saneline) operating at local rates.

Thorn Initiative
http://www.thorn-initiative.org.uk

Thorn is a training course for mental health staff who wish to gain skills in psychosocial interventions and the care of those with severe mental illness. The website has a variety of links, a reading list and other useful resources for training staff.

Service user- and carer-led organisations

Depression Alliance
http://www.depressionalliance.org.uk

Depression Alliance offers support and advice for people experiencing depression.

Hearing Voices Network

http://www.hearingvoices.org.uk

> This is a user-led group which helps people who are hearing voices. An information pack and mailing list of self-help groups around the UK are available.

MDF The BiPolar Organisation

http://www.mdf.org.uk   Tel: 08456 340 540

> This is a national user-led organisation for those whose lives are affected by manic depression, including relatives and friends.

Mental Health Foundation

http://www.mentalhealth.org.uk

> The Mental Health Foundation commissions and publishes helpful user-led research and campaigns for service improvements.

Mind

http://www.mind.org.uk   Tel: 0845 766 0163

> Mind is the foremost mental health charity providing information for service users, carers, family and friends, researchers, students and the public. It publishes Openmind, which reaches about 25 000 readers.

National Voices Forum

http://www.voicesforum.org.uk

> National Voices Forum describes itself as a 'UK user led organisation run by mad people for mad people'.

Rethink

> http://www.rethink.org   National advice service Tel: 0208 974 6814
> This was formerly the National Schizophrenia Fellowship and is the largest non-statutory provider of mental health services. Its site is for service users, relatives and professionals, has useful links and a small amount of information in other languages.

Zito Trust

http://www.zitotrust.co.uk

> This website describes improvements in the provision of community care for people with severe mental illness. The Trust offers support to victims of failures of care and supports research and training in this field.

Early intervention and youth-friendly sites

Early Psychosis Prevention and Intervention Centre (EPPIC)
http://www.eppic.org.au

> EPPIC aims to facilitate early detection and treatment of psychosis. This long-established and comprehensive Australian website for those trying to cope with first-time psychosis contains useful information sheets for users and carers.

Get Connected
http://www.getconnected.org.uk

> Get Connected is a UK website which aims to help young people make contact with the most effective source of help for a wide range of problems and difficulties.

IRIS – Initiative to Reduce the Impact of Schizophrenia
http://www.iris-initiative.org.uk

> This is another very useful website about reaching people early in their illness. The national Early Intervention Programme can be contacted at earlyintervention@rethink.org

Steady – Support and Training for Elation and Depression in Youth
http://www.steady.org.uk

> Steady is an offshoot of MDF and is specifically aimed at the needs of young people (aged 18–25 years), with an emphasis on learning self-management.

Benefits information

Barton Hill Advice Service
http://www.bhas.org.uk

> This provides free guides to welfare benefits and is especially good for information on disability living allowance.

Department of Work and Pensions
http://www.dwp.gov.uk   Benefits enquiry line Tel: 0800 882200

Information for carers

Beacon of Hope
http://www.lightship.org

> Beacon of Hope is a website providing information for partners of those with mental illness.

Carers UK

http://www.carersuk.org   CarersLine Tel: 0808 808 7777

This was formerly the Carers National Association.

Caring about Carers

http://www.carers.gov.uk

This is the Government website for carers and provides good information on carers' assessments.

Crossroads

http://www.crossroads.org.uk   Tel: 0845 450 0350

Crossroads is an organisation providing trained carer support workers who offer respite breaks in carers' own homes.

Princess Royal Trust for Carers

http://www.carers.org

The Princess Royal Trust for Carers is a carers' organisation with over 100 carers' centres in the UK.

Prodigy

http://www.prodigy.nhs.uk/schizophrenia

The prodigy website has a large amount of information about schizo-phrenia, which is in a form useful for sharing with relatives.

Schizophrenia.com

http://www.schizophrenia.com

A website set up by a carer providing in-depth information, support and education related to schizophrenia.

Young Carers

http://www.youngcarers.hants.org.uk

This website provides information for young carers under 18 years.

YoungMinds

http://www.youngminds.org.uk   Parents information service Tel: 0800 018 2138

YoungMinds is the website of the national charity which aims to improve the mental health of all young people.

Information on medication

Electronic British National Formulary

http://www.bnf.org

An online version of the *British National Formulary*, which takes a bit of getting used to but is very useful and quick once it becomes familiar.

NWMHP Pharmacy Medicine Information
http://www.nmhct.nhs.uk/pharmacy

This provides a drug information site for service users.

UK Medicines Information
http://www.ukmi.nhs.uk

This website provides information on medication and is principally for healthcare professionals in primary and secondary care.

United Kingdom Psychiatric Pharmacy Group
http://www.ukppg.org.uk

This is a useful site for information and patient information leaflets which can be downloaded.

Reading list

Lindsey Kemp and Theresa Tattan

Each chapter in the book contains a rich resource of references on that topic. Here is a list of general interest, beginning with some of the classic papers from the founders of rehabilitation psychiatry.

Classics

Berrios, G. E. & Freeman, H. (1991) *150 Years of British Psychiatry 1841–1991*. London: Gaskell.

Ekdawi, M. & Conning, A. (1994) *Psychiatric Rehabilitation – A Practical Guide*. London: Chapman & Hall.

Hume, C. A. & Pullen, I. (1986) *Rehabilitation in Psychiatry: An Introductory Handbook*. London: Churchill Livingstone.

Murphy, E. (1991) *After the Asylums: Community Care for the Mentally Ill*. London: Faber & Faber.

Porter, R. (2002) *Madness: A Brief History*. Oxford: Oxford University Press.

Shepherd, G. (1984) *Institutional Care and Rehabilitation*. Boston, MA: Longman.

Shepherd, G. (1990) *Theory and Practice of Psychiatric Rehabilitation*. Chichester: John Wiley & Sons.

Tuke, S. (1813) *Description of the Retreat: An Institution near York for Insane Persons*. Reprinted (1996) with an introduction by Richard Hunter and Ida Macalpine and a foreword by Kathleen Jones. London: Process Press.

Watts, F. & Bennett, D. (1991) *Theory and Practice of Psychiatric Rehabilitation*. Chichester: John Wiley & Sons.

Wing, J. K. & Morris, B. (1981) *Handbook of Psychiatric Rehabilitation Practice*. Oxford: Oxford Medical Publications.

First-person accounts

Chamberlin, J. (1978) *On Our Own: Patient Controlled Alternatives to the Mental Health System*. New York: McGraw-Hill.

Clay, S. (1994) The wounded prophet. In *Recovery: The New Force in Mental Health* (eds Ohio Department of Mental Health). Columbus, OH: Ohio Department of Mental Health.

Coleman, R. (1999) *Recovery: An Alien Concept*. Gloucester: Hansell Publishing.

Deegan, P. (1988) Recovery: the lived experience of rehabilitation. *Psychosocial Rehabilitation Journal*, **11**, 11–19.

Deegan, P. (1996) Recovery as a journey of the heart. *Psychiatric Rehabilitation Journal*, **19**, 91–97.

Jamieson, K. R. (1995) *An Unquiet Mind: A Memoir of Moods and Madness*. New York: Alfred A. Knopf.

Leete, E. (1989) How I perceive and manage my illness. *Schizophrenia Bulletin*, **8**, 605–609.

Lovejoy, M. (1984) Recovery from schizophrenia: a personal odyssey. *Hospital and Community Psychiatry*, **35**, 809–812.

North, C. (1988) *Welcome, Silence: My Triumph over Schizophrenia*. London: Simon & Schuster.

Unzicker, R. (1989) On my own: a personal journey through madness and re-emergence. *Psychosocial Rehabilitation Journal*, **13**, 70–77.

Woolis, R. (1992) *When Someone you Love has a Mental Illness: A Handbook for Family, Friends and Caregivers*. New York: Jeremy P. Tarcher/Putnam.

Carers and families

Barraclough, C. & Tarrier, N. (1997) *Families of Schizophrenic Patients, Cognitive Behavioural Intervention*. Gateshead: Atheneum Press.

Ramsay, R., Gerada, G., Mars, S., *et al* (2001) *Mental Illness, A Handbook for Carers*. London: Jessica Kingsley.

Wilkinson, G., Kendrick, A. & Moore, B. (2000) *A Carers Guide to Schizophrenia*. London: Royal Society of Medicine.

Rehabilitation and recovery

Brown, C. (2003) *Recovery and Wellness: Models of Hope and Empowerment for People with Mental Illness*. New York: Haworth Press.

Corrigan, P. & Giffort, D. W. (eds) (1998) Building teams and programmes for effective psychiatric rehabilitation. In *New Directions for Mental Health Services*, pp. 79–88. San Francisco, CA: Jossey Bass Wiley.

Corrigan, P. & McCracken, S. (2003) *Interactive Staff Training: Rehabilitation Teams that Work*. Kluwer Academic Publishing.

Ekdawi, M. & Conning, A. (1994) *Psychiatric Rehabilitation – A Practical Guide*. London: Chapman & Hall.

Finch, J. & Moxley, D. (eds) (2003) *Source Book for Rehabilitation and Mental Health Practice*. Dordrecht: Kluwer Academic Publishing.

Flexer, R. & Soloman, P. (1993) *Psychiatric Rehabilitation in Practice*. Guildford: Butterworth Heinemann.

Gamble, C. & Brennan, G. (2000) *Working with Severe Mental Illness*. Oxford: Ballière Tindall.

Goldstein, G. & Beers, S. R. (1998) *Rehabilitation*. Dordrecht: Kluwer Academic.

Hemphill, B. (1991) *Rehabilitation in Mental Health: Goals and Objectives for Independent Living*. Thorofare, NJ: Slack Inc.

Hughes, R. A. (1999) *Best Practices in Psychosocial Rehabilitation*. Columbia, MD: International Association of Psychosocial Rehabilitation Services.

Hume, C. A. (1993) *Rehabilitation for Mental Health Problems: An Introductory Handbook*. London: Churchill Livingstone.

Katz, N. (1992) *Psychiatric Rehabilitation*. St Louis, MO: Warren H. Green.

Kuehnel, T. (1990) *Resource Book for Psychiatric Rehabilitation*. Philadelphia, PA: Lippincott Williams & Wilkins.

Lieberman, R. P. (1991) *Handbook of Psychiatric Rehabilitation*. Oxford: Pergamon Press.

Lieberman, R. P. (1992) *Effective Psychiatric Rehabilitation*. San Francisco, CA: Jossey Bass.

Lieberman, R. P. (ed.) (1998) *Psychiatric Rehabilitation of Chronic Mental Patients*. Arlington, VA: American Psychiatric Press.

Pilling, S. (1991) *Rehabilitation and Community Care*. London: Routledge.

Pratt, C., Gill, K., Barrett, N., *et al* (1999) *Psychiatric Rehabilitation*. Oxford: Academic Press.

Royal College of Psychiatrists (2003) *Rehabilitation and Recovery Now* (Council Report CR121). London: Royal College of Psychiatrists.

Spaulding, W. (2003) *Treatment and Rehabilitation of Severe Mental Illness: A Comprehensive Approach*. New York: Guilford Press.

Therapeutic

Cullari, S. (1996) *Treatment Resistance: A Guide for Practitioners*. Allyn & Bacon.

Hodges, J. R. (1994) *Cognitive Assessment for Clinicians*. Oxford: Oxford Medical Publications.

Mortimer, A. & Spence, S. (2001) *Managing Negative Symptoms of Schizophrenia*. London: Science Press.

Reveley, M. A. & Deakin, J. F. W. (2000) *The Pharmacology of Schizophrenia*. London: Arnold.

Rowan, T. & O'Hanlon, W. H. (1998) *Solution Orientated Therapy for Chronic and Severe Mental Illness*. Chichester: John Wiley & Sons.

Vocational rehabilitation

Ciardiello, J. & Bell, M. (eds) (1998) *Vocational Rehabilitation of Persons with Prolonged Psychiatric Disorder*. Baltimore, MD: John Hopkins University Press.

Royal College of Psychiatrists (2003) *Employment Opportunities and Psychiatric Disability* (Council Report CR111). London: Royal College of Psychiatrists.

Schizophrenia

Goldstein, G. (1998) *Neuropsychology (Human Brain Function: Assessment and Rehabilitation)*. Dordrecht: Kluwer Academic Publishing.

Harris, M. & Bergman, H. (eds) (1993) *Case Management for Mentally Ill Patients: Theory and Practice*. London: Taylor & Francis.

Keefe, R. & McEvoy, J. (2001) *Negative Symptom and Cognitive Deficit Treatment Response In Schizophrenia*. Arlington, VA: American Psychiatric Press.

Lewis, S. & Buchanan, R. (2002) *Fast Facts Schizophrenia* (2nd edn). Abingdon: Health Press.

Lieberman, J. A. & Murray, R. M. (2001) *Comprehensive Care of Schizophrenia: A Textbook of Clinical Management*. London: Martin Dunitz.

Mueser, K. & Tarrier, N. (1998) *Handbook of Social Functioning in Schizophrenia*. Boston, MA: Allyn & Bacon.

National Institute for Clinical Excellence (2003) *Core Interventions in the Treatment and Management of Schizophrenia in Primary and Secondary Care*. London: NICE.

Royal College of Psychiatrists (2001) *The Management of Schizophrenia Part 1: Pharmacological Treatments* (Occasional Paper OP51). London: Royal College of Psychiatrists.

Sharma, T. & Harvey, P. (2000) *Cognition in Schizophrenia: Impairments and Treatment Strategies*. Oxford: Oxford University Press.

Wykes, T., Tarrier, N. & Lewis, S. (1998) *Outcomes and Innovation in Psychological Treatment of Schizophrenia*. Chichester: John Wiley & Sons.

Dual diagnosis

Dennison, S. J. (2003) *Handbook of Dual Diagnosis*. Philadelphia, PA: Lippincott Williams & Wilkins.

Henrickson, E., Schmal, M. S. & Ekleberry, S. (eds) (2004) *Treating Co-occurring Disorders: A Handbook for Health and Substance Misuse Professionals*. New York: Haworth Press.

O'Connel, D. & Beyer, E. (eds) (2002) *Managing the Dual Diagnosis Patient: Current Issues and Clinical Approaches*. New York: Haworth Press.

Rosental, R. N. (2003) *Dual Diagnosis (Key Readings In Addiction Psychiatry)*. London: Brunner-Routledge.

Watkins, T. R. (2000) *Dual Diagnosis: An Integrated Approach to Treatment*. London: Sage.

Index

Compiled by Linda English